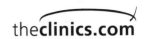

SURGICAL CLINICS
OF NORTH AMERICA

Current Management of Inflammatory Bowel Disease

GUEST EDITOR
Joseph J. Cullen, MD

CONSULTING EDITOR
Ronald F. Martin, MD

June 2007 • Volume 87 • Number 3

SAUNDERS

An Imprint of Elsevier, Inc.
PHILADELPHIA   LONDON   TORONTO   MONTREAL   SYDNEY   TOKYO

W.B. SAUNDERS COMPANY
A Division of Elsevier Inc.

1600 John F. Kennedy Blvd., Suite 1800, Philadelphia, PA 19103-2899

http://www.theclinics.com

SURGICAL CLINICS OF NORTH AMERICA
June 2007
Editor: Catherine Bewick

Volume 87, Number 3
ISSN 0039–6109
ISBN-10: 1-4160-4371-3
ISBN-13: 978-1-4160-4371-3

Reprints. For copies of 100 or more of articles in this publication, please contact the commercial Reprints Department Elsevier Inc., 360 Park Avenue South, New York, New York 10010-1710. Tel. (212) 633-3813, Fax: (212) 462-1935, email: reprints@elsevier.com.

The ideas and opinions expressed in *The Surgical Clinics of North America* do not necessarily reflect those of the Publisher. The Publisher does not assume any responsibility for any injury and/or damage to persons or property arising out of or related to any use of the material contained in this periodical. The reader is advised to check the appropriate medical literature and the product information currently provided by the manufacturer of each drug to be administered to verify the dosage, the method and duration of administration, or contraindications. It is the responsibility of the treating physician or other health care professional, relying on independent experience and knowledge of the patient, to determine drug dosages and the best treatment for the patient. Mention of any product in this issue should not be construed as endorsement by the contributors, editors, or the Publisher of the product or manufacturers' claims.

Surgical Clinics of North America (ISSN 0039–6109) is published bimonthly by Elsevier Inc., 360 Park Avenue South, New York, NY 10010-1710. Months of publication are February, April, June, August, October, and December. Business and Editorial Offices: 1600 John F. Kennedy Blvd., Suite 1800, Philadelphia, PA 19103-2899. Customer Service Office: 6277 Sea Harbor Drive, Orlando, FL 32887-4800. Periodicals postage paid at New York, NY and additional mailing offices. Subscription prices are $220.00 per year for US individuals, $347.00 per year for US institutions, $110.00 per year for US students and residents, $270.00 per year for Canadian individuals, $424.00 per year for Canadian institutions, $286.00 for international individuals, $424.00 per year for international institutions and $143.00 per year for Canadian and foreign students/residents. To receive student/resident rate, orders must be accompanied by name of affiliated institution, date of term, and the *signature* of program/residency coordinator on institution letterhead. Orders will be billed at individual rate until proof of status is received. Foreign air speed delivery is included in all *Clinics* subscription prices. All prices are subject to change without notice. POSTMASTER: Send address changes to *Surgical Clinics*, Elsevier Periodicals Customer Service, 6277 Sea Harbor Drive, Orlando, FL 32887-4800. **Customer Service: 1-800-654-2452 (US). From outside of the US, call 1-407-345-1000.**

The *Surgical Clinics of North America* is also published in Spanish by McGraw-Hill Interamericana Editores S.A., P.O. Box 5-237 06500 Mexico D.F. Mexico; and in Portuguese by Interlivros Edicoes Ltda., Rua Comandante Coelho 1085, CEP 21250, Rio de Janeiro, Brazil; and in Greek by Paschalidis Medical Publications, Athens Greece.

The *Surgical Clinics of North America* is covered in *Index Medicus, EMBASE/Excerpta Medica, Current Contents/Clinical Medicine, Current Contents/Life Sciences, Science Citation Index*, and *ISI/BIOMED*.

Printed in the United States of America.

CONSULTING EDITOR

RONALD F. MARTIN, MD, Staff Surgeon, Marshfield Clinic, Marshfield, Wisconsin; Lieutenant Colonel, Medical Corps, United States Army Reserve

GUEST EDITOR

JOSEPH J. CULLEN, MD, Professor of Surgery, University of Iowa Carver College of Medicine, Iowa City, Iowa

CONTRIBUTORS

ANIS A. AHMADI, MD, Inflammatory Bowel Disease Fellow, Inflammatory Bowel Diseases Program, Division of Gastroenterology, Department of Medicine, University of Florida, Gainesville, Florida

KEVIN E. BEHRNS, MD, Robert H. Hux Professor of Surgery, Department of Surgery, Division of General and GI Surgery, University of Florida, Gainesville, Florida

JUAN C. CENDAN, MD, Assistant Professor of Surgery, Department of Surgery, Division of General and GI Surgery, University of Florida, Gainesville, Florida

JOSEPH J. CULLEN, MD, Professor of Surgery, University of Iowa Carver College of Medicine, Iowa City, Iowa

BOBBY V.M. DASARI, MS, MRCS, Clinical Fellow in Colorectal Surgery, Royal Victoria Hospital, Belfast, United Kingdom

DAVID E. ELLIOTT, MD, PhD, Division of Gastroenterology and Hepatology, Department of Internal Medicine, University of Iowa Carver College of Medicine, Iowa City, Iowa

KIMBERLY EPHGRAVE, MD, FACS, Professor of Surgery, University of Iowa Hospitals and Clinics, Iowa City, Iowa

KEITH R. GARDINER, MD, MCH, FRCS, Consultant Colorectal Surgeon, Royal Victoria Hospital; and Honorary Senior Lecturer in Surgery, The Queen's University of Belfast, Belfast, United Kingdom

ANNA HINDLE, MD, Surgical Resident, George Washington University, Washington, DC

M. NEDIM INCE, MD, Division of Gastroenterology and Hepatology, Department of Internal Medicine, University of Iowa Carver College of Medicine, Iowa City, Iowa

AMANDA M. METCALF, MD, Professor of Surgery, Department of Surgery, Roy J. and Lucille A. Carver College of Medicine, University of Iowa Hospitals and Clinics, Iowa City, Iowa

FRANK A. MITROS, MD, Frederick W. Stamler Professor of Pathology, Department of Pathology, Roy J. and Lucille A. Carver College of Medicine, Iowa City, Iowa

TODD PONSKY, MD, Chief Resident, Pediatric Surgery, Children's National Medical Center, Washington, DC

STEVEN POLYAK, MD, Assistant Professor, Inflammatory Bowel Diseases Program, Division of Gastroenterology, Department of Medicine, University of Florida, Gainesville, Florida

ANTHONY SANDLER, MD, Chief, Pediatric Surgery, Children's National Medical Center, Washington, DC

SCOTT R. STEELE, MD, FACS, Colon and Rectal Surgery, Department of Surgery, Madigan Army Medical Center, Fort Lewis, Washington

ROBERT W. SUMMERS, MD, Clifton Professor of Internal Medicine and Director of Clinical Activities, Division of Gastroenterology/Hepatology, Department of Internal Medicine, University of Iowa Carver College of Medicine, Iowa City, Iowa

CYRUS P. TAMBOLI, MD, FRCPC, Assistant Professor, Department of Internal Medicine, Division of Gastroenterology, University Hospitals and Clinics, University of Iowa Roy J. and Lucille A. Carver College of Medicine, Iowa City, Iowa

REBECCA THORESON, MD, Department of Surgery, University of Iowa College of Medicine, University of Iowa Hospitals and Clinics; and Veterans Affairs Medical Center, Iowa City, Iowa

ANDREW D. VANDERHEYDEN, MD, Resident in Pathology, Department of Pathology, Roy J, and Lucille A. Carver College of Medicine, Iowa City, Iowa

CONTENTS

inflammatory cytokines (anti-TNFα antibodies) have been used successfully to treat IBD. Recent advances have also identified mucosal regulatory pathways.

Chronic idiopathic inflammatory bowel diseases (IBD) include Crohn's disease (CD), ulcerative colitis (UC), and colonic IBD type unclassified (IBDU). This article focuses upon currrent medical therapies for adult CD and UC, and is organized according to therapy for the corresponding disease type, stage, and severity.

The treatment of inflammatory bowel disease (IBD) is undergoing rapid and profound change. Entirely new approaches are being developed that reflect a greater understanding of how to control the inflammatory process. These began with inflixumab therapy for Crohn's disease. Additional tumor necrosis antibodies will soon be employed, and other biological agents are being investigated. Probiotics, helminth ova therapy, alternative and complementary treatments, leukocytophoresis, and bone-marrow and stem-cell transplantation are additional exciting regimens that are being explored. Although some of these approaches provide marked improvement in these parameters, others are unproven or fraught with adverse effects and complications. Still, control of ulcerative colitis and Crohn's is improving with more changes likely to come.

Patients with chronic colitis from inflammatory bowel disease (IBD) have an increased risk of colorectal cancer (CRC). Previously, to ameliorate this, prophylactic total colectomy was offered to patients who had chronic ulcerative colitis (UC); however, research has identified less invasive management options through better understanding of the pathogenesis of cancer in chronic inflammation, a more uniform histologic diagnosis by pathologists, and proper surveillance colonoscopy techniques. This article reviews the pathogenesis of neoplasia in IBD, and then reviews the risk factors for CRC in IBD, surveillance guidelines and their limitations, surveillance techniques, ileal pouch dysplasia, and chemoprevention. Although data for CRC risk in Crohn's disease (CD) are not as extensive, it has been suggested that the risks are comparable to UC.

FORTHCOMING ISSUES

RECENT ISSUES

SURGICAL
CLINICS OF
NORTH AMERICA

Surg Clin N Am 87 (2007) xi–xii

Foreword

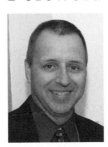

Ronald F. Martin, MD
Consulting Editor

To paraphrase my former senior partner in surgery and mentor, Walter B. Goldfarb, MD, in regard to the thought process of surgeons, "Ronnie, if we were cognitive we wouldn't know what to think." Despite Dr. Goldfarb's quick-witted and self-deprecating humor, he is probably one of the most cognitive persons I know. But he does bring up an interesting point on whether surgeons think and how.

I am sure that surgeons think—they think a lot and they think fast—primarily out of necessity. To consider how we think is another matter altogether. In my opinion, the best example of early modern surgical thinking is the evolution of gastric surgery. The leap form structural thinking about anatomic relationships alone to the consideration of structure and function relationships is what allowed for the development of modern gastric surgery—and its near disappearance. The understanding of humoral and neural stimulation of acid production and gastric motor function has set the stage for some of the great careers in surgical history. The further understanding of physiology and pathophysiology has allowed for mechanical alteration of a physiologic process and subsequent pharmacologic modification of acid secretion and treatment of infectious contributors to ulcer disease states. If one were to draw a parallel from physics, this would be roughly equivalent to the change from Newtonian mechanics to Einstein's theory of relativity.

The development of thought on inflammatory bowel disease may be similar but sufficiently different in some ways. Inflammatory bowel disease treatment primarily relied upon ablative surgical therapy and has long since been of keen interest to surgeons. With the advent of flexible fiber-optic

0039-6109/07/$ - see front matter © 2007 Published by Elsevier Inc.
doi:10.1016/j.suc.2007.04.001

endoscopy and better pharmacologic agents, the emphasis on primary management of patients who have inflammatory bowel disease has shifted to nonoperative management. As one reads the collection of articles in this issue, one will readily conclude that the level of discourse at this time for these problems is on a molecular level, and that our knives, strings, and staplers are reserved for prevention of neoplastic disease and management of pharmacologic failure in many cases. For a surgeon to think of inflammatory bowel disease with our current level of understanding as a collection of diseases that require only our operative abilities would be to woefully miss the point. One could draw again a rough parallel from physics that the molecular and subcellular approach to inflammatory bowel disease is analogous to quantum mechanics in that we deal with small particles and probabilities to guide our thinking.

As in physics, we in surgery continue to seek a "Grand Unified Theory"—coincidence that it is "GUT" by acronym? you decide—that bridges the gaps between immunologic and molecular management, prophylactic operative management, and ablative management of neoplastic or structural failure.

Dr. Cullen and colleagues have provided us with an outstanding collection of articles that expertly and coherently view the fundamental issue with inflammatory bowel disease from multiple vantage points. This is one collection of clinical problems that truly needs to be understood from the DNA level to the gross anatomic to the human personal level. I thank Dr. Cullen and his cocontributors for an excellent issue.

Ronald F. Martin, MD
Department of Surgery
Marshfield Clinic
1000 North Oak Avenue
Marshfield, WI 54449, USA

E-mail address: martin.ronald@marshfieldclinic.org

SURGICAL
CLINICS OF
NORTH AMERICA

ELSEVIER
SAUNDERS

Surg Clin N Am 87 (2007) xiii–xiv

Preface

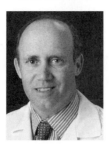

Joseph J. Cullen, MD
Guest Editor

Management of inflammatory bowel disease has undergone a tremendous evolution in the last 70 years. Operative management of Crohn's disease has progressed from surgeons advocating a bypass operation, which was considered much safer for a disease with high mortality for resection, to increased enthusiasm for resection after the advent of antibiotics and recognition of the cancer risk in the bypassed segment, to the latest innovation of strictureplasty. For ulcerative colitis, the advent of proctocolectomy with Brooke ileostomy was a great initial surgical milestone that has advanced to the creation of continent anorectal pouches to maintain anorectal function. In addition to the surgical advances in inflammatory bowel disease, our understanding of the mechanisms of these diseases and options for medical therapeutics has also developed. Introduction of the anti-tumor necrosis factor agent infliximab has added to the armamentarium of the gastroenterologist in treating refractory Crohn's disease.

This issue of *Surgical Clinics of North America* is devoted to inflammatory bowel disease, and will be a reference for both medical and surgical disciplines involved in the treatment of patients with Crohn's disease or ulcerative colitis. Both medical and surgical therapy and complications of inflammatory bowel disease are discussed, along with potential new therapeutic options based on the mechanism of understanding of these diseases. Additionally, there is the ever-increasing dilemma of pathological diagnosis of inflammatory bowel disease as either Crohn's or ulcerative colitis, which is important for surgeons and gastroenterologists involved in the subsequent treatment.

doi:10.1016/j.suc.2007.03.007

Many of the authors have academic clinical practices that are devoted to various aspects of treating patients with inflammatory bowel disease, whereas others have active research laboratories devoted to studying the mechanisms involved in inflammatory bowel disease. I would like to thank the authors for taking time out of their busy practices or research laboratories for their invaluable contributions to this issue.

Joseph J. Cullen, MD
Professor of Surgery
University of Iowa Carver College of Medicine
4605 JCP
Iowa City, IA 52242 USA

E-mail address: joseph-cullen@uiowa.edu

ELSEVIER
SAUNDERS

SURGICAL
CLINICS OF
NORTH AMERICA

Surg Clin N Am 87 (2007) 575–585

Pathophysiology of Inflammatory Bowel Disease: An Overview

Rebecca Thoreson, MD[a,b], Joseph J. Cullen, MD[a,b,*]

[a]Department of Surgery, University of Iowa College of Medicine, 4605 JCP,
University of Iowa Hospitals and Clinics, Iowa City, IA 52242, USA
[b]Veterans Affairs Medical Center, Highway 6 West, Iowa City, Iowa, 52241, USA

Inflammatory bowel disease, Crohn's disease, and ulcerative colitis are considered idiopathic diseases affecting the gastrointestinal tract. These two diseases are often considered together because of multiple similarities, including gastrointestinal inflammation, waxing and waning severity and symptoms, and unknown etiology. However, they have separate symptoms and microscopic characteristics as well as patterns within the gastrointestinal tract (Table 1).

The incidence of inflammatory bowel disease varies according to geographic location. Higher rates are typically found in the more developed countries of Scandinavia, northern Europe, and North America, with lower rates in Asia, Africa, and South America. However the incidence is increasing in the less-developed countries as they become more industrialized, implicating environment, diet, and cultural practices as potential risk factors. Other epidemiologic studies have shown that inflammatory bowel disease typically affects young people; however, there is a bimodal incidence with a large peak in the second or third decade of life followed by a smaller peak later in life. The bimodal distribution is seen more consistently with ulcerative colitis than with Crohn's disease [1].

Etiology

Numerous environmental factors have been studied that influence inflammatory bowel disease, including smoke exposure, diet, oral contraceptives, and nonsteroidal anti-inflammatory agents. There also may be microbial

* Corresponding author. Department of Surgery, University of Iowa College of Medicine, 4605 JCP, University of Iowa Hospitals and Clinics, Iowa City, IA 52242.
  E-mail address: joseph-cullen@uiowa.edu (J.J. Cullen).

Table 1
Key features of ulcerative colitis and Crohn's disease

	Ulcerative colitis	Crohn's disease
Area affected	Colon only	Mouth to anus
Distribution	Continuous	Skip lesions
Histologic features	Mucosa/submucosa, crypt abscesses; superficial ulcers	Transmural granulomas, aphthoid ulcers
Macroscopic features	Mucosal friability, psuedopolyps, loss of haustra (chronic)	Cobblestoning, fistulas fissures
Typical symptoms	Rectal bleeding Diarrhea—often bloody, abdominal pain, weight loss	Abdominal pain, diarrhea, fever, weight loss, fistulas

influences along with immunologic dysregulation. In addition, there is evidence that genetic factors also play a role. Finally, the combination and interaction of genetics, environmental influences, and immunologic abnormalities may play the most important role.

Genetics

Studies comparing the prevalence of inflammatory bowel disease among different ethnic groups suggest genetic tendencies. Inflammatory bowel disease is seen two to four times greater in the Jewish population as compared with other ethnic groups. Ashkenazi Jews have the greatest risk within the Jewish population. Other epidemiologic studies have shown higher rates in whites, lower rates in African Americans, and the lowest rates in Asians [2].

The prevalence of inflammatory bowel disease is also increased in relatives of those who have Crohn's disease and ulcerative colitis. A Danish study found that the risk increases 2 to 13 times for offspring of patients who have inflammatory bowel disease as compared with the general population. For patients who have ulcerative colitis, the occurrence of inflammatory bowel disease in their offspring was 6.26%; for patients who have Crohn's disease, the occurrence was 9.2% [3]. The increased familial risk is similar to other diseases including type 1 and type 2 diabetes, schizophrenia, and celiac disease; the genetic risk ratio is higher for Crohn's disease than ulcerative colitis [4].

Twin studies are another way to determine a genetic contribution for a disease. If a disease were entirely due to genetics, the concordance rates in monozygotic/identical twins would be higher (and should be approaching 100%) than dizygotic/nonidentical twins (which should be approaching 50%). If the disease was dependent only on extrinsic or acquired factors, the concordance rates would be similar among both types of twins. For Crohn's disease, studies have found concordance rates of 20% to 50% in monozygotic twins and less than 10% in dizygotic twins, emphasizing a definite genetic component. With ulcerative colitis, this genetic component was found to be weaker but still present with concordance rates of 16% in monozygotic twins and 4% in dizygotic twins [4].

Numerous studies have demonstrated that genetics do play a role in the manifestation of inflammatory bowel disease. However, classic Mendelian inheritance patterns are not seen. Thus inflammatory bowel disease cannot be credited to a single gene locus. Numerous areas of possible linkage have been identified. Some of the main areas of linkage being studied are chromosomes 16 (IBD1), 12 (IBD2), 6 (IBD3—the HLA region), and 14 [2]. The IBD1 locus on chromosome 16 contributes to susceptibility to Crohn's disease only [5]. Further studies have shown associations with mutations in a gene located in this area of linkage, which encodes for a protein, NOD2 (also known as CARD 15—capsase activating recruitment domain). This protein activates NF-κB and also responds to bacterial lipopolysaccharides. When mutated and in the presence of bacterial lipopolysaccharides, NOD2 no longer activates NF-κB, and the response to bacterial lipopolysaccharides is greatly reduced [6]. These studies not only show the genetic association but also a possible disease mechanism. Another region studied extensively is IBD3 on chromosome 6. This is an area that includes the HLA complex and has been linked with Crohn's disease and ulcerative colitis. This region has several genes involved in the host inflammatory response [7]. Another area linked specifically to Crohn's disease is on chromosome 5q (IBD5). This area contains the cytokine gene cluster [8]. Studies continue to look for further areas of linkage as well as identifying significant genes in the disease process.

Environmental influences

Smoking is one environmental factor that has been shown to have an effect on inflammatory bowel disease. Cigarette smoking has different effects with Crohn's disease than ulcerative colitis. For ulcerative colitis, the risk for current smokers is less than for those who have never smoked. The risk decreases further with an increasing number of cigarettes smoked [9]. Upon smoking cessation, however, the risk increases to higher than that of nonsmokers. An opposite effect is seen with Crohn's disease. Smoking doubles the risk of Crohn's disease. No dose-dependent response is seen, and ex-smokers continue to carry a slightly lower but increased risk [10].

Another relationship is seen with appendectomies. There have been reports of a low rate of appendectomy among patients who have ulcerative colitis. A Swedish study found that there was an inverse relationship between ulcerative colitis and appendectomy when the appendectomy was done for inflammatory conditions. This relationship did not hold true when appendectomies were performed for nonspecific abdominal pain. This was also only true for patients who underwent appendectomies before 20 years of age [11]. Because of this observation, there have been proposals that appendectomy has immune-modulating effects and protects against ulcerative colitis. A possible explanation for this finding is that the appendix is largely lymphoid, and removing it may alter the balance of regulatory and effector T cells.

Infectious possibilities

It has been proposed that another contribution to inflammatory bowel disease is one of infectious origin. Many different bacteria have been suspected of being involved in the pathogenesis of inflammatory bowel disease. The inflammation seen with the disease may be a result of a dysfunctional but appropriate response to an infectious source. Numerous bacteria have been proposed as being causes, but most of these have not been fully supported in studies. In Crohn's disease, *Mycobacterium paratuberculosis*, *Pseudomonas* species, and *Listeria* species have all been suggested as probable causes; however, convincing evidence is lacking. In ulcerative colitis, other bacteria have been implicated. These include *Bacillus* species, adhesive *E. coli*, and *Fusobacterium varium*. Again there is not enough compelling evidence for any of these species [12]. Further organisms are continuing to be studied in regard to contributing to the pathogenesis of the two diseases.

Immunologic factors

In Crohn's disease and ulcerative colitis, there are chronic inflammatory changes in the gastrointestinal tract. These are mediated by different immunologic factors for each disease, although they are both a consequence of T-cell activation. Crohn's disease inflammation is thought to be triggered by Th1 cells, which organize cell-mediated immune response. The cytokine IL-12 is increased in the mucosa in Crohn's disease. This leads to increased Th1 response as well as increase IFN-γ. IFN-γ, in turn, further up-regulates macrophages leading of a cycle of uncontrolled inflammation [13]. Loss of regulation of these excessive activated Th1 cells and macrophages also leads to activation of matrix metalloproteinases, by way of IFN-γ and TNF-α, which cause tissue damage [14]. Another explanation for this unregulated inflammation is that the T cells in Crohn's disease are resistant to normal apoptosis, leading to further development of the inflammatory cycle [15]. The cytokine expression is different comparing ulcerative colitis and Crohn's disease. In ulcerative colitis, the inflammation is thought to be regulated by Th2-cells, which mediate B cells and antibody responses; however this has not been proven. It has been shown that there is increased expression of IL-5, which is a Th2 cytokine, but IL-4, another Th2 cytokine, is not increased [16]. The Th2 contribution may be helping the antibody response, because in ulcerative colitis, there is an increase in IgG plasma cells presumably mediated by T cells [17].

Clinical features of Crohn's disease

The hallmark of Crohn's disease is one of chronic inflammation of the gastrointestinal tract without evidence of infection. It is generally a chronic condition with a relapsing nature. There are often periods of remission, but it may also manifest as chronic continuous symptoms. Unlike ulcerative colitis, Crohn's disease can occur anywhere along the gastrointestinal tract from the mouth to the anus. However, there are three main sites of involvement: the small intestine alone, the colon alone, or combined small and large intestine involvement. The terminal ileum is the most commonly affected area and is involved in two thirds of the patients. Numerous studies have been done regarding the clinical patterns. Overall, the combined small and large intestine pattern is seen in 26% to 48%. The small intestine only pattern is seen in 11% to 48%, and the colon only involvement is seen in 19% to 51% [18]. Further breaking down the patterns, one study found that involvement of the terminal ileum and colon together was the most common pattern, occurring in 55% of patients. Other areas of the small intestine excluding the terminal ileum were involved in only 3% of the cases studied [19]. The duodenum, esophagus, stomach, and mouth may also be involved. However, these are uncommon and rarely occur without concurrent disease activity in the small bowel and/or colon. The different patterns of disease can then lead to different patterns of clinical manifestations as described below.

Clinical symptoms by location

The clinical symptoms of Crohn's disease can vary significantly depending on the disease location. The predominant symptoms in Crohn's disease are typically abdominal pain and diarrhea. These are present in more than 70% of all patients at diagnosis [18]. Other common symptoms include fever and weight loss. Other symptoms that may depend on location of disease are bloody stools, strictures, and fistula to skin or adjacent organs.

Esophageal involvement is rare and has been reported in 0.2% of patients who have Crohn's disease. It is almost always seen with disease elsewhere in the gastrointestinal tract. Esophageal involvement includes aphthous ulcers or deeper ulcerations, stenosis, or pseudopolyps. These patients generally have esophageal symptoms, including dysphagia, odynophagia, heartburn, or chest pain [20].

Gastroduodenal involvement is slightly more common than esophageal involvement but is still rare. It has been reported in 0.5% to 4% of patients who have Crohn's disease. The large majority of patients have coexisting distal disease, and the duodenal disease generally has a more benign course than distal disease [21]. The most common site is the duodenal bulb, which is usually associated with disease proximally in the antrum or distally in the latter parts of the duodenum [22]. Common symptoms include upper abdominal pain, weight loss, nausea and vomiting, and occasionally hematemesis. The abdominal pain is usually epigastric and can mimic peptic ulcer disease symptoms. Stricture is the main pathologic finding, which can subsequently lead to obstruction. Fistulas are fairly rare and, when seen within the duodenum, usually originate from distal disease. Histologically, acute and chronic inflammation is usually seen. Granulamatous inflammation is also often seen [21]. Other common features are edema, aphthous ulcerations, and irregular mucosal thickening [21,22].

Similar clinical patterns are seen in the three main patterns of disease: small intestine alone, the colon alone, or combined small and large intestine involvement. However there may be significant differences in the clinical symptoms [23]. Patients who had colonic disease had more rectal bleeding: 46% compared with 22% for ileocolic and 10% for small intestine alone. Another difference noted was in rectal fistula. Also, those who had ileocolic and colonic alone disease had more rectal fistula: 21% and 19% compared with only 5% in those who had small intestine only involvement. Other common symptoms with no statistical difference between the three main patterns of disease include diarrhea, abdominal pain, and malnutrition.

This same study also found differences in complications between the three main patterns of disease [23]. Internal fistulas occurred more in those who had ileocolic disease (34%) as compared with small intestine alone (17%) and colon alone (16%). Perianal fistulas were also seen more commonly in the ileocolic pattern (38%) as well as the colonic pattern (36%) compared with only 14% in those who had a small intestine pattern. Intestinal obstruction was found in 44% of those who had ileocolic disease and 35% in those who had with small intestine pattern, but only 17% in those who had colon only disease. Another more rare complication was megacolon, which was seen mostly in those who had only colonic disease. The extraintestinal manifestation of arthritis was also seen more in those who had colonic disease.

Weight loss in patients who have Crohn's may have multiple causes. Partial obstruction can lead to food avoidance due to pain, which contributes to the weight loss. Occasionally there may be persistent pain, and this is due to acute inflammation or abscesses rather than partial obstruction. Another mechanism of weight loss is malabsorption and malnutrition if the small bowel is extensively involved. Other complications of small bowel disease are fistulas that often involve the vagina, skin, or bladder.

Crohn's colitis can manifest as rectal bleeding with other common symptoms of abdominal pain along with diarrhea. Also, strictures may occur, leading to obstruction and distention. Toxic megacolon may also occur; however, this is more commonly seen in ulcerative colitis.

Perianal involvement occurs with inflammation and fistulization within anal crypt glands. Skin tags, fissures, and perianal scarring occur. Symptoms include pain, purulent drainage, and difficulties with defecation.

Extraintestinal manifestations may also occur involving the dermatologic system, ocular system, joints, or the hepatobiliary system. Dermatologically, patients can have erythema nodosum and pyoderma gangrenosum. Eye involvement can include uveitis and episcleritis. Ankylosing spondylitis, sacral ileitis, and peripheral polyarthropathy are possible joint manifestations. In the hepatobiliary system, primary sclerosing cholangitis can occur, but this is more often seen with ulcerative colitis. Most of these symptoms correlate with bowel disease activity except for primary sclerosing cholangitis and ankylosing spondylitis.

Histologic features

Crohn's disease is characterized microscopically by transmural inflammation anywhere along the gastrointestinal tract. Lymphoid aggregates spread across all layers of the bowel wall but primarily in mucosa and submucosa, which is practically diagnostic for Crohn's disease. Mucosal inflammation is seen with neutrophils infiltrating into the epithelial layer, which overlay these mucosal lymphoid aggregates. Progression leads to neutrophils infiltrating into crypts, forming crypt abscess, and finally destructing the crypt. The crypt destruction leads to atrophy of the colon. Chronic damage may also been seen in the form of villus blunting in the small intestine. Ulcerations are common and are often seen on a background of normal mucosa. Noncaseating granulomas are also characteristic. These are sarcoid-like granulomas, which may be found within areas of active disease or areas of uninvolved bowel.

Gross features

A main feature of Crohn's disease is apthous ulcers. These are small areas of mucosal ulceration that develop over lymphoid aggregates and are seen as red spots or mucosal depressions. They may enlarge and become stellate. These may also combine and become longitudinal ulcerations usually along the mesenteric side of the bowel wall. They may then further develop into a network of long ulcerations surrounding spared edematous mucosa leading to cobblestone appearance. These ulcerations may also perforate the submucosa and make channels through the bowel wall, leading to fistulas, sinuses, or abscesses. Acute inflammation of the bowel wall is seen as boggy and edematous. Chronic inflammation results in a thickened and leathery appearance due to fibrotic scarring. The bowel lumen may be narrowed due to the edema and inflammation. Because of its transmural nature, strictures may also form due to fibrosis within the bowel wall. Fistulas may also form to adjacent organs or skin. The inflammation extending through the bowel wall may also involve the mesentery and surrounding lymph nodes. Creeping fat may be seen when the mesentery wraps around the bowel surface. There may also be a sharp demarcation between the involved areas and uninvolved areas leading to skip lesions.

Clinical features of ulcerative colitis

Ulcerative colitis is characterized as noninfectious inflammation of the gastrointestinal tract, limited to the rectum and colon. It is a relapsing and remitting disorder with disease-free intervals alternating with periods of symptomatic inflammation. Although usually grouped together with Crohn's disease, there are many differences between the two. In ulcerative colitis, the inflammation is limited to the mucosa and submucosa, rather than the transmural inflammation seen in Crohn's disease. Unlike Crohn's disease, ulcerative colitis is a continuous disease with no skip lesions between areas of disease. The rectum is almost always involved, and the disease may continue proximally from there. Although the small intestine may be involved in cases of "backwash ileitis," ulcerative colitis is confined to the colon. Four major categories of colonic involvement have been defined. *Proctitis* is rectum-only involvement. *Proctosigmoiditis* includes the rectal involvement with extension into the sigmoid region. *Left-sided colitis* refers to disease extending from rectum continuously to the splenic flexure. *Pancolitis* is inflammation past the splenic flexure, potentially extending to the cecum [24]. In adults, 55% present with proctitis, 30% with left-sided colitis, and 15% with pancolitis [25].

Clinical features

Patients may have differing symptoms based on the extent of their disease. In general, there is a relapsing pattern whereby symptoms may persist for days, weeks, or months and then subside with asymptomatic periods lasting for months, years, or even decades. Typical symptoms include rectal bleeding or bloody diarrhea, abdominal pain, fever, weight loss, and malaise. Proctitis symptoms include bloody stools, tenesmus, and/or painful straining. Urgency and frequency may also be present as well as incontinence of stool. Those who have disease extending more proximal generally have similar symptoms but may also have lower abdominal pain and, in more severe cases, nausea, vomiting, and weight loss. Other signs of chronic disease include malnutrition, weight loss, and anemia.

Extraintestinal manifestations may also be seen with ulcerative colitis, similar to Crohn's disease. These include ocular lesions like iritis and uveitis. Dermatologic symptoms include pyoderma gangrenosum and erythema nodosum. Typically pyoderma gangrenosum is more often associated with ulcerative colitis than Crohn's disease and erythema nodosum more with Crohn's disease. However this is not evident in all studies [26]. Joint symptoms may also be seen ranging from peripheral arthralgias and arthritis to ankylosing spondylitis. Primary sclerosing cholangitis is another major extraintestinal manifestation that is more commonly seen in ulcerative colitis.

Toxic megacolon is a severe life-threatening complication of ulcerative colitis. It occurs more often in ulcerative colitis than Crohn's disease and is mostly seen in patients who have proctitis. It is often seen within the first few months of diagnosis. It is characterized by nonobstructive colonic dilatation with systemic toxicity. Symptoms include abdominal distension, abdominal tenderness, fever, increased white blood cell count, anemia, hypotension, or altered level of consciousness [27]. Inflammation is seen throughout the bowel wall with necrosis and degeneration of the myocytes. When the disease progresses, the bowel wall may become so thin due to distension and necrosis that it perforates.

The development of colorectal cancer is seen more in ulcerative colitis than Crohn's disease. Ulcerative colitis increases the risk of colorectal cancer compared with the noninflammatory bowel disease population. The risk of cancer increases with an increase in the extent of the disease. One Swedish population study found that the relative risk was increased for pancolitis (14.8) as compared with left-sided colitis (2.8). Those who had proctitis alone did not have a significant increased risk of cancer. A younger age at diagnosis of ulcerative colitis also seems to increase the risk of cancer [28].

Histologic features

In ulcerative colitis, the inflammation is limited to the mucosa and submucosa. In active disease, neutrophils can be found infiltrating the crypts, forming crypt abscesses. Superficial erosions or ulcerations occur and can penetrate deeper into the submucosa in more severe disease. Active disease also results in decreased goblet cell mucin, whereas crypts become more indistinct, shorter, and decreased in number. The destroyed crypts of the active diseased state regenerate with Paneth's cells, which normally are not seen past the hepatic flexure.

Gross features

On gross examination, the main feature noted in ulcerative colitis is that of continuity. The inflammatory changes extend continuously from the rectum. There are no skip lesions as in Crohn's disease. In active disease, the mucosa is generally erythematous and friable. Superficial ulcers are often observed and pseudopolyps are characteristic of severe disease. These are areas of normal but edematous mucosa bulging around the diseased inflamed mucosa. Chronic changes may also be seen. Loss of haustra and mucosal folds are evidence of chronic inactive disease. With repeated outbreaks of active disease, there may be layering of the muscularis mucosa. This leads to hypertrophy of the muscularis mucosa with fibrosis and a decrease in the diameter of the colon, which may eventually lead to stricture. In patients who have pancolitis, backwash ileitis may also be seen consisting of inflammatory changes seen in the terminal ileum in conjunction with inflammation extending to the cecum.

Summary

Ulcerative colitis and Crohn's disease are two distinct diseases with similar characteristics and symptoms. As of now, they are linked together under the heading of inflammatory bowel disease. Table 1 details the major pathologic differences between the two disease entities.

References

[1] Sandler R, Loftus E Jr. Epidemiology of inflammatory bowel disease. In: Sartor R, Sandborn W, editors. Kirsner's inflammatory bowel diseases. 6th edition. Philadelphia: Saunders; 2004. p. 245–62.

[2] Ahmad T, Satsangi J, Mcgovern D, et al. Review article: the genetics of inflammatory bowel disease. Aliment Pharmacol Ther 2001;15:731–48.

[3] Orholm M, Fonager K, Sorensen HT. Risk of ulcerative colitis and Crohn's disease among offspring of patients with chronic inflammatory bowel disease. Am J Gastroenterol 1999; 94(11):3236–8.

[4] Halme L, Paavola-Sakki P, Turunen U, et al. Family and twin studies in inflammatory bowel disease. World J Gastroenterol 2006;12(23):3668–72.

[5] Hugot JP, Laurent-Puig P, Gower-Rousseau C, et al. Mapping of a susceptibility locus for Crohn's disease on chromosome 16. Nature 1996;379:821–3.

[6] Ogura Y, Bonen D, Inohara N, et al. A frameshift mutation in NOD2 associated with susceptibility to Crohn's disease. Nature 2001;411:603–6.

[7] Ahmad T, Marshall S, Jewell D. Genetics of inflammatory bowel disease: the role of the HLA complex. World J Gastroenterol 2006;12(23):3628–35.

[8] Rioux J, Daly M, Silverberg M, et al. Genetic variation in the 5q31 cytokine gene cluster confers susceptibility to Crohn disease. Nat Genet 2001;29:223–8.

[9] Franceschi S, Panza E, Vecchia C, et al. Nonspecific inflammatory bowel disease and smoking. Am J Epidemiol 1987;125(3):445–52.

[10] Lindberg E, Tysk C, Andersson K, et al. Smoking and inflammatory bowel disease. A case control study. Gut 1988;29:352–7.

[11] Andersson R, Olaison G, Tysk C, et al. Appendectomy and protection against ulcerative colitis. N Engl J Med 2001;344(11):808–14.

[12] Ohkusa T, Nomura T, Sato N. The role of bacterial infection in the pathogenesis of inflammatory bowel disease. Intern Med 2004;43(7):534–9.

[13] Pallone F, Monteleone G. Interleukin 12 and Th1 responses in inflammatory bowel disease. Gut 1998;43:735–6.

[14] Shanahan F. Crohn's disease. Lancet 2002;359:62–9.

[15] Boirivant M, Marini M, Di Felice G, et al. Lamina propria T cells in Crohn's disease and other gastrointestinal inflammation show defective CD2 pathway-induced apoptosis. Gastroenterology 1999;116:557–65.

[16] Fuss I, Neurath M, Boirivant M, et al. Disparate CD4$^+$ lamina propria (LP) lymphokine secretion profiles in inflammatory bowel disease. J Immunol 1996;157:1261–70.

[17] Macdonald TT, Monteleone G, Pender SLF. Recent developments in the immunology of inflammatory bowel disease. Scand J Immunol 2000;51:2–9.

[18] Munkholm P, Binder V. Clinical features and natural history of Crohn's disease. In: Sartor R, Sandborn W, editors. Kirsner's inflammatory bowel diseases. 6th edition. Philadelphia: Saunders; 2004. p. 289–300.

[19] Mekhjian HS, Switz DM, Melnyk CS, et al. Clinical features and natural history of Crohn's disease. Gastroenterology 1979;77:898–906.

[20] Decker GAG, Loftus EV Jr, Pasha T, et al. Crohn's disease of the esophagus: clinical features and outcomes. Inflamm Bowel Dis 2001;7(2):113–9.

[21] Nugent FW, Roy MA. Duodenal Crohn's disease: an analysis of 89 cases. Am J Gastroenterol 1989;84(3):249–54.

[22] Yamamoto T, Allan RN, Keighley MRB. An audit of gastroduodenal Crohn disease: clinicopathologic features and management. Scand J Gastroenterol 1999;34:1019–24.

[23] Farmer RG, Hawk WA, Turnbull RB Jr. Clinical patterns in Crohn's disease: a statistical study of 615 cases. Gatroenterology 1975;68(4):627–35.

[24] Cantor M, Bernstein CN. Clinical course and natural history of ulcerative colitis. In: Sartor R, Sandborn W, editors. Kirsner's inflammatory bowel diseases. 6th edition. Philadelphia: Saunders; 2004. p. 280–8.

[25] Ghosh S, Shand A, Ferguson A. Regular review ulcerative colitis. BMJ 2000;320:1119–23.

[26] Bernstein CN, Blanchard JF, Rawsthorne P, et al. The prevalence of extraintestinal disease in inflammatory bowel disease: a population-based study. Am J Gastroenterol 2001;96(4): 1116–22.

[27] Sheth SG, LaMont JT. Toxic megacolon. Lancet 1998;351:509–13.

[28] Ekbom A, Helmick C, Zack M, et al. Ulcerative colitis and colorectal cancer. N Engl J Med 1990;323:1228–33.

SURGICAL
CLINICS OF
NORTH AMERICA

Surg Clin N Am 87 (2007) 587–610

Operative Management of Small Bowel Crohn's Disease

Keith R. Gardiner, MD, MCh, FRCS (Gen)[a,b,*],
Bobby V.M. Dasari, MS, MRCS[a]

[a]Royal Victoria Hospital, Grosvenor Road, Belfast, BT12 6BA, UK
[b]The Queen's University of Belfast, Belfast, UK

Historical aspects

When Crohn, Ginzburg, and Oppenheimer first described "regional enteritis," they believed that a cure for this disease could only be possible with complete surgical resection. High morbidity, mortality, and recurrence rates led to a trend toward bypass surgery, however. This procedure carried a lower mortality rate but could be complicated by the development of an infected mucocele or a cancer in the bypassed segment. There was therefore a return to resectional surgery.

Over the last 25 years, there have been moves toward more conservative surgery (strictureplasty and conservative resection), nonsurgical management (percutaneous drainage of abscesses, endoluminal dilatation of strictures, antibiotic management of microperforations), and an exploration of the usefulness of minimal access surgery (laparoscopic or laparoscopic assisted).

Frequency of surgical intervention

Surgery is an important component of management of Crohn's disease, with studies showing that 70% to 90% of patients require surgical intervention at some point in the course of the disease [1,2]. The need for surgery depends on site and duration of disease. In patients who have ileocecal disease, the probability of requiring surgery within 5 years of onset is 75% and reaches 90% after 10 years of symptoms. For patients who have ileal disease

* Corresponding author. Royal Victoria Hospital, Grosvenor Road, Belfast, BT12 6BA, UK.
  E-mail address: keith.gardiner@belfasttrust.hscni.net (K.R. Gardiner).

0039-6109/07/$ - see front matter © 2007 Published by Elsevier Inc.
doi:10.1016/j.suc.2007.03.011

only, the probability of requiring surgery is 50% at 5 years and 70% at 10 years [3]. Patients who have small bowel Crohn's disease and raised antibody concentrations to microbial antigens have an increased risk for requiring small bowel surgery [4]. Seiderer and colleagues [5] have shown that genotyping (identification of CARD15 variant 1007fs) can predict the need for surgery in patients who have Crohn's disease and symptoms suggestive of small bowel strictures.

Philosophy of surgical approach

Crohn's disease is now considered a panenteric disease and is therefore not curable. Surgery carries with it a relatively high rate of major complications and recurrence, and a variable amount of diarrhea and metabolic upset because of a shortened bowel [6,7]. These observations have led to a philosophy of reserving surgery for patients who experience complications of their disease or in whom medical therapy has failed or not been tolerated.

There is an alternative philosophy of the use of surgery at an earlier stage in the course of the disease before serious septic complications develop [8]. This approach is based on the complication rates following surgery for non-complicated Crohn's disease (12%) being much lower than those encountered when operating on advanced Crohn's disease (49%) when the disease is usually complicated by abscess or fistula formation [8].

Indications for surgery

Many patients require surgery for complications of their disease, most commonly recurrent intestinal obstruction because of strictures and perforations (abscesses, fistulas, free perforation) and less commonly because of major hemorrhage, failure to thrive, cancer, obstructive uropathy, and extraintestinal manifestations. The ileocecal region and small bowel are the most common sites requiring surgery. Duodenal involvement occurs in only 1% to 3% of patients who have Crohn's disease, with surgery being required for strictures, fistulas, or bleeding.

Intestinal obstruction

Intestinal obstruction is a frequent primary indication for surgery; it may be caused by a single narrow stricture (Fig. 1) or a series of strictures and present acutely or with chronic symptoms [9]. Acute small bowel obstruction usually follows ingestion of high-residue, indigestible fiber products, such as raw fruits or vegetables. This type of obstruction usually resolves with nonoperative management. Surgery is indicated when an obstructive episode fails to resolve, when there are frequent bouts of obstruction, or when the obstruction is associated with a septic response, an intra-abdominal mass,

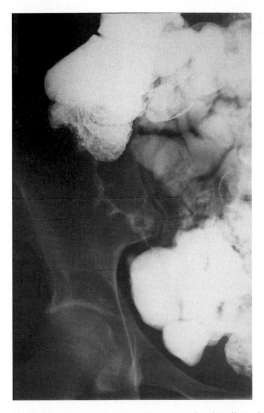

Fig. 1. Small bowel series showing recurrent stricture proximal to ileocolonic anastomosis.

fistula, or malnutrition. Surgery usually involves a resection, or rarely ileostomy formation or internal bypass. Chronic obstruction is typified by recurring episodes that do not respond to long-term medical therapy and usually require elective surgery. Surgery generally involves a resection, but one or more strictureplasties are an option if the patient has had previous intestinal resections or has multiple strictures.

Alternatives to surgery for intestinal strictures

Endoscopy and hydrostatic balloon dilatation of strictures has been used as an alternative to either resection or strictureplasty in selected patients who have short (< 10 cm) solitary small bowel (or colonic) primary or anastomotic strictures. Dilatation is usually used for strictures in the terminal ileum that are not complicated by fistula or abscess formation and that can be accessed at colonoscopy. High technical success rates (66% to 100%) have been reported [10,11]. Complications (8% to 25%) include hemorrhage and perforation [11,12]. Repeat dilatations are necessary in 60% of patients [11]. Primary strictures tend to be longer, associated with more ulceration, and have a higher risk for perforation and recurrence after dilatation than is described with anastomotic strictures [12]. Endoscopic stricture dilatation would therefore seem to have more of a role for solitary (recurrent) strictures at an ileocolonic anastomosis.

Postdilatation intralesional steroid injections have also been described that were associated with a reduced recurrence rate [13]. Bickston and colleagues [14] have reported an undernourished patient who had small bowel obstruction attributable to a Crohn's stricture of the terminal ileum that was successfully treated by insertion of a metallic enteral endoprosthesis.

Intra-abdominal abscesses

Up to 25% of patients who have Crohn's disease present with intra-abdominal abscesses at some point in their life [15]. Abscesses can develop because of a local perforation, in association with a fistula, or postoperatively because of intra-abdominal contamination or anastomotic leakage. Abscesses can be classified as intraperitoneal, interloop, intramesenteric, or retroperitoneal.

Abscesses may present as a tender abdominal mass but clinical features may be indistinguishable from an exacerbation of the disease. CT and ultrasound scanning may aid the diagnosis; however, abscesses may only be confirmed at laparotomy in up to 50% patients [16]. Surgery is often difficult in patients who have abscesses because they may be nutritionally depleted, steroid dependent, or immunocompromised. Surgery usually involves resection of bowel and drainage of abscesses. Anastomosis may be considered if there are local and systemic factors that are conducive to healing of an intestinal anastomosis [17] but a temporary stoma and later restoration of intestinal continuity is often necessary.

Interloop abscesses are usually found at the time of resection when bowel loops are separated. Intramesenteric abscesses may be drained by intraoperative needle aspiration. It has been recommended that the involved segment should be excluded by bringing both ends to the skin surface as mucous fistulas and performing enteroenterostomy between proximal and distal segments, rather than risk peritoneal contamination and difficulty with the vascular pedicle by performing intestinal resection at that stage [18].

Alternatives to surgery for intra-abdominal abscesses

If the patient is hemodynamically stable and the abscess has been diagnosed preoperatively, percutaneous drainage is an option. Intraperitoneal, pelvic, and retroperitoneal abscesses may all be suitable for percutaneous drainage under CT (Fig. 2) or ultrasonographic guidance. This may change a two-stage procedure (initial resection and stoma; later restoration of intestinal continuity) to a one-stage procedure with definitive resection and anastomosis [19]. Not all patients may need a subsequent resection [20]. A sinogram should be performed by way of the drainage catheter a week later to investigate for enteric communication. If no enteric communication is demonstrated, the catheter can be removed and the patient followed for

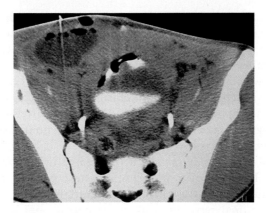

Fig. 2. CT scan showing percutaneous drainage of Crohn's-related abscess in right iliac fossa.

recurrence. If the abscess cavity had an enteric communication, complete resolution is unlikely without resection. Garcia and colleagues [21] studied 51 patients who had intra-abdominal abscesses complicating Crohn's disease and found that fewer patients developed recurrent abscesses after initial surgical drainage and resection (12%) than patients treated by percutaneous drainage alone (56%). Gutierrez and colleagues [22] compared percutaneous drainage with open surgical drainage in 66 patients who had intra-abdominal abscesses in Crohn's disease. They found no difference in time to resolution of infection. One third of the patients treated with percutaneous drainage required surgery within 1 year.

Free perforation

Free perforation is a rare complication of Crohn's disease and typically occurs during an acute exacerbation of chronic disease just proximal to a strictured intestinal segment. Urgent laparotomy is required, with resection of the involved segment being preferred to simple closure with suture because associated mortality is reduced 10-fold to approximately 4% [23].

Fistulas

Fistulas are commonly found (35%) in patients operated on for Crohn's disease but were the primary indication in only 6.3% of patients [24]. Patients may present with fistulas but they are more commonly recognized as postoperative complications (leak from anastomosis or strictureplasty site). Fistulas may be classified as internal (enteroenteric, enterovesical, or enterovaginal) or external (enterocutaneous). The same patient may have several types of fistula.

Enteroenteric fistulas are the most common internal fistula and may cause few symptoms unless associated with obstruction or intra-abdominal abscess. An enteroenteric fistula is an indication for surgery when it causes a bypass of a sizable portion of intestine with consequent diarrhea and mal-absorption. Treatment is by primary resection and anastomosis in most cases, unless the patient is poorly nourished or there is excess intraoperative blood loss or unresolved sepsis. Surgical resection involves resection of the fistula source—which is most often the terminal ileum (with anastomosis)—and performing a wedge excision and closure of the adjacent segment that has been secondarily involved [18]. For ileosigmoid fistulas, simple suture closure of the sigmoid may be vulnerable to leakage; limited sigmoid colonic resection and anastomosis is recommended [18].

Enterovesical fistulas may present with pneumaturia or repeated urinary tract infections. Diagnosis is by cystogram, cystoscopy, or CT scan. Surgery is the appropriate treatment and involves separation of the small bowel from the bladder, intestinal resection with anastomosis, and débridement and closure of the bladder, leaving a urinary catheter in for 10 days. Cystography before catheter removal can be used to confirm bladder integrity.

Enterovaginal fistulas usually occur in patients who have undergone a hysterectomy. They are treated by surgical resection and anastomosis of the fistula source and débridement and closure of the vagina with omental interposition between the intestinal anastomosis and vaginal closure [18].

Enterocutaneous fistulas usually occur postoperatively as a result of anastomotic breakdown or at a later stage because of recurrent disease (Fig. 3). Most open onto the anterior abdominal wall through a previous incision. Spontaneous fistulas may develop in close proximity to an

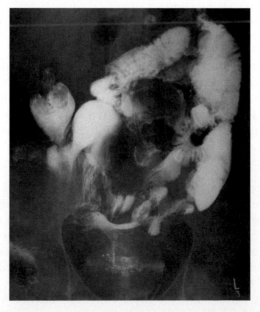

Fig. 3. Small bowel series showing multiple strictures and enterocutaneous fistulas to midline wound and to right iliac fossa.

ileostomy in 1% of patients and usually indicate a short stricture or recurrent disease. The fistula itself is not an indication for surgery; initial efforts are directed toward elimination of sepsis, protection of the skin, restoration of nutrient and electrolyte deficiencies, and establishment of fistula anatomy before planning a definitive procedure [25]. Early surgery (defunctioning ileostomy) may be necessary for an early postoperative fistula.

All fistulas are initially associated with sepsis, although discharge through the abdominal wall may satisfactorily drain the sepsis. CT and ultrasound scans may aid identification and percutaneous drainage of any associated abscess. Surgical drainage of the abscess may be necessary if the abscess cavity is inaccessible or multiloculated, and for those patients who show persistent sepsis despite percutaneous drainage. The surrounding skin needs to be protected at an early stage to prevent contact dermatitis. This procedure may be possible with a stoma bag or require wound drainage bags and suction. Nutritional support needs to be considered at an early stage with the options being oral/enteral nutrition with a high-protein, low-residue feed (if the fistula site is distal), or parenteral nutrition or fistuloclysis (feeding into distal bowel by way of fistula site) if the fistula is proximal. Proton pump inhibitors and somatostatin analogs are often used in an attempt to reduce gastric acid production and pancreatic secretion, respectively. Definition of the fistula tract usually involves oral contrast studies (small bowel series or small bowel enema), fistulography, and CT scanning.

Definitive surgery should be delayed for at least 3 months to allow time for spontaneous closure and for resolution of obliterative peritonitis. Fistulas are unlikely to close if they are associated with recurrent disease, distal obstruction, or persistent infection, or if there is mucocutaneous continuity or discontinuity of bowel ends. A decision may be made not to operate if the fistula has a low output and the operative risk is high. Surgery involves complete mobilization of the bowel, resection of the fistulizing segment, and anastomosis.

Alternatives to surgery for fistulas

Prolonged parenteral nutrition may be necessary to correct undernutrition before surgery can be contemplated. Immunosuppressants, such as azathioprine, 6-mercaptopurine, and cyclosporine, have all been evaluated in the setting of enterocutaneous fistulas. Favorable results have been reported for the use of 6-mercaptopurine for external and internal fistula: almost 40% of fistulas closed after a 6-month period of treatment [26,27]. There is a high recurrence rate following withdrawal of treatment, however. Long-term treatment with oral cyclosporine produces an improvement in enterocutaneous fistulas in 40% of patients [28,29], but side effects are common and there is a tendency for the fistulas to recur when the drug is withdrawn.

Infliximab has been evaluated in patients who have Crohn's disease and enterocutaneous fistulas. The ACCENT-1 study showed a rapid response to three infusions of infliximab in 46% of patients, but the duration of the effect was limited to only 3 to 4 months [30]. The ACCENT-2 study treated 306 patients who had actively draining enterocutaneous fistulas with three infliximab infusions [31]. Sixty-nine patients responded (22%) and these patients were then treated with further infusions of infliximab (or placebo) every 8 weeks. At the end of the trial the response rate (discontinuation of fistula drainage in more than 50% fistulas) to infliximab was 46% compared with a response rate to placebo of 23%; complete response rate (all fistulas closed) was 36% for infliximab and 19% for placebo. The most common side effect was abscess formation in association with the fistula.

Failed medical treatment

Medical therapy is initiated for most patients suffering from disease symptoms unless presentation mandates emergency surgery. Medical therapy is considered to have failed if:

Symptoms cannot be controlled with the maximum possible doses
Disease progresses (worsening symptoms or new complications) while on maximum medical therapy
Significant treatment-related side effects occur
There is noncompliance with medication

Failure of medical therapy has been found to be the most common indication for surgery in some series.

Hemorrhage

Massive hemorrhage is an uncommon indication (0.9%–1.4%) for surgery. Other causes, such as coagulopathy and peptic ulcer, need to be excluded. Surgery is indicated in patients who are hemodynamically unstable, those who continue to bleed after receiving four to six units of blood, and those who have recurrent major hemorrhage. Preoperative or intraoperative mesenteric angiography may aid in localizing the bleeding source, especially if there is multisite disease [32,33]. The involved segment requires resection with or without anastomosis depending on hemodynamic stability. If there is difficulty in identifying the responsible segment, wide resection may be necessary. One third of patients who have Crohn's disease experience recurrent hemorrhage, usually within 3 years of the original episode.

Alternatives to surgery for massive hemorrhage

Mesenteric angiography and intra-arterial infusion of vasopressors [34] or embolization [35,36] have been recently used in an attempt to avoid surgical resection.

Malignancy

Cancer is an uncommon complication of small bowel Crohn's disease (0.3%) and may be multifocal and poorly differentiated. The risk for small bowel cancer is increased 12- to 60-fold in patients who have small bowel Crohn's disease compared with the general population [37]. Predisposing factors include long duration of disease, early age of onset, smoking, diffuse disease, and bypassed intestinal segments [38]. Bypassed segments are impossible to keep under surveillance and are therefore best resected. Concern about the potential to develop cancer at the site of longstanding strictures has led to the recommendation that stricture biopsies should be undertaken when strictureplasty is being performed [39,40]. The presence of a neoplasm may be suggested in a patient who has longstanding Crohn's disease who develops an unresolving obstruction [41]. In most patients who have small bowel cancer complicating Crohn's disease, the neoplasm is found incidentally at surgery. Surgical resection is indicated but the outcome is poor [41] with a mean survival of 6 months for small bowel cancers [38].

Obstructive uropathy

The right ureter may be compressed or obstructed by an ileocecal phlegmon or an associated abscess with consequent hydronephrosis. Urinary symptoms are often absent and the obstructive uropathy is frequently diagnosed by CT scanning. The obstructive uropathy is usually relieved by intestinal resection [42]. If the ileocecal segment is densely fixed in position, a proximal defunctioning ileostomy may be necessary to allow the inflammation to reduce, with a subsequent resection [42].

Failure to thrive

Growth retardation is seen in 26% of children affected by Crohn's disease [43]. This finding may be attributable to malabsorption, nutritional deficiencies, and corticosteroid therapy. If a prepubertal patient remains undernourished despite adequate medical therapy and nutritional supplementation, operative intervention is recommended. Surgery for growth retardation is not beneficial after the onset of puberty.

Gastroduodenal disease

Symptomatic gastroduodenal disease occurs in 0.5% to 4% of patients who have Crohn's disease and is usually associated with disease at other sites. The most common indications for intervention are strictures, hemorrhage, and fistulas. Duodenal strictures may be bypassed (gastrojejunostomy), subjected to strictureplasty (depending on their site), or dilated (hydrostatic balloon). Strictureplasty may be preferable to bypass because it decreases the chances of stomal ulceration and diarrhea. Hemorrhage is usually managed by upper gastrointestinal endoscopy and adrenaline injection, rarely necessitating duodenotomy and underrunning of the bleeding source. Fistulas generally arise from small bowel disease and therefore surgical intervention includes small bowel resection (and anastomosis) and closure of the duodenum. Pettit and Irving [44] have recommended that it is safer to close this secondary duodenal defect with the aid of a jejunal serosal patch, or to use a Roux-en-Y duodenojejunostomy.

Preparation for surgery

Preparation for surgery entails counseling of the patient; documentation of extent of disease and presence of sepsis; consideration of bowel preparation, antibiotic, and venous thromboembolism prophylaxis (subcutaneous heparin, compression stockings); correction of fluid, electrolyte, and nutritional deficiencies; review of medication (corticosteroids and immunosuppressants); and marking of possible stoma sites.

Counseling of the patient includes discussion of disease extent, indications for surgery, alternatives to surgery, possible findings at surgery, intraoperative assessment and decision making (extent of resection, use of strictureplasty, formation of stoma), postoperative pain relief, expected discharge date, possible complications (bleeding, intra-abdominal and wound infections, intestinal injury, anastomotic leakage, fistula formation, respiratory atelectasis and infection, venous thromboembolism, incisional hernia, adhesive intestinal obstruction) and long-term outcome (possibility of recurrent disease, need for adjuvant therapy, symptomatic consequences of intestinal resection, nutritional deficiencies).

The extent of disease can be documented by small bowel series, colonoscopy (or barium enema), gastroscopy (if there are upper gastrointestinal symptoms), or isotope-labeled white cell scanning. It is wise to repeat studies preoperatively if the most recent imaging is more than 1 year old. There is evidence that newer modalities (enteroscopy, CT enterography, wireless capsule endoscopy, magnetic resonance enteroclysis) may improve detection of intestinal disease and strictures [45–49]. Blood tests (C-reactive protein, white cell count), CT scanning, and isotope-labeled white cell scan may also give useful information about the presence of septic complications [50,51].

Bowel preparation should be considered if there is any suggestion of colonic involvement, but may not be possible or well tolerated if there are obstructive symptoms. Prophylactic antibiotics (third-generation cephalosporin and metronidazole) should be given at induction and for up to 24 hours. A treatment regime (5 days of antibiotics) may be necessary if there is significant intraoperative contamination.

Patients who have small bowel Crohn's disease may be undernourished because of oral intake failure and malabsorption. Common nutritional disturbances are weight loss, hypoalbuminemia, anemia, and deficiencies of zinc, selenium, iron, vitamin A, vitamin D, and folic acid. Severely undernourished patients may benefit from preoperative nutrition support by either enteral or parenteral nutrition.

Stoma sites are best marked by specialist stoma care nurses who discuss the site with the patient considering visibility at the summit of the infraumbilical fat pad, within the surface markings of rectus abdominis muscle, and remote from old scars, skin creases, and bony prominences.

Drugs need to be reviewed so that anticoagulants are omitted; immunosuppressants may also need to be discontinued if there is leukopenia, and corticosteroids may need to be given to cover the perioperative stress in patients at risk for adrenal suppression (systemic steroid therapy within the last 6 months). No relationship between perioperative use of infliximab or immunosuppressants and the development of postoperative complications has been found [52].

Surgical approach

Surgical assessment and resection for Crohn's disease can now be performed laparoscopically—or with laparoscopic assistance—and by the traditional open approach. Laparoscopic surgery offers the possibilities of less postoperative morbidity, a faster recovery of pulmonary and intestinal function, better cosmesis, less narcotic use, shorter length, reduced costs of hospital stay, and reduced time to resumption of work. For patients who have Crohn's disease, laparoscopic surgery may also reduce intra-abdominal adhesions and abdominal wall injury seen in patients requiring repeated surgery. A laparoscopic approach can be used in Crohn's disease to create stomas, for ileocolonic resection, small bowel resection, and strictureplasty [53]. Concerns regarding the use of the laparoscopic approach have been a risk for underestimating the extent of the disease and an inability to complete the operation because of the presence of a thickened mesentery, inflammatory masses, abscesses, and fistulas.

The laparoscopic approach for ileocolonic resection usually involves mobilization of the terminal ileum and right colon; this can be performed medial to lateral or vice versa. The ileocolic pedicle is usually divided at an early stage to release the affected bowel from the retroperitoneum. A small 4- to 8-cm midline incision allows exteriorization of the specimen, control of remaining mesenteric blood vessels, bowel division, and extracorporeal anastomosis. Total intracorporeal resection and anastomosis have been described [54,55]. Extracorporeal resection and anastomosis may be safer and more rapid, however, and allows reliable examination of the total small bowel [53].

There is evidence of reduced surgical stress and faster recovery of pulmonary function after a laparoscopic approach. The laparoscopic approach was found to have no effect on recurrence rate or quality of life [56–58]. Lowney and colleagues [56] found that all disease recurrences were at the preanastomotic site, which did not substantiate the hypothesis that occult segments of disease were being missed as a result of the laparoscopic approach. Bergamaschi and colleagues [59] reported a reduced incidence of obstructive episodes over a 5-year period despite a similar preanastomotic recurrence rate; this may be because of a lower rate of adhesion formation and a reduced rate of ventral hernias.

Tilney and colleagues [60] in a meta-analysis showed that there was no significant difference in blood loss, anastomotic leak rate, or incidence of wound or chest infection, bowel obstruction, or formation of intra-abdominal abscesses between open and laparoscopic approaches in Crohn's disease. The operative times were significantly longer in the laparoscopic group. The laparoscopic group had a faster return of intestinal function and a shorter duration of hospital stay, however.

There is a large variation in the reported conversion rates for laparoscopic surgery for Crohn's disease (2%–40%). The conversion rate is likely to depend on patient selection, time constraints, and surgeon experience [61]. In a prospective study involving 69 consecutive patients, Alves and colleagues [62] found that recurrent episodes of Crohn's disease and the presence of intra-abdominal abscesses or fistulas were independent risk factors for conversion. Conversion was not found to increase morbidity or mortality, however [62], and therefore some authors believe that the presence of a mass or fistula are not contraindications to a laparoscopic approach [2,63]. The benefits of a laparoscopic approach begin to be lost when large incisions are needed for resection and anastomosis, which is more likely to be the case with larger, complex masses [2,64]. When a laparoscopic approach was used for recurrent Crohn's disease, the conversion rate (21%) and morbidity (10%) were higher than for those who had no prior surgery [65]. A laparoscopic approach may still be recommended if conversion is necessary; these patients do as well as those undergoing primary open surgery [66].

A fast-track multimodal rehabilitation approach has now been applied to open ileocolonic resections for Crohn's disease with a reduction in hospital stay and low morbidity and readmission rates [67]. This type of approach achieves similar rates of recovery of intestinal function and duration of hospital stay to those published using a laparoscopic approach. The main advantages of laparoscopic surgery over open surgery thus may be cosmesis and a reduction in wound complications because of the smaller size of the wounds [68].

Principles of open laparotomy for Crohn's disease

Consideration is necessary regarding positioning of the patient, maintaining body temperature, intraoperative venous thromboembolism prophylaxis, choice of incision, and intraoperative assessment and decision-making. The choice regarding position is between supine or modified lithotomy positions. The argument in favor of a modified lithotomy position is that any portion of the bowel can be involved and a sigmoid colon resection (and anastomosis) may be necessary. An infraumbilical midline skin incision gives good access to the small bowel and the ileocecal region and avoids potential stoma sites in the right and left iliac fossae. The midline incision can be reopened for recurrent disease, but may need to be extended to gain access if there is small bowel adherent to the existing scar.

A full exploration of the abdominal cavity is necessary to identify sites of disease and length of normal small bowel. It is not uncommon to find that the disease is more extensive than preoperative imaging had suggested. Sites of disease can be identified by visual inspection (fat wrapping, inflammatory changes, wall thickening, mesenteric thickening, adherence to adjacent organs), palpation (induration, thickening of the mesenteric edge, luminal narrowing), and intraoperative endoscopy [69,70]. Strictures may be identified by palpation or by the use of intraluminal Foley catheter, bougie, ball bearing, or plastic sphere. Bleeding sites may be identified by intraluminal endoscopy or intraoperative mesenteric angiography.

Intraoperative decision making involves whether to resect, perform strictureplasty, bypass, or defunction by stoma. Decisions regarding resection include the extent of resection, the margins of resection beyond the disease margins, preservation of the ileocecal valve, and type of anastomosis (stapled or hand-sewn; end-to-end, end-to-side, or side-to-side).

Bypass, stoma, resect, or strictureplasty

Bypass operations were introduced in the 1950s because of an associated reduced mortality rate, but have largely been abandoned because of the risk for continued disease activity and malignancy. A bypass procedure is still an option if an ileocolonic phlegmon is densely adherent onto iliac vessels or ureter, however, with a definitive resection being performed a few months later when the acute inflammation has subsided.

An ileostomy may be formed to defunction distal disease in association with a resection when an anastomosis is unsafe (undernourished patient, systemic steroid therapy, intra-abdominal sepsis), or if there is a simultaneous resection of colon and rectum. There is a significantly lower early recurrence rate after formation of ileostomy than after anastomosis [71].

Strictureplasty was introduced by Katariya and colleagues [72] who applied the technique to tuberculous strictures of the small intestine, to preserve intestinal length and reduce the risk for developing a short bowel syndrome in patients who would otherwise have undergone massive resection for these strictures. Lee and Papaioannou [73] applied the technique to patients who had Crohn's strictures of the small bowel. Since then strictureplasty has been used in patients who have short fibrous Crohn's strictures, in whom the technique has been shown to conserve intestinal length, relieve obstructive symptoms, promote weight gain, and enable reduction or withdrawal of steroid therapy. Strictureplasty has also been performed on recurrent strictures at ileocolonic anastomoses [74].

Sites of strictureplasty generally heal well with a low incidence of suture line breakdown; this may be because the blood supply to the involved segment of bowel remains untouched. There is radiologic, endoscopic, histopathologic, and operative evidence that active Crohn's disease regresses at the site of strictureplasty, especially when a large anastomosis has been performed [75,76]. The Cleveland Clinic [77] has reported a 5-year recurrence rate of 28% in a series of 698 strictureplasties in 162 patients with the recurrent strictures being found at the previous strictureplasty site in only 5% of patients. Because of the concern that a cancer may complicate a longstanding stricture and go unrecognized, it has been recommended that an intraoperative full-thickness biopsy should be taken from stricture sites during strictureplasty.

Indications for strictureplasty are: patients who have symptomatic fibrous strictures in the presence of diffuse disease, previous extensive intestinal resections (> 100 cm) or recent resection (within 1 year). Contraindications to strictureplasty are: patients who have small bowel perforation, malnutrition, or hypoalbuminemia; and strictures that are all located within a short segment, are very long (> 20 cm), or are found at the site of a fistula, an acute inflammatory mass, or in close proximity to a segment that needs to be resected.

Strictureplasty can be performed by several different techniques. Heinecke-Mikulicz and Finney are the two most commonly performed, Heinecke-Mikulicz strictureplasty being used for strictures less than 10 cm in length and Finney for strictures of 10 to 20 cm. In the Heinecke-Mikulicz technique, a linear antimesenteric incision is made through the stricture and extending for 3 cm on either side followed by closure of the wound transversely with a single-layer interrupted suture. In the Finney method, the strictured bowel is arranged in a U shape and the stricture is opened on the antimesenteric margin and closed side-to-side. Tichansky and colleagues [75] have reported a lower reoperation rate in patients whose strictures were subjected to Finney rather than Heineke-Mikulicz strictureplasty.

With regard to resection, the main debate has focused on whether patients should have a limited or extensive resection and on the influence of microscopic involvement of the resection limits on subsequent recurrence. Berman and Krause [78] reported a lower recurrence rate after radical resection (29%) when compared with a conservative procedure (84%) after a 7.5- to 9.5-year follow-up. A large randomized controlled trial comparing limited (2 cm) and extended (12 cm) margins showed no relationship between recurrence and resection margins, however [79]. Hamilton and colleagues [80] compared recurrence rates in patients who underwent resection based on visual inspection with those in whom the resection margin was based on frozen section evaluation. There was no difference in clinical recurrence rates or reoperation rates after 10 years of follow-up. Glehen and colleagues [81] have reported that small bowel length (as measured at laparotomy) is significantly shorter in patients who have Crohn's disease than in controls. Limited resection is therefore the procedure of choice; frozen section evaluation of resection margins does not influence recurrence rates.

Anastomoses may be performed by hand-sewn or stapled techniques and a variety of configurations have been described (end-to-end, end-to-side, and side-to-side). Stapled anastomoses have been reported to be associated with a lower morbidity [82], lower anastomotic leak rate [83], and lower reoperation rate [82], but these findings were not reported in all studies. Concerns about the use of staplers are related to a greater risk for bleeding in thickened bowel in patients who have undergone resection and anastomosis for chronic intestinal obstruction. Indeed, this thickened proximal bowel wall may exceed the specifications of the stapling device and therefore hand-sewn anastomosis may be safer. A hand-sewn anastomotic technique that is interrupted and single layer is less likely to cause luminal narrowing and is therefore preferred.

Regarding configuration of the anastomosis, a standard end-to-end anastomosis produces the narrowest lumen and so may make anastomotic recurrence more likely to be symptomatic. A retrospective study showed fewer symptomatic recurrences and lower operation rate in patients treated by a wide-stapled anastomosis compared with end-to-end sutured anastomosis [82]. Most studies have shown no effect of anastomotic configuration on recurrence rate, however.

Intraoperative challenges

During the course of laparotomy for Crohn's disease, the surgeon may encounter an inflammatory mass, an unexpected abscess, an internal fistula, thickened mesentery, enlarged lymph nodes, or multisite disease. It is usually easier to deal with these situations if the affected bowel and associated mass can be delivered into the wound. The challenge then is to separate non-diseased bowel from diseased bowel without causing injury to normal bowel or to its vascular supply. This is usually achieved by a combination of blunt and sharp dissection.

For ileocolonic fistulas, the terminal ileum is usually the offending segment. Intraoperative colonoscopy may help to determine whether the colon is diseased (and therefore requiring resection) or secondarily affected. For ileo-ileal fistulas, the secondary site may be débrided and primarily sutured. For ileo-colonic fistulas, the secondary site can be treated by wedge excision or limited resection.

The mesentery of the ileocecal region affected by Crohn's disease is usually thickened and friable; care is needed during division to prevent significant blood loss or the development of a large mesenteric hematoma. It is often difficult to fashion convenient pedicles to ligate and it is usually safer to serially clamp the mesentery and to ligate using sutures. If diffuse jejunoileal disease is encountered, the site and extent of the disease should be documented but only disease that is currently causing a complication should be dealt with surgically to avoid major intestinal resection and the development of short bowel syndrome.

Outcome of surgery

Outcome of surgery can be classified according to mortality, morbidity, quality of life, and recurrence. In the Mount Sinai experience, postoperative (30-day) mortality rate was 3.2% with sepsis the most common cause [84]. In a long-term study, sepsis and severe electrolyte imbalance attributable to short bowel syndrome were the most common causes of death related to Crohn's disease [85]. Major postoperative complications occur in 10% to 20% of patients, the most common complications being bowel obstruction, intra-abdominal and wound infections, anastomotic leakages, and fistulas [6,75,84]. Serious postoperative complications are more likely if there is pre-existing intra-abdominal sepsis or preoperative immune suppression because of steroid use [6]. Post-strictureplasty intestinal hemorrhage may occur in as many as 10% of patients and if it is persistent may require surgery. Preoperative mesenteric angiography may help identify the source and avoid having to open or resect multiple intestinal segments that had been subjected to strictureplasty.

Later complications of small bowel resection for Crohn's disease include cholelithiasis; urolithiasis; fluid, electrolyte, mineral, and vitamin deficiencies; undernutrition; and diarrhea. Short bowel syndrome is unavoidable in a small percentage of patients who have Crohn's disease as a result of recurrent resection of affected small intestine and inflammatory destruction of remaining small bowel [86]. Agwunobi and colleagues [87] reported that most patients who had Crohn's disease developed intestinal failure as a result of multiple unplanned laparotomies for intra-abdominal sepsis (61%), with extensive primary surgery (17%) and uncomplicated sequential resection (22%) causing the remainder. Short bowel syndrome can be classified according to the anatomic configuration (jejunum-jejunostomy; jejunum-jejunocolonic anastomosis) and results in a variable degree of intestinal failure. Patients who have moderate intestinal failure require parenteral fluid and electrolyte supplementation; those who have severe intestinal failure require parenteral administration of fluid, electrolytes, and nutrition. Patients on home parenteral nutrition are at risk for severe complications, such as line-related sepsis, venous thromboembolism, and metabolic liver and bone disease.

Many patients who have Crohn's disease have physical and mental limitations on their quality of life, with depression reported in 33% to 100% of patients. Low quality-of-life scores with active disease improve to normal when remission is obtained by surgery [88]. Thaler and colleagues [57] found that quality of life was significantly reduced in patients who had Crohn's disease at long-term followup irrespective of surgical approach (laparoscopic versus open).

Recurrent disease after surgery

Surgery aims to overcome complications of Crohn's disease or to improve quality of life when medical treatment has failed, but does not cure Crohn's disease because of its panenteric nature. After intestinal resection and anastomosis, recurrence rates increase progressively with time after the surgery [89]. The risk for recurrence depends on the age of patient at initial surgery, site of the disease, extent of disease, disease pattern (stricturing or perforating), and postsurgical behavior (cigarette smoking). There is controversy regarding the effect, if any, of anastomotic configuration on the risk for recurrence.

Recurrence can be defined as endoscopic, radiologic, symptomatic, or requiring reoperation. Following ileocecal resection with anastomosis for terminal ileal disease, longitudinal endoscopic studies have shown that inflammation typically recurs within 12 months of resection [90]. The relevance of endoscopic recurrence has been queried; however, there is evidence that endoscopic recurrence often predicts later symptomatic recurrence and that endoscopic severity predicts future disease activity [91].

Overall, the risk for recurrence following intestinal resection and anastomosis is in the region of 29% to 35% at 5 years, 52% to 55% at 10 years, 60% to 75% at 15 years, and rising to 94% at 25 years [7,89]. The presence of a symptomatic recurrence does not mandate surgery. The rates of recurrence requiring re-resection have been reported to be 25% to 35% at 5 years and 40% to 70% at 15 years [92,93]. The risk for recurrence is higher for ileocolonic disease (50% at 5 years, 53% at 13 years) than for ileal disease [3,92], and higher for perforating disease than nonperforating disease [94]. An effect of disease pattern on recurrence rate has not been a universal finding, however [95].

Smoking increases the risk for recurrent disease as defined on endoscopy, by symptomatology, and in those requiring reoperation [96]. The 6-year recurrence-free rate after surgery is 60% for nonsmokers, 41% for ex-smokers, and 27% for smokers. The likelihood of recurrence correlates with the number of cigarettes smoked and the duration of smoking and is especially high in female smokers who have small bowel disease [97].

Crohn's disease tends to recur in the proximal limb of an ileo-ileal or ileo-colonic anastomosis, although as many as one third of recurrences occur separately from it [98]. Fewer recurrences occur at strictureplasty than at resection sites [98]. When disease recurs, old notes and radiologic studies need to be reviewed and an up-to-date assessment made of remaining small and large bowel using contrast examinations and colonoscopy. CT scanning is useful if intra-abdominal sepsis is suspected and nuclear medicine imaging may help to determine whether symptoms are attributable to disease recurrence or postoperative adhesions.

Indications for surgery in patients who have recurrent disease are the same as for those who have primary surgery: failed medical therapy and acute or chronic complications. There is concern that reoperative surgery for Crohn's disease leads to the development of short bowel syndrome; this often leads to a more cautious approach and strictureplasty is often favored. Resection is usually undertaken for intra-abdominal sepsis and fistula formation, however.

Postoperative advice and treatment

Having achieved remission by surgical intervention, the next challenge is to maximize the period of symptom-free remission. Cessation of smoking is the postoperative intervention with the best evidence of effect on maintenance of remission, the relapse rate in ex-smokers being reduced by approximately 40% [96]. Esaki and colleagues [99] showed that postoperative enteral nutrition (>1200 kcal/day) reduced postsurgical recurrence, especially in patients who had penetrating disease and in those who had disease confined to the small bowel. There has been a lot of interest in prophylaxis against postoperative recurrence using aminosalicylates, antibiotics, corticosteroids, thiopurines, and probiotics. Many of the studies have used an endpoint of endoscopic recurrence to assess response to prophylactic treatment, rather than symptomatic recurrence, which would be a more useful clinical endpoint.

There have been several placebo-controlled trials of mesalazine as a prophylactic treatment with conflicting results. Meta-analysis has shown an advantage for Pentasa at a dose of 4 g/d, but only in patients who have isolated ileal disease [100]. Metronidazole (20 mg/kg/d for 3 months) reduces symptomatic and endoscopic relapse at 1 year [101]. The side-effect profile (nausea, vomiting, rashes, peripheral neuropathy) means that this antibiotic cannot be used long-term, however. With regard to steroids, prednisolone was found to have no prophylactic effect. Budesonide (6 mg/d) reduced endoscopic but not clinical recurrence at 1 year in patients who had inflammatory disease but not in those who had fibrostenotic disease [102]. Budesonide at a 3-mg dose was no better than placebo in preventing endoscopic recurrence in patients after ileal or ileocecal resection, however [103].

Thiopurines (azathioprine and 6-mercaptopurine) are effective steroid-sparing agents in active Crohn's disease but have a significant range of side effects and require regular toxicity monitoring. Studies in children (1 mg/kg/d) and adults (50 mg/d) have shown that 6-mercaptopurine is more effective than aminosalicylates (or placebo/no medication) in preventing postoperative recurrence [104,105]. Domenech and colleagues [106] found that azathioprine was more effective than aminosalicylates in reducing clinical and endoscopic recurrence rates after surgical resection. Two other studies found no difference in efficacy between azathioprine (at a dose of 2 mg/kg/d or 50 mg/d) and aminosalicylates in preventing postsurgical recurrence [107,108]. Alves and colleagues [109] have shown that immunosuppressive drugs (one of azathioprine, 6-mercaptopurine, or methotrexate) reduce the rate of postoperative recurrence and the need for further surgery after a second ileocolonic anastomotic recurrence.

Trials assessing probiotic therapy have shown that neither Lactobacillus G nor Lactobacillus johnsonii LA1 was more effective than placebo in maintaining remission following intestinal resection [110,111].

Rutgeerts [112] has stratified postoperative patients into those at low (nonsmoker, first operation, and fibrostenosis) and high (female smoker, smoker; at least one previous operation; perforating disease and extensive disease) risk for recurrence. For patients at higher risk who have exclusively ileal disease, Pentasa at a dose of 4 g/d is a reasonable choice with minimal side effects. For patients who have extensive disease needing repeated operations, or with perforating disease, treatment with a thiopurine (azathioprine at 2–2.5 mg/kg/d or 6-mercaptopurine at 1–1.5 mg/kg/d) would seem a pragmatic approach.

Summary

Despite advances in medical treatment, most patients who have Crohn's disease of the small intestine need surgery at some point during the course of their disease. Surgery is currently indicated for intractable disease and complications of the disease (strictures, abscesses, fistulas, hemorrhage). There is increasing interest in nonsurgical and minimal access strategies of dealing with complicated disease, however. These new approaches may enable postponement of surgery to a more favorable time, or conversion of a two-stage procedure involving a stoma to a one-stage resection with anastomosis. A continuing challenge is prevention of disease recurrence postoperatively.

References

[1] Mekhijan HS, Sweitz DM, Watts HD, et al. National cooperative Crohn's disease study: factors determining recurrence of Crohn's disease after surgery. Gastroenterology 1979; 77:907–13.

[2] Canin-Endres J, Salky B, Gattorno F, et al. Laparoscopically assisted intestinal resection in 88 patients with Crohn's disease. Surg Endosc 1999;13:595–9.

[3] Fazio VW, Wu JS. Surgical therapy for Crohn's disease of the colon and rectum. Surg Clin North Am 1997;77:197–210.

[4] Mow WS, Vasiliauskas EA, Lin YC, et al. Association of antibody responses to microbial antigens and complications of small bowel Crohn's disease. Gastroenterology 2004;126: 414–24.

[5] Siederer J, Brand S, Herrmann KA, et al. Predictive value of the CARD variant 1007fs for the diagnosis of intestinal stenoses and the need for surgery in Crohn's disease in clinical practice: results of a prospective study. Inflamm Bowel Dis 2006;12:1114–21.

[6] Post S, Betzler M, von Ditfurth B, et al. Risks of intestinal anastomoses in Crohn's disease. Ann Surg 1991;213:37–42.

[7] Chardavoyne R, Flint GW, Pollack S, et al. Factors affecting recurrence following resection for Crohn's disease. Dis Colon Rectum 1986;29:495–502.

[8] Hulten L. Surgical treatment of Crohn's disease of the small bowel or ileocecum. World J Surg 1988;12:180–5.

[9] Michelassi F, Balestracci T, Chappell R, et al. Primary and recurrent Crohn's: experience with 1379 cases. Ann Surg 1991;214:230–8.

[10] Morini S, Hassan C, Lorenzetti R, et al. Long-term outcome of endoscopic pneumatic dilatation in Crohn's disease. Dig Liver Dis 2003;35:893–7.

[11] Ferlitsch A, Reinisch W, Puspok A, et al. Safety and efficacy of endoscopic balloon dilation for treatment of Crohn's disease strictures. Endoscopy 2006;38:483–7.

[12] Nomura E, Takagi S, Kikuchi T, et al. Efficacy and safety of endoscopic balloon dilation for Crohn's strictures. Dis Colon Rectum 2006;49:S59–67.

[13] Singh VV, Draganov P, Valentine J. Efficacy and safety of endoscopic balloon dilation of symptomatic upper and lower gastrointestinal Crohn's disease strictures. J Clin Gastroenterol 2005;39:298–9.

[14] Bickston SJ, Foley E, Lawrence C, et al. Terminal ileal stricture in Crohn's disease: treatment using a metallic enteral endoprosthesis. Dis Colon Rectum 2005;48:1081–5.

[15] Ribeiro MB, Greenstein AJ, Yamazaki Y, et al. Intra-abdominal abscess in regional enteritis. Ann Surg 1991;21:32–6.

[16] Michelassi F, Fichera A. Indications for surgery in inflammatory bowel disease. In: Kirsner JB, editor. Inflammatory bowel disease. 5th edition. Philadelphia: WB Saunders; 2000. p. 616–25.

[17] Jawhari A, Kamm M, Ong C, et al. Intraabdominal and pelvic abscess in Crohn's disease; results of non-invasive and surgical management. Br J Surg 1998;85:367–71.

[18] Strong S, Fazio VW. The surgical management of Crohn's disease. In: Kirsner JB, editor. Inflammatory bowel disease. 5th edition. Philadelphia: WB Saunders; 2000. p. 658–709.

[19] Lambiase RE, Deyoe L, Cronan JJ, et al. Percutaneous drainage of 335 consecutive abscesses: results of primary drainage with 1 year follow-up. Radiology 1992;184:167–79.

[20] Sahai A, Belair M, Gianfelice D, et al. Percutaneous drainage of intra-abdominal abscesses in Crohn's disease. Am J Gastroenterol 1997;92:275–8.

[21] Garcia JC, Persky SE, Bonis PA, et al. Abscesses in Crohn's disease: outcome of medical versus surgical treatment. J Clin Gastroenterol 2001;32:409–12.

[22] Gutierrez A, Lee H, Sands BE. Outcome of surgical versus percutaneous drainage of abdominal and pelvic abscesses in Crohn's disease. Am J Gastroenterol 2006;101:2283–9.

[23] Greenstein AJ, Sachar DB, Mann D, et al. Spontaneous free perforation and perforated abscess in 30 patients with Crohn's disease. Ann Surg 1987;205:72–6.

[24] Michelassi F, Stella M, Balestracci T, et al. Incidence, diagnosis and treatment of enteric and colorectal fistulae in patients with Crohn's disease. Ann Surg 1993;218:660–6.

[25] Irving M, O'Dwyer ST. Surgical management of anastamotic leakage and intraabdominal sepsis. In: Fielding P, Dudley H, editors. Rob and Smith's operative surgery. 5th edition. New York: Butterworth-Heinemann; 1993. p. 93–104.

[26] Korelitz BI, Present DH. Favorable effect of 6-mercaptopurine on fistulas of Crohn's disease. Dig Dis Sci 1985;30:58–64.

[27] Margolin ML, Korelitz BI. Management of bladder fistulas in Crohn's disease. J Clin Gastroenterol 1989;11:399–402.

[28] Hanauer SB, Smith MB. Rapid closure of Crohn's fistulas with continuous intravenous cyclosporine A. Am J Gastroenterol 1993;88:646–9.

[29] Present DH, Lichtiger S. Efficacy of cyclosporine in treatment of fistula of Crohn's disease. Dig Dis Sci 1994;39:374–80.

[30] Present DH, Rutgeerts P, Targan S, et al. Infliximab for the treatment of fistulas in patients with Crohn's disease. N Engl J Med 1999;340:1398–405.

[31] Sands BE, Anderson FH, Bernstein CN, et al. Infliximab maintenance therapy for fistulizing Crohn's disease. N Engl J Med 2004;350:876–85.

[32] Cirocco WC, Reilly JC, Rusin LC. Life-threatening hemorrhage and exsanguinations from Crohn's disease. Report of four cases. Dis Colon Rectum 1995;38:85–95.

[33] Remzi FH, Dietz DW, Unal E, et al. Combined use of preoperative provocative angiography and highly selective methylene blue injection to localize an occult small-bowel bleeding site in a patient with Crohn's disease: report of a case. Dis Colon Rectum 2003;46: 260–3.

[34] Ozuner G, Fazio VW. Management of gastrointestinal bleeding after strictureplasty for Crohn's disease. Dis Colon Rectum 1995;38:297–300.

[35] Kazama Y, Watanabe T, Akahane M, et al. Crohn's disease with life-threatening hemorrhage from terminal ileum: successful control with superselective arterial embolization. J Gastroenterol 2005;40:1155–7.

[36] Sze DY. Targeted drug delivery for refractory hemorrhagic Crohn disease. J Vasc Interv Radiol 2006;17:163–7.

[37] Kronberger IE, Graziadei IW, Vogel V. Small bowel adenocarcinoma in Crohn's disease: a case report. World J Gastroenterol 2006;12:1317–20.

[38] Michelassi F, Testa G, Pomidor WJ, et al. Adenocarcinoma complicating Crohn's disease. Dis Colon Rectum 1993;36:654–61.

[39] Marchetti F, Fazio VW, Ozuner G. Adenocarcinoma arising from a strictureplasty site in Crohn's disease. Dis Colon Rectum 1996;39:1315–21.

[40] Jaskowiak NT, Michelassi F. Adenocarcinoma at a strictureplasty site in Crohn's disease: report of a case. Dis Colon Rectum 2001;44:284–7.

[41] Solem CA, Harmsen WS, Zinsmeister AR, et al. Small intestinal adenocarcinoma in Crohn's disease: a case-control study. Inflamm Bowel Dis 2004;10:32–5.

[42] Siminovitch JM, Fazio VW. Ureteral obstruction secondary to Crohn's disease: a need for ureterolysis? Am J Surg 1980;139:95–8.

[43] Telander RL, Schmeling DJ. Current surgical management of Crohn's disease in childhood. Semin Pediatr Surg 1994;3:19–27.

[44] Pettit S, Irving M. The operative management of fistulating Crohn's disease—experience with 100 consecutive cases. Surg Gynecol Obstet 1988;167:223–8.

[45] Higgins PD, Caoili E, Zimmermann M, et al. Computed tomographic enterography adds information to clinical management in small bowel Crohn's disease. Inflamm Bowel Dis 2006; [Epub PMID 17206719].

[46] Leighton JA, Legnani P, Seidman EG. Role of capsule endoscopy in inflammatory bowel disease: where we are and where we are going. Inflamm Bowel Dis 2006; [Epub PMID 17206673].

[47] Girelli CM, Porta P, Malacrida V, et al. Clinical outcome of patients examined by capsule endoscopy for suspected small bowel Crohn's disease. Dig Liver Dis 2007;39(2):148–54 [Epub PMID 17196893].

[48] Negaard A, Sandvik L, Mulahasanovic A, et al. Magnetic resonance enteroclysis in the diagnosis of small-intestinal Crohn's disease: diagnostic accuracy and inter and intra-observer agreement. Acta Radiol 2006;47:1008–16.

[49] Triester SL, Leighton JA, Leontiadis GI, et al. A meta-analysis of the yield of capsule endoscopy compared to other diagnostic modalities in patients with non-stricturing small bowel Crohn's disease. Am J Gastroenterol 2006;101:954–64.

[50] Booya F, Fletcher JG, Huprich JE, et al. Active Crohn's disease: CT findings and interobserver agreement for enteric phase CT enterography. Radiology 2006;241: 787–95.

[51] Almer S, Granerus G, Strom M, et al. Leukocyte scintigraphy compared to intraoperative small bowel enteroscopy and laparotomy findings in Crohn's disease. Inflamm Bowel Dis 2006; [Epub PMID 17206712].

[52] Colombel JF, Loftus EV Jr, Tremaine WJ, et al. Early postoperative complications are not increased in patients with Crohn's disease treated perioperatively with infliximab or immunosuppressive therapy. Am J Gastroenterol 2004;99:878–83.

[53] Casillas S, Delaney CP. Laparoscopic surgery for inflammatory bowel disease. Dig Surg 2005;22:135–42.

[54] Ludwig KA, Milsom JW, Church JM, et al. Preliminary experience with laparoscopic intestinal surgery for Crohn's disease. Am J Surg 1996;171:52–5.

[55] Dutta BS, Rothenberg JC, Bealer J. Total intracorporeal laparoscopic resection of Crohn's disease. J Pediatr Surg 2003;38:717–9.

[56] Lowney JK, Dietz DW, Birnbaum EH, et al. Is there any difference in recurrence rates in laparoscopic ileocolic resection for Crohn's disease compared with conventional surgery? A long-term follow up study. Dis Colon Rectum 2005;491:58–63.

[57] Thaler K, Dinnewitzer A, Oberwalder M, et al. Assessment of long-term quality of life after laparoscopic and open surgery for Crohn's disease. Colorectal Dis 2005;7:375–81.

[58] Maartense S, Dunker MS, Slors JF, et al. Laparoscopic-assisted versus open ileocolic resection for Crohn's disease: a randomized trial. Ann Surg 2006;243:143–9.

[59] Bergamaschi R, Pessaux P, Armaud JP. Comparison of conventional and laparoscopic ileocolic resection for Crohn's disease. Dis Colon Rectum 2003;46:1129–33.

[60] Tilney HS, Constantinides VA, Heriot AG, et al. Comparison of laparoscopic and open ileocecal resection for Crohn's disease: a metaanalysis. Surg Endosc 2006;20: 1036–44.

[61] Evans J, Poritz L, MacRae H. Influence of experience on laparoscopic ileocolic resection for Crohn's disease. Dis Colon Rectum 2002;45:1595–600.

[62] Alves A, Panis Y, Bouhnik Y, et al. Factors that predict conversion in 69 consecutive patients undergoing laparoscopic ileocaecal resection for Crohn's disease: a prospective study. Dis Colon Rectum 2005;48:2302–8.

[63] Hasegawa H, Watanabe M, Nishibori H, et al. Laparoscopic surgery for recurrent Crohn's disease. Br J Surg 2003;90:970–3.

[64] Bauer JJ, Harris MT, Grunmbach NM, et al. Laparoscopic-assisted intestinal resection for Crohn's disease. Dis Colon Rectum 1995;38:712–5.

[65] Wu J, Birnbaum E, Kodner I, et al. Laparoscopic-assisted ileocolic resections in patients with Crohn's disease: are abscesses, phlegmons, or recurrent disease contraindications? Surgery 1997;122:682–8.

[66] Casillas S, Delaney CP, Senagore AJ, et al. Does conversion of a laparoscopic colectomy adversely affect patient outcome? Dis Colon Rectum 2004;47:1680–5.

[67] Andersen J, Kehlet H. Fast track open ileo-colic resections for Crohn's disease. Colorectal Dis 2005;7:394–7.

[68] Milsom JW. Laparoscopic surgery in the treatment of Crohn's disease. Surg Clin North Am 2005;85:25–34.

[69] Lescut D, Vanco D, Bonniere P, et al. Perioperative endoscopy of the whole small bowel in Crohn's disease. Gut 1993;34:647–9.

[70] Esaki M, Matsumoto T, Hizawa K, et al. Intraoperative enteroscopy detects more lesions but is not predictive of postoperative recurrence in Crohn's disease. Surg Endosc 2001;15: 455–9.

[71] Heimann TM, Greenstein AJ, Lewis B, et al. Prediction of early symptomatic recurrence after intestinal resection in Crohn's disease. Ann Surg 1993;218:294–8.

[72] Katariya RN, Sood S, Rao PG, et al. Strictureplasty for tubercular strictures of the gastrointestinal tract. Br J Surg 1977;64:496–8.

[73] Lee ECG, Papaioannou N. Minimal surgery for chronic obstruction in patients with extensive or universal Crohn's disease. Ann R Coll Surg Engl 1982;64:229–33.

[74] Tjandra JJ, Fazio VW. Strictureplasty for ileocolic anastomotic strictures in Crohn's disease. Dis Colon Rectum 1993;36:1099–103.

[75] Tichansky D, Cagir B, Yoo E, et al. Strictureplasty for Crohn's disease: meta-analysis. Dis Colon Rectum 2000;43:911–9.

[76] Tonelli F, Fedi M, Paroli GM, et al. Indications and results of side-to-side isoperistaltic strictureplasty in Crohn's disease. Dis Colon Rectum 2004;47:494–501.

[77] Ozuner G, Fazio VW, Lavery IC, et al. How safe is strictureplasty in the management of Crohn's disease. Am J Surg 1996;171:57–60.

[78] Bergman L, Krause U. Crohn's disease: a long-term study of the clinical course in 186 patients. Scand J Gastroenterol 1977;12:937–44.

[79] Fazio VW, Marchetti F, Church JM, et al. Effect of resection margins on the recurrence of Crohn's disease in the small bowel. A randomised controlled trial. Ann Surg 1996;224: 563–71.

[80] Hamilton SR, Reese J, Pennington L, et al. The role of resection margin frozen section in the surgical management of Crohn's disease. Surg Gynecol Obstet 1985;160:57–62.

[81] Glehen O, Lifante JC, Vignal J, et al. Small bowel length in Crohn's disease. Int J Colorectal Dis 2003;18:423–7.

[82] Munoz-Juarez M, Yamamoto T, Wolff BG, et al. Wide-lumen stapled anstomosis vs conventional end-to-end anastomosis in the treatment of Crohn's disease. Dis Colon Rectum 2001;44:20–6.

[83] Resegotti A, Astegiano M, Farina E, et al. Side-to-side stapled anastomosis strongly reduces anastomotic leak rates in Crohn's disease surgery. Dis Colon Rectum 2005;48: 464–8.

[84] Greenstein AJ, Meyers S, Sher L, et al. Surgery and its sequelae in Crohn's colitis and ileocolitis. Arch Surg 1981;116:285–8.

[85] Harper PH, Fazio VW, Lavery IC, et al. The long-term outcome in Crohn's disease. Dis Colon Rectum 1987;30:174–9.

[86] Krupnick AS, Morris JB. The long-term results of resection and multiple resections in Crohn's disease. Semin Gastrointest Dis 2000;11:41–51.

[87] Agwunobi AO, Carlson GL, Anderson ID, et al. Mechanisms of intestinal failure in Crohn's disease. Dis Colon Rectum 2001;44:1834–7.

[88] Casellas F, Lopez-Vivancos J, Badia X, et al. Impact of surgery for Crohn's disease on health-related quality of life. Am J Gastroenterol 2000;95:177–82.

[89] Trnka YM, Glotzer DJ, Kasdon EJ, et al. The long-term outcome of restorative operation in Crohn's disease: influence of location, prognostic factors and surgical guidelines. Ann Surg 1982;196:345–55.

[90] Lochs H, Mayer M, Fleig WE, et al. Prophylaxis of postoperative relapse in Crohn's disease with mesalamine. European Cooperative Crohn's disease Study VI. Gastroenterology 2000;118:264–73.

[91] Rutgeerts P, Geboes K, van Trappen G, et al. Predictability of the postoperative course of Crohn's disease. Gastroenterology 1990;99:956–63.

[92] Whelan G, Farmer RG, Fazio VW, et al. Recurrence after surgery in Crohn's disease: relationship to location of disease (clinical pattern) and surgical indication. Gastroenterology 1985;88:1826–33.

[93] Bernell O, Lapidus A, Hellers G. Risk factors for surgery and postoperative recurrence in Crohn's disease. Ann Surg 2000;231:38–45.

[94] Lautenbach E, Berlin J, Lichtenstein G. Risk factors for early postoperative recurrence of Crohn's disease. Gastroenterology 1998;115:259–67.

[95] McDonald PJ, Fazio VW, Farmer RG, et al. Perforating and nonperforating Crohn's disease: an unpredictable guide to recurrence after surgery. Dis Colon Rectum 1989;32: 117–20.

[96] Cottone M, Rosselli M, Orlando A, et al. Smoking habits and recurrence in Crohn's disease. Gastroenterology 1994;106:643–8.

[97] Yamamoto T, Keighley MR. Smoking and disease recurrence after operation for Crohn's disease. Br J Surg 2000;87:398–404.
[98] Fichera A, Lovadina S, Rubin M, et al. Patterns and operative treatment of recurrent Crohn's disease: a prospective longitudinal study. Surgery 2006;140:649–54.
[99] Esaki M, Matsumoto T, Hizawa K, et al. Preventive effect of nutritional therapy against postoperative recurrence of Crohn's disease, with reference to findings determined by intra-operative enteroscopy. Scand J Gastroenterol 2005;40:1431–7.
[100] Sutherland LR. Mesalamine for the prevention of postoperative recurrence: is nearly there the same as being there? Gastroenterology 2000;119:436–8.
[101] Rutgeerts P, Hiele M, Geboes K, et al. Controlled trial of metronidazole treatment for prevention of Crohn's recurrence after ileal resection. Gastroenterology 1995;108:1617–21.
[102] Hellers G, Cortot A, Jewell D, et al. Oral budesonide for prevention of postsurgical recurrence in Crohn's disease. The IOIBD Budesonide Study Group. Gastroenterology 1999; 116:294–300.
[103] Ewe K, Bottger T, Buhr HJ, et al. Low-dose budesonide treatment for prevention of postoperative recurrence of Crohn's disease: a multicentre randomized placebo-controlled trial. German Budesonide Study Group. Eur J Gastroenterol Hepatol 1999;11:277–82.
[104] Kader HA, Raynor SC, Young R, et al. Introduction of 6-mercaptopurine in Crohn's disease in Crohn's disease patients during the perioperative period; a preliminary evaluation of recurrence of disease. J Pediatr Gastroenterol Nutr 1997;25:93–7.
[105] Hanauer SB, Korelitz BI, Rutgeerts P, et al. Postoperative maintenance of Crohn's disease remission with 6-mercaptopurine, mesalamine, or placebo: a 2-year trial. Gastroenterology 2004;127:723–9.
[106] Domenech E, Scala L, Bernal I, et al. Azathioprine and mesalazine in the prevention of postsurgical recurrence of Crohn's disease: a retrospective study. Gastroenterol Hepatol 2004;27:563–7.
[107] Nos P, Hinojosa J, Aguilera V, et al. Azathioprine and 5-ASA in the prevention of postoperative recurrence of Crohn's disease. Gastroenterol Hepatol 2000;23:374–8.
[108] Ardizzone S, Maconi G, Sampietro GM, et al. Azathioprine and mesalamine for prevention of relapse after conservative surgery for Crohn's disease. Gastroenterology 2004;127: 730–40.
[109] Alves A, Panis Y, Joly F, et al. Could immunosuppressive drugs reduce disease recurrence rate after second resection for Crohn's disease? Inflamm Bowel Dis 2004;10:491–5.
[110] Prantera C, Scribano ML, Falasco G, et al. Ineffectiveness of probiotics in preventing recurrence after curative resection for Crohn's disease: a randomised controlled trial with Lactobacillus GG. Gut 2002;51:405–9.
[111] Marteau P, Lemann M, Seksik P, et al. Ineffectiveness of Lactobacillus johnsonii LA1 for prophylaxis of postoperative recurrence in Crohn's disease: a randomised, double blind, placebo controlled GETAID trial. Gut 2006;55:842–7.
[112] Rutgeerts P. Crohn's disease recurrence can be prevented after ileal resection. Gut 2002;51: 152–3.

ELSEVIER
SAUNDERS

SURGICAL
CLINICS OF
NORTH AMERICA

Surg Clin N Am 87 (2007) 611–631

Operative Management of Crohn's Disease of the Colon Including Anorectal Disease

Scott R. Steele, MD, FACS

Colon & Rectal Surgery, Department of Surgery, Madigan Army Medical Center,
Fort Lewis, WA 98431, USA

Inflammatory bowel disease (IBD) is an idiopathic, ulcerogenic, inflammatory condition of the gastrointestinal tract, including Crohn's disease and ulcerative colitis. Despite being included under the broad umbrella of IBD, Crohn's disease differs distinctly from ulcerative colitis. Because Crohn's disease occurs anywhere along the alimentary tract from the mouth to the anus and is marked by multiple recurrences, surgical excision is not a curative procedure. In fact, up to 90% of patients require at least one operation during their lifetime [1]. The surgeon must then not only take into account the appropriate treatment of the acute problem at hand but also balance the ramifications of that therapy with potential future exacerbations in what is most often a palliative procedure. Surgeons therefore need to be exceedingly aware of the indications, surgical options, and expected outcomes for the patient who has Crohn's disease. Furthermore, although the precise cause of the disease remains unknown, our understanding of the principles guiding surgical treatment has expanded greatly and continues to evolve.

Crohn's disease of the colon and rectum

Clinical presentation

Crohn's disease most commonly affects the terminal ileum and cecum, followed by colonic, small bowel, and finally perianal disease. Although

---

No outside financial support or provision of supplies was solicited or received in connection with this work.

This is an original work by the above author. The opinions expressed are the author's and author's alone. They do not necessarily reflect the opinion of the US Government, the US Department of Defense, or Madigan Army Medical Center.

E-mail address: docsteele@hotmail.com.

0039-6109/07/$ - see front matter. Published by Elsevier Inc.
doi:10.1016/j.suc.2007.03.006
surgical.theclinics.com

isolated colonic disease can occur in approximately 25% of patients, it is most often seen in conjunction with terminal ileal disease or with concomitant perianal disease [2]. The distribution within the colon remains at a consistent pattern, with approximately one third of patients having total colonic involvement, 40% showing segmental disease, and approximately 30% having disease only on the left side [3]. In general terms, Crohn's disease falls into one of three broad categories: fistulizing, fibrotic (stricturing), or inflammatory. Regardless of the type, the most common symptoms patients who have colorectal involvement experience are abdominal pain, rectal bleeding, and malnutrition [2]. In addition, patients can experience diarrhea, hip and pelvic pain from abscess and fistulas, and obstructive symptoms. Unlike ulcerative colitis, rectal bleeding is not a common presenting symptom [4]. Physical examination may have a paucity of findings, although perianal disease and extracolonic manifestations, such as oral ulcerations, skin lesions, and joint problems, may be present.

Diagnosis

Patients presenting with the above symptoms often undergo extensive radiologic work-up. In the past, contrast studies, such as a barium enema, would identify patterns of extensive longitudinal and transverse linear ulcerations creating a cobblestone and nodular pattern, skip lesions, and strictures [5]. CT scan has largely replaced the barium enema, although the luminal findings remain the same. In addition, CT may demonstrate extraluminal findings, such as segmental thickening of the colon with mesenteric fat stranding, terminal ileal or small bowel thickening, and abscesses [6,7]. Endoscopic evaluation and biopsy remain the gold standard, and patients should undergo complete colonoscopy with evaluation of the terminal ileum [8]. Early changes of the colon include aphthous ulcerations, erosions, and serpiginous ulcers all in a skip-type pattern. As the full-thickness inflammatory cycle continues, these ulcerated areas progress, enlarge, and coalesce forming the cobblestone-type pattern. Finally, other patients may show strictures that may be difficult to navigate for the endoscopist. Biopsy results showing granulomas are classic for Crohn's disease, although this is only found in 25% to 42% of patients, and may only represent a marker of more virulent disease [9]. In addition, long-standing ulcerative colitis may show granulomas on biopsy, thus enhancing the difficulty of differentiating the two conditions at times [10]. Other, albeit not exclusive, histologic evidence of Crohn's disease is architectural distortion of the crypts (ie, varying size, shape, symmetry), ulcerations, and skip areas [11]. The patient should also undergo an upper gastrointestinal and small bowel follow-through evaluation to exclude concomitant gastroduodenal and small bowel involvement. Finally, MRI and video capsule endoscopy are being used more to aid in the diagnosis and evaluation of patients who have Crohn's disease [12,13].

Medical management

Although not the focus of this article, medical treatment of Crohn's disease is a largely expanding field with ever-improving outcomes. Most importantly and often underemphasized, nutritional support remains paramount, whether the enteral route can be used or total parenteral nutrition is required. Most patients have been tried on antibiotics, aminosalicylates, corticosteroids, or other immunosuppressive medications to include biologic agents, such as anti-tumor necrosis factor antibodies, 6-mercaptopurine, or azathioprine. Surgeons should be aware of the various treatment regimens because medical therapy is often a lifelong requirement and may affect perioperative decision making (ie, pulse dose steroids, wound healing).

Indications for surgery

Regardless of the disease location, operative indications in Crohn's disease remain remarkably consistent. In broad terms, indications for operative management are for failure of medical therapy or complications from the disease. These indications include intractable disease (ie, steroid dependency), fistula, abscess, obstruction (stricture), growth retardation, perforation, extraintestinal disease, and malignancy. Acute large-volume bleeding in Crohn's disease is not as common as ulcerative colitis, but may occasionally occur. As stated, despite improvements in medical therapy, more than 75% of patients require surgery at some point in their lives [14,15]. In fact, failure of medical management is still the most common reason for surgery in patients who have Crohn's disease of the colon [15,16]. Fortunately, with improvements in medical therapy, elective operations have increased from 70% in the 1970s to 81% from 1992 through 2002 [17], although rates of hospitalization still double those of ulcerative colitis [18].

Specific conditions and surgical options

Overview

Patients who have terminal ileum and cecal or right colonic disease are the most common anatomic distribution encountered in practice, accounting for approximately 40% of those patients undergoing surgery [3]. Classically, these patients present with obstructive symptoms or those mimicking acute appendicitis. In either case, resection of the diseased segment with ileocolonic anastomosis is the preferred option. Traditionally, those patients presenting with symptoms of appendicitis undergoing laparotomy and discovered to have Crohn's disease would undergo an appendectomy if the cecum was normal, or withhold on resection and undergo medical treatment only. In a study by Weston and colleagues [19], 50% of patients undergoing ileocolic resection required no further surgery as a result of their Crohn's disease. This finding was significantly less than 92% requiring further surgery in those undergoing appendectomy only, including 65% requiring an operation within the subsequent 3 years. The authors concluded that early ileocolic resection may be in the patient's best interests to avoid further problems. If possible, it is important to save as much of the right colon as possible to preserve the water absorption capability and lessen problems with diarrhea.

Isolated involvement of the colon occurs in up to 25% to 30% of patients. Just like Crohn's disease of the small intestine, preservation of bowel length with the goal of maintaining normal function is paramount in patients who have colonic disease [20]. Extent of resection depends on multiple factors, including extent and duration of disease, ability to exclude malignancy, rectal compliance, sphincter function, and prior resections. Similar to the small bowel, segmental resection is common with ileocolonic or colocolonic anastomosis found to be safe and easy to perform [21]. In those patients who have pancolitis, total abdominal colectomy with ileorectal anastomosis or total proctocolectomy with end ileostomy are commonly performed. Total proctocolectomy with ileal pouch–anal anastomosis (IPAA) is rarely done, but more commonly occurs in the setting of a misdiagnosis of ulcerative colitis. Proctectomy is more often required secondary to ongoing symptoms, such as pelvic sepsis, poor function, or rarely hemorrhage. When performing a proctectomy for Crohn's disease, it is important to consider the potential for a delayed- or nonhealing perineal wound. An intersphincteric approach, maximizing the amount of healthy muscle and tissue to close, lessens the chances of this difficult and highly morbid problem to occur. In those unfortunate patients who do develop a chronic perineal fistula or sinus, ensuring the patient does not have recurrent disease with a fistula from bowel followed by a conservative approach with local wound care is the preferred initial approach. Many of these patients require more extensive procedures with debridement and flap closure with gracilis muscle or other well-vascularized tissue [22,23].

Fistulas

The large bowel is occasionally the site of fistulous disease with patients who have Crohn's disease. It is important to determine the site of origin of the fistula, because often the colon is secondarily involved with active inflammation in the stomach, duodenum, or small bowel. In cases that require surgical therapy, often the colon may need only debridement and closure of the fistula site. Evaluation of the colonic mucosa is therefore important, because active inflammation at the site may predispose to healing problems and may require segmental resection. Primary colonic involvement can result in transmural inflammation and fistulous communication with other bowel [24], lung [25], skin [26], bladder [27], or vagina [28]. In these cases, the colon often requires segmental resection with closure of the secondarily involved organ. Occasionally the inflammatory process is so intense that safe dissection is not possible and the entire phlegmon needs to be resected en bloc. Lapidus and colleagues [3] have shown that in patients who have Crohn's disease, a fistula is associated with an increased lifetime probably of undergoing surgical resection (relative risk = 1.7). The question of this trend continuing in the era of monoclonal antibodies against tumor necrosis factor (TNF) was investigated by Portiz and colleagues [29]. In a study of 26 patients receiving infliximab for fistulizing Crohn's disease (perianal, enterocutaneous, rectovaginal, peristomal, and intra-abdominal fistulas), 6 patients (23%) had a complete response to infliximab, 12 patients (46%) had a partial response, and 8 patients (31%) had no response to the medication. Fourteen (54%) patients still required surgery (10 bowel resections and 4 perianal procedures), and 6 additional patients refused surgery. Of the 6 patients who had closure of the fistula with infliximab, 5 had perianal or rectovaginal, not intra-abdominal. Almost 75% of patients still required surgery or had continued open fistulas. The surgeon therefore must continue to understand the principles of resection for fistula disease, because most patients, especially with intra-abdominal fistulas, may still need surgical intervention.

Obstruction and stricture

Obstruction as a result of colonic stricture occurs in up to 17% of patients [30]. Because of transmural inflammation, it is not uncommon to have luminal narrowing within the colon, especially with repeated flares. Malignancy may be present in approximately 7% of colonic strictures, however [30]. It is often difficult to differentiate malignant from benign strictures on a strictly clinical basis. All colonic strictures should therefore be evaluated by endoscopy and biopsy. Should malignancy be present, appropriate resection following standard oncological principles is mandatory. Other benign Crohn's strictures, especially at prior anastomotic sites, are often amenable to dilation [31]. In 20 patients who underwent dilation for either colonic or ileocolonic anastomotic strictures, Nomura and colleagues [32] found initial symptomatic relief in 75% of patients following the first dilation. Approximately one third of patients developed recurrent strictures in the first 2 years. Complications of dilation included fistula, fever, bleeding, and perforation. Although medical therapy is useful in other aspects of the disease, these strictures are often fibrotic in nature and nonresponsive, thus requiring resection for symptomatic strictures even when found to be benign. Strictures at sites of prior anastomoses may be secondary to recurrent disease or technical problems from the first surgery. To prevent this, there is some evidence that stapled side-to-side anastomosis in patients who have Crohn's disease have a decreased rate of postoperative strictures and leaks [33–36]. In a study including 72 ileocolic and 7 colocolic resection and anastomoses, only 2% of those patients who underwent stapled side-to-side anastomosis developed recurrent symptoms at 46 months, versus 43% of those undergoing hand-sewn end-to-end repair [37]. It is unknown whether these differences are related to technical problems, such as relative obstruction at the anastomotic site or ischemia leading to stenosis, but it does emphasize how the surgeon can potentially influence disease recurrence.

Hemorrhage

Hemorrhage in Crohn's disease is much less common than in ulcerative colitis [38]. Although patients who have Crohn's disease may develop occasional bloody diarrhea, massive lower GI bleeding rarely occurs and when present may be secondary to deep ulcerations, toxic colitis, or an underlying mass. Patients require continued resuscitation, correction of any coagulopathy, and transfusion as indicated. Endoscopy is the most useful diagnostic and therapeutic maneuver for bleeding from a colonic or terminal ileal source [39]. Often medical therapy or endoscopic therapy can control bleeding. Should bleeding continue or recur, segmental resection is preferred when the site of the hemorrhage is localized, and is required in up to 40% in some series of acute lower gastrointestinal bleeding [40]. In the setting of nonlocalizable disease, every effort should be made to identify the source of bleeding should the patient's clinical condition permit. This effort may include upper and lower endoscopy, nuclear medicine imaging, angiography, or small bowel evaluation (push endoscopy, video capsule endoscopy, or small bowel follow-through). In the unstable or nonlocalizable lower source, a subtotal colectomy with end ileostomy may be required [41].

Toxic colitis

Toxic colitis in the patient who has Crohn's disease is similar to ulcerative colitis. Even in patients who have had a thorough resuscitation, intravenous steroids or other immunosuppressants, and maximal nutritional support, emergent surgical intervention may be required. Indications for operative intervention include free perforation, worsening acidosis, clinical deterioration, or lack of improvement with medical management. In the operating room the colon is inflamed and friable, and the surgeon must be careful to avoid perforation and spillage of colonic contents. In the past, many patients underwent the Turnbull et al [42] procedure—a loop ileostomy and decompressive transverse and possible sigmoid colostomy. Although this procedure rarely is performed today, it may still play a role in the sickest of patients as a temporizing procedure only. Although primary anastomosis is an option, patients should most often undergo a subtotal colectomy with end ileostomy, which has been shown to be safe with low rates of morbidity and mortality [43]. The dilemma of what to do with the rectal stump remains. Options include dividing the colon more proximally in the distal sigmoid, with construction of a mucus fistula or implantation into the subcutaneous space [44], or local reinforcement of the rectal remnant. In a study of 62 cases of colectomy and stump closure involving ulcerative colitis and patients who have Crohn's disease in the setting of toxic colitis, leakage occurred in 3 of 9 patients who had a short rectal stump versus only 1 of 53 patients who had a rectal stump above the peritoneal reflection [45]. In another study of 147 patients who had intra-abdominal closure of the rectal stump, only 3 patients (2%) developed pelvic abscess that were able to be drained percutaneously, and none had stump blowout [46].

Although described as the procedure of choice in the 1970s [47], rarely does a patient who has toxic colitis undergo a proctocolectomy with end ileostomy in the acute phase, because it is associated with a much higher morbidity and mortality. In a study of 70 patients who had toxic megacolon, only 4 patients underwent proctocolectomy, with 3 of the 4 (75%) developing surgical complications, compared with 4 of 49 (8%) of those undergoing subtotal colectomy [48]. Should the patient have a rectal perforation or persistent hemorrhage despite subtotal colectomy, proctectomy at a subsequent procedure may be performed.

Dysplasia & malignancy

The development of malignancy with long-standing Crohn's disease is increased 4 to 20 times that of the average population [49,50]. Although in the past it was believed to be a lower risk than ulcerative colitis [51], a plethora of studies have shown Crohn's colitis to have equivalent risk for cancer [52–54]. Many authors have examined the risk factors associated with development of malignancy, and extent of colonic disease (at least one third) and disease duration (>8 years) are most often associated with an increased relative risk [55]. Age at diagnosis of Crohn's disease has had inconsistent findings, with some authors finding older age at diagnosis [55] versus others identifying younger age (<30 years old) with increased risk for neoplasm [56]. The malignancies, however, tend to present at a younger age and are more often multiple and left sided [57]. In a retrospective review of 222 patients undergoing surgical resection for Crohn's colitis, Maykel and colleagues [55] found the incidence of dysplasia was 2.3% and adenocarcinoma was 2.7%. Of those 11 patients, only 3 were identified preoperatively, demonstrating the difficulty of following these patients who have long-standing Crohn's colitis.

Endoscopic surveillance strategies to detect malignancy have had mixed results [58,59]. In a recent Cochrane Review, surveillance colonoscopy has not been shown to affect survival in these patients, despite detecting the cancers earlier [60]. Still, recommendations for surveillance in patients who have Crohn's colitis mimic those for ulcerative colitis, with surveillance beginning 8 to 10 years after disease onset for pancolitis and approximately 15 years for left-sided disease, with colonoscopy increasing from every 3 years during the second decade of disease to annual endoscopic evaluation after 30 years of colitis [61]. Even when detected, dysplasia can be difficult to diagnose and grade histologically. Substantial evidence indicates that diagnosis of dysplasia in the setting of active colitis, or within a polyp in a setting of colitis (dysplasia-associated lesion or mass [DALM]), carries a significant risk for malignancy and is a strong indication for resection [62,63]. Low-grade dysplasia outside the setting of a DALM and even in areas of flat mucosa warrants close follow-up, although the need for immediate resection remains unproved [64,65]. Treatment of malignancy in the patient who has Crohn's disease is similar to that of the general population, with ligation of the primary blood supply along with the resection of the corresponding mesentery. With synchronous lesions occurring in up to 10% [49] and reports of metachronous lesions [66,67], consideration should be given to a subtotal colectomy with ileorectal anastomosis.

Special situations

Extent of resection

For those patients who have rectal sparing in the setting of Crohn's colitis, a total abdominal colectomy with ileorectal anastomosis (TAC-IRA) is an appropriate option. Because patients who have Crohn's disease are prone to diarrhea, it is important to perform a thorough evaluation of the rectal capacity and sphincter function to minimize the chances of fecal incontinence postoperatively. Whether or not to perform segmental resection or TAC-IRA in the patient who has Crohn's colitis continues to be a matter of debate. Bernell and colleagues [21] reviewed a series of 833 patients who had Crohn's colitis and found a higher rate of recurrence at 10 years for those undergoing TAC-IRA (58%) versus those undergoing a segmental resection (47%). Andersson and associates [68] confirmed these findings in a study of 57 patients in which the re-resection rates were similar, although those undergoing segmental resection had less symptomatic recurrence and overall improved bowel function. In contrast to the above findings, Tekkis [69] performed a meta-analysis of all studies between 1998 and 2002 encompassing 488 patients and demonstrated no significant differences in overall recurrence rate, complications, or need for a permanent stoma. Time to recurrence was longer in the TAC-IRA group by 4.4 years ($P < .001$), however. The authors concluded that subtotal colectomy may be better for patients who have two or more segments involved, yet the issue remains unresolved. Further complicating this matter, patients who have diffuse disease, including proctitis, after undergoing total proctocolectomy with ileostomy, have been shown to be less likely to require medications 1 year after resection and have an increased time interval to first recurrence than either subtotal or segmental colectomy [70]. One thing remains certain: once a decision is made to perform a colonic segmental resection, length of resection margins does not influence the risk for relapse. Only resection to grossly normal bowel is required [71].

Diverting stoma and bypass

Diverting stoma or bypass procedures are not performed as much as in the past; however, they may be required in select situations. A diverting stoma is useful for patients who have severe rectal and perianal disease to help resolve active inflammation while trying to maximize medical therapy. Although the disease often has recurrence following restoration of intestinal continuity, diversion remains a valuable tool for patients who have severe fistulous disease or in patients undergoing attempt at repairs (endorectal advancement flap) either concomitantly or before the surgical procedure. Bypass procedures are an option in the septic patient who has a large terminal ileal-ascending colon phlegmon with involvement of retroperitoneal structures in which mobilization or resection brings about concerns for proper identification and protection of the ureter and vascular structures. In this case diversion or bypass can allow resolution of the inflammation followed by resection and restoration of continuity at a later date. The cumulative risk for permanent ileostomy continues to be high, with a study of 507 patients showing a 25% rate at a follow-up of 10 years [3]. This finding highlights the severity of the disease and underscores the need to counsel patients in depth regarding potential complications and outcomes.

Ileal pouch–anal anastomosis in Crohn's disease

IPAA in the patient who has Crohn's disease still should be the rare exception. The common scenario in which this occurs is the patient who has a firm diagnosis of ulcerative colitis who undergoes a total proctocolectomy with IPAA and then subsequently is diagnosed with Crohn's disease. Another common scenario is the patient who has indeterminate colitis who after extensive counseling elects to undergo a restorative proctectomy. Different authors have examined this scenario, each with similar outcomes, but have come to different conclusions. In a European study, 41 patients, including 26 who had a preoperative diagnosis of Crohn's disease, underwent elective IPAA over a 13-year period. No patient had a prior history of perineal or active small bowel disease. Of the 20 patients followed for at least 10 years, 35% developed Crohn's disease–related complications, such as pouchitis, abscesses, and pouch-anal fistulas, with 2 patients (10%) requiring pouch excision. The authors proposed that restorative proctocolectomy can be considered in patients meeting select criteria [72]. Hartley and colleagues [73] from the Cleveland Clinic identified 60 patients who underwent IPAA for presumed ulcerative colitis and were subsequently determined to have Crohn's disease. Approximately one third of these patients developed recurrent Crohn's disease, with 10% undergoing pouch excision, and an additional patient needing permanent diversion. Although 50% of patients still had urgency and 40% had persistent continence issues, the authors concluded that most patients having an intact functioning pouch had symptoms controlled with medication, supported pouch placement in selected patients with Crohn's disease. In contrast, Braveman and colleagues [74] from the Lahey Clinic retrospectively looked at 32 patients who had a postoperative diagnosis of Crohn's disease following pouch construction. They identified complications in 93%, including fistula (63%), pouchitis (50%), and anal stricture (38%), resulting in diversion or pouch excision in 29% of patients. Of those patients who had a functioning pouch, one half continued to require medication to treat active Crohn's disease. The authors recommended that no patient who has Crohn's disease should undergo pouch construction. Brown and associates [75] also recommend that

Crohn's disease should remain a contraindication to pouch construction, because more than one half of their 36 patients who had Crohn's disease following restorative proctocolectomy required diversion or pouch excision compared with only 10% of indeterminate colitis and 6% of ulcerative colitis. In addition, 64% of Crohn's patients developed pouch-related complications. Finally, Reese and colleagues [76] looked at 10 studies with 225 patients who had Crohn's disease undergoing restorative proctocolectomy and found patients who had Crohn's disease developed more anastomotic strictures, higher pouch failure, and higher rates of urgency than ulcerative colitis or indeterminate colitis patients. Whether or not improvements in future medications to control postoperative symptoms or future diagnostic techniques will determine which Crohn's patients can have successful outcomes with IPAA remains to be determined.

Anorectal Crohn's disease

Clinical presentation

Bissel [77] was the first to recognize the anorectal component of Crohn's disease, nearly 2 years after its original description, and approximately 30 years before the identification of a colonic component. Since that time, anorectal disease has been recognized as one of the most challenging aspects of the patient who has Crohn's disease. The most common perianal manifestations include edematous (elephant ear) skin tags, hemorrhoids, blue discoloration of the anus, recurrent abscesses, and fistulas. Fissures are also common—most often multiple, off the midline, deep, and with associated large skin tags. Patients who have long-standing Crohn's disease often have stenosis or stricture of the anal opening associated with chronic inflammation. Although isolated perianal disease is the presenting symptom in only 10% to 15% of patients [78], it is seen in up to 90% [79] of patients overall and more common in those who have concomitant rectal or colonic disease [3,80].

Diagnosis and evaluation

Direct observation of the perianal area identifies disease, such as skin tags, external fistula openings, and fissures. All patients should also undergo digital rectal examination and anoscopy to aid in diagnosis, especially those patients who do not have a known history of Crohn's disease. A thorough physical examination to identify any extraintestinal manifestations should also be performed. As an adjunct, flexible or rigid sigmoidoscopy can also be done to evaluate the rectum and sigmoid colon. Although clinical evidence of Crohn's disease as manifested by the large skin tags, fissures, or multiple fistulas are seen as hallmarks of disease, a biopsy should be performed to aid in diagnosis. In the perianal area local septic processes and tenderness may require an examination under anesthesia to fully identify the extent of the disease. Endorectal ultrasound, CT, and MRI have also proven as useful radiologic adjuncts for the patient who has perianal disease to help diagnose and delineate fistula and abscesses [79,81,82]. Finally, patients presenting with perianal disease consistent with Crohn's disease should undergo a full alimentary tract evaluation with endoscopic and radiologic evaluation.

Medical treatment

Medical therapy for anorectal disease is similar to other intestinal therapies. Antibiotics, such as ciprofloxacin and Flagyl, are often used as first-line agents [83]. Steroids, aminosalicylates, and the immunosuppressive medications 6-mercaptopurine and azathioprine are easier and safer to use with the ability to monitor levels [84]. Immunomodulators, such as monoclonal anti-TNF antibodies and azathioprine, have been found to heal up to 71% of perianal fistulas and 79% of ulcers and fissures in patients who have Crohn's disease [85]. The field continues to expand with other biologic therapies, such as TNF-binding neutralizing fusion proteins and interleukins, and other immunomodulators, such as thalidomide, tacrolimus, and mycophenolate mofetil, with varying results to date [86]. Regardless of the medical therapy these patients are undergoing, a distinguishing characteristic of the surgical treatment of perianal disease in patients who have Crohn's disease is to consider whether or not they are symptomatic. Because this disease process is hallmarked by recurrence, aggressive intervention in the asymptomatic patient is unwarranted and potentially dangerous.

Specific conditions and surgical options

Anal skin tags and hemorrhoids

Patients who have perianal Crohn's disease consisting of the large edematous, blue-colored tags are unfortunately often misdiagnosed with hemorrhoids and undergo excision with poor results. Although these lesions may cause difficulty with hygiene and irritation, they are present in up to 70% of Crohn's patients who have perianal disease and are most often asymptomatic [87]. Before embarking on resection, surgeons should be aware of the propensity for poor wound healing, especially with the underlying diarrhea seen in Crohn's disease. Patients should be counseled as to the risk for nonhealing wounds, continence problems, and need for conservative treatment with warm sitz baths and antidiarrheal medications. Although Taylor et al [88] noted that granulomas may be found in the anal skin tags this is rarely needed to help confirm diagnosis of Crohn's disease. Internal hemorrhoids in Crohn's disease tend to be less symptomatic and are best treated medically [89], despite evidence that selected patients who have severe hemorrhoidal symptoms nonresponsive to medical management can safely undergo hemorrhoidectomy with adequate healing [90].

Anorectal abscess

Approximately 50% to 60% of all Crohn's disease patients who have perianal disease experience at least one perianal abscess [91], with up to 60% having a recurrent abscess within 2 years [92]. Treatment of simple abscesses normally involves only incision and drainage. It is important to place the incision as close to the anal verge as possible, while still achieving adequate drainage, to consider the potential for development of a future anal fistula. Alternatively, a small pessar mushroom-tipped catheter may be placed in the cavity, thus evacuating the abscess and allowing the cavity to close around the catheter. Patients may also have an abscess in the presence of fistula disease, in which case concomitant drainage of the abscess and seton placement is the preferred option. It is important for the surgeon to identify all foci of sepsis and provide adequate drainage, including seton placement when needed. This drainage not only avoids the development of systemic symptoms, but prevents local destruction of the tissues, thus preserving sphincter function.

Anal fistula

Perianal fistulas are one of the most difficult management scenarios in this patient population. Because the disease process is hallmarked by extensive recurring inflammation, perianal fistulas are often deep, eroding through sphincter muscle and associated with extensive scarring. They can have high blind tracts, originate at levels well above the dentate line, and are often found in conjunction with rectal inflammation. Just as in fistulas in patients who do not have Crohn's disease, the therapy is intimately associated with the anatomy and degree of sphincter involvement. In Crohn's disease, however, the surgeon must also take into account rectal compliance, concomitant proctitis, and the potential for chronic diarrhea. Anything that impairs overall continence, such as an aggressive fistulotomy, or creates a wound that may not heal, must be avoided. With this in mind, in the absence of overt proctitis, low-lying fistulas with minimum sphincter involvement can safely be treated with fistulotomy [91]. When the fistula is higher or more complex, preoperative imaging studies, such as MRI or endorectal ultrasound, are useful to identify not only the anatomy but also any associated undrained abscess collections that need to be addressed. Surgical options for fistulas include setons, endoanal advancement flaps, and fistula plugs. Many patients who have fistulous disease require chronic indwelling setons, such as silastic vessel loops. Patients should be periodically re-examined to ensure that there is adequate drainage and to examine for the rare development of malignancy. Endorectal advancement flaps can be used selectively in patients who have Crohn's disease. In a study of 31 consecutive endorectal advancement flaps on 26 patients, Joo and colleagues [93] had a 71% success rate at a mean follow-up of 17.3 months. Diverting stoma was only used in 6 patients, with 4 of those patients having successful closure. The authors also found that only 25% (2/8) of patients who had active small bowel disease had successful eradication of the fistula versus 20 of 23 (87%) who did not have small bowel disease. This finding highlights the need for consideration of a diverting stoma until the flap has healed, and optimal control of all active disease before attempted repair. Even the addition of fibrin glue to endorectal flap repair has been unable to improve results [94]. The Surgisis fistula plug has had some success with one study of 20 patients showing 80% closure rate, with single tracts having the best results [95]. Unfortunately, even in this era of monoclonal antibodies against TNF, severe anal fistulas may still require permanent defunctioning stomas or proctectomy [96].

Rectovaginal and anovaginal fistula

These fistulas are particularly problematic in the patient who has Crohn's disease. Many of these fistulas are associated with deep erosions and intense inflammation, rectal wall and rectovaginal fibrosis, and associated sphincter damage. Surgical options therefore may be even more difficult. It is important to identify the source of the fistula, because occasionally a presumed rectovaginal fistula may originate from small bowel. After treating the patient medically for Crohn's disease, the surgeon must pay particular attention to look for abscess that may need to be drained initially. Many patients unfortunately require diversion in this setting before any definitive repair. In a study of 48 women who had a low anovaginal fistula from Crohn's disease, 9 patients had severe disease and required proctocolectomy and ileostomy, 4 needed setons only, and the remaining 35 underwent flap procedures [97]. Eight of 9 patients requiring diverting ileostomies successfully healed, and they achieved an overall initial success rate of 54%. Five patients had to undergo repeat flap procedures, all of which were successful. Endorectal flap can thus be used in this patient population, even without diverting stomas, although patient selection is crucial. Infliximab has had mixed results as isolated therapy, with short-term 14-week closure rates of 45% [98], whereas other studies demonstrated the presence of rectovaginal fistulas as a poor predictor for response to infliximab [99,100].

Anal fissure

Patients who have Crohn's disease and anal fissures are a particular challenge. These fissures are often painless. Patients presenting with a predominant complaint of pain should raise the suspicion for an underlying abscess and prompt an examination under anesthesia. Concomitant perianal pathology is present in more than half of patients [101] with approximately one third having multiple fissures [102]. Although most authors suggest conservative management with adequate fiber and fluid intake, control of diarrhea, stool softeners, and sitz baths, other authors have advocated a more aggressive surgical approach. In a study of 56 patients who had Crohn's disease and anal fissures, Fleshner and colleagues [102] found that 49% of patients healed with medical therapy alone. Of those who failed medical management, 10 of 15 (67%) patients healed their fissure when treated surgically with a lateral internal sphincterotomy (LIS). In addition, 25% of patients who had unhealed fissures that did not undergo LIS went on to develop an abscess or fistula from the base of the fissure, leading the authors to propose a more liberal use of LIS for fissures not responding to medical therapy. In another study of 25 patients who had Crohn's disease with symptomatic fissures, 22 had completely healed their fissure by 2 months following sphincterotomy. At a mean follow-up of 7.5 years, no patient had a direct complication from operative therapy and only 3 eventually required proctectomy for severe recurrent disease [90]. Despite these reports, given the continence risks associated with surgery, medical management is the preferred initial therapy in patients who have Crohn's-related fissures. Surgical intervention should be reserved for those patients who have minimal active anorectal inflammation who have failed conservative therapy. Division of sphincter muscle should be kept to a minimum.

Anorectal stenosis and strictures

Repeated bouts of inflammation may also lead to anal strictures or stenosis. Symptoms include difficulty or pain with bowel movements and decreasing size of stools. Physical examination should evaluate for presence of infection or malignancy with corresponding biopsies or cultures as indicated. Many patients have concomitant fissures or other perianal disease. Most patients who have Crohn's disease with stenosis initially respond to dilation. In a study of 44 patients, Linares et al [103] found that the site of the stricture was rectal in 22, anal in 14, and both in the remaining 11 patients. More than 95% had concomitant proctitis, and although a single dilation was successful in 15 patients, multiple dilations were necessary in 18 other patients. Emphasizing the recurrent severe nature in these patients, 19 of the 44 (43%) ultimately required proctocolectomy and 3 additional patients underwent diversion. Diversion alone is occasionally necessary [104], yet this may lead to worsening anal stenosis with retention of purulent intraluminal fluid leading to systemic symptoms [105]. Although anoplasty and endorectal advancement flap have been described for patients who have high anal or low rectal stenosis [106], it should be avoided in patients who have active proctitis.

Anorectal malignancy

Although rare, adenocarcinoma and squamous cell carcinoma arising in the setting of long-standing Crohn's fistulas has been described [107,108] as well as in defunctionalized rectal stumps [109]. Ky et al [107] described seven patients who had malignancy arising in the setting of chronic fistulas in patients who had Crohn's disease, with deaths occurring despite proper follow-up. Because evaluation is limited by the extent and severity of the disease and painful examination, malignancy may be difficult to detect. Any change in symptoms or inability to exclude malignancy should therefore mandate examination under anesthesia with appropriate biopsies and curette of the fistula tracts with histologic examination. Sjodahl et al [110] has recommended that annual surveillance examination with proctoscopy of the anorectal region should start after 15 years of disease for those patients who have extensive colitis, chronic severe anorectal disease, rectal remnant after diversion, anorectal stricture, or any bypassed segment in a patient who has sclerosing cholangitis. Patients who are diagnosed with malignancy should undergo appropriate resection with chemoradiation therapy as indicated.

Special situations

Control of the proximal bowel

There remains controversy regarding the exact role proximal bowel disease has on anorectal manifestations. Sweeney and colleagues [111] found that a large majority of patients respond without surgery. In 42 of 61 patients the anal fissure healed solely with medical therapy directed toward their intestinal disease. The remaining patients either developed further anal lesions (16%) or had their fissures removed along with a proctectomy for severe perianal disease. The authors proposed a more conservative nonoperative approach, reserving surgery for cases in which suppurative anorectal complications developed [111]. In a study of 127 patients who had perianal disease, McKee and Keenan [78] also found that the treatment and outcome of patients who had perianal Crohn's disease was in large part determined by the extent and severity of the proximal intestinal involvement. Finally, in a multicenter study of six databases from the United States and Europe, Sachar evaluated 1686 cases of isolated Crohn's ileitis and 1655 cases of Crohn's colitis to determine if there was a correlation specifically for abdominal fistulas and perianal fistula disease. There was a varying association with perianal disease and ileitis across the centers, although Crohn's colitis had a significant association. Control of the proximal bowel thus seems to have an impact on lessening perianal symptoms.

Diversion and proctectomy

In severe cases of nonhealing fissures or fistulas, the physician should always question the underlying diagnosis. A thorough history and physical examination focusing on secondary manifestation of the systemic disease (not only Crohn's disease, but tuberculosis, HIV, and so forth) is mandatory. Cultures should be sent to look for an underlying infectious or immunodeficiency syndrome. In addition, a formal examination under anesthesia with biopsies to exclude malignancy and directed cultures is also helpful. If that is all normal and Crohn's disease is the sole problem, there is evidence that fecal diversion alone may heal perianal disease, at least temporarily. In a study of 31 patients, 25 (81%) had early complete remission of their lesions, including all 3 patients who had deep anal ulcers. Each of these patients developed a late relapse between 11 and 54 months later, however. At present, diversion is not widely accepted as a therapy for refractory Crohn's disease fissures, although this must be kept in mind as a potential maneuver to quell unremitting inflammation [112]. One of the most common reasons for diversion is continued perineal sepsis. Although diversion may be successful to help with symptoms in up to 80%, relapse with the stoma in place occurs in most of those patients, and unfortunately restoration of intestinal continuity rarely occurs [112]. In a study of 86 patients who had Crohn's disease undergoing 344 operations, 49% ultimately required permanent diversion with predictors of need being active colonic disease and anal canal stricture [104].

Proctectomy is required in up to 25% of patients who have perianal disease, although it is often secondary to the extent and severity of concomitant distal colonic and rectal involvement [78]. McKee and Keenan [78] found that proctectomy was needed in 32 of 99 patients who had concomitant colitis and perianal disease, but in none of the 28 patients who had perianal disease alone. Patients should be counseled that even with the wide range and success of current medications, this unpredictable disease may result in untoward and unwanted outcomes for both patient and surgeon alike.

Summary

Crohn's disease remains a complex disease process with many different manifestations in the colon, rectum, and anus. Although advances in medical therapy continue to evolve and change the way that patients are treated, surgeons still play a major role in disease management. Because of its recurring nature, surgeons must adhere to the dictums of dealing with the complications of the disease versus aiming for cure and focus on maximization of patient functional outcome while minimizing complications.

References

[1] Whelan G, Farmer RG, Fazio VW, et al. Recurrence after surgery in Crohn's disease. Relationship to location of disease (clinical pattern) and surgical indication. Gastroenterology 1985;88(6):1826–33.
[2] Farmer RG, Hawk WA, Turnbull RB Jr. Clinical patterns in Crohn's disease: a statistical study of 615 cases. Gastroenterology 1975;68(4 Pt 1):627–35.
[3] Lapidus A, Bernell O, Hellers G, et al. Clinical course of colorectal Crohn's disease: a 35-year follow-up study of 507 patients. Gastroenterology 1998;114(6):1151–60.
[4] Renison DM, Forouhar FA, Levine JB, et al. Filiform polyposis of the colon presenting as massive hemorrhage: an uncommon complication of Crohn's disease. Am J Gastroenterol 1983;78(7):413–6.
[5] Kelvin FM, Oddson TA, Rice RP, et al. Double contrast barium enema in Crohn's disease and ulcerative colitis. AJR Am J Roentgenol 1978;131(2):207–13.
[6] Orel SG, Rubesin SE, Jones B, et al. Computed tomography vs barium studies in the acutely symptomatic patient with Crohn disease. J Comput Assist Tomogr 1987;11(6):1009–16.
[7] Berliner L, Redmond P, Purow E, et al. Computed tomography in Crohn's disease. Am J Gastroenterol 1982;77(8):548–53.

 [8] Fefferman DS, Farrell RJ. Endoscopy in inflammatory bowel disease: indications, surveillance, and use in clinical practice. Clin Gastroenterol Hepatol 2005;3(1):11–24.
 [9] Morpurgo E, Petras R, Kimberling J, et al. Characterization and clinical behavior of Crohn's disease initially presenting predominantly as colitis. Dis Colon Rectum 2003; 46(7):918–24.
[10] Mahadeva U, Martin JP, Patel NK, et al. Granulomatous ulcerative colitis: a re-appraisal of the mucosal granuloma in the distinction of Crohn's disease from ulcerative colitis. Histopathology 2002;41(1):50–5.
[11] Le Berre N, Heresbach D, Kerbaol M, et al. Histological discrimination of idiopathic inflammatory bowel disease from other types of colitis. J Clin Pathol 1995;48(8):749–53.
[12] Rieber A, Wruk D, Potthast S, et al. Diagnostic imaging in Crohn's disease: comparison of magnetic resonance imaging and conventional imaging methods. Int J Colorectal Dis 2000; 15(3):176–81.
[13] Lashner BA. Sensitivity-specificity trade-off for capsule endoscopy in IBD: is it worth it? Am J Gastroenterol 2006;101(5):965–6.
[14] Penner RM, Madsen KL, Fedorak RN. Postoperative Crohn's disease. Inflamm Bowel Dis 2005;11(8):765–77.
[15] Hancock L, Windsor AC, Mortensen NJ. Inflammatory bowel disease: the view of the surgeon. Colorectal Dis 2006;8(Suppl 1):10–4.
[16] Michelassi F, Balestracci T, Chappell R, et al. Crohn's disease. Experience with 1379 patients. Ann Surg 1991;214(3):230–8 [discussion: 238–40].
[17] Siassi M, Weiger A, Hohenberger W, et al. Changes in surgical therapy for Crohn's disease over 33 years: a prospective longitudinal study. Int J Colorectal Dis 2007;22(3):319–24.
[18] Bernstein CN, Nabalamba A. Hospitalization, surgery, and readmission rates of IBD in Canada: a population-based study. Am J Gastroenterol 2006;101(1):110–8.
[19] Weston LA, Roberts PL, Schoetz DJ Jr, et al. Ileocolic resection for acute presentation of Crohn's disease of the ileum. Dis Colon Rectum 1996;39(8):841–6.
[20] Wolff BG. Resection margins in Crohn's disease. Br J Surg 2001;88(6):771–2.
[21] Bernell O, Lapidus A, Hellers G. Recurrence after colectomy in Crohn's colitis. Dis Colon Rectum 2001;44(5):647–54 [discussion: 654].
[22] Hurst RD, Gottlieb LJ, Crucitti P, et al. Primary closure of complicated perineal wounds with myocutaneous and fasciocutaneous flaps after proctectomy for Crohn's disease. Surgery 2001;130(4):767–72 [discussion: 772–3].
[23] Scammell BE, Keighley MR. Delayed perineal wound healing after proctectomy for Crohn's colitis. Br J Surg 1986;73(2):150–2.
[24] El H II, Abdul-Baki H, El-Zahabi LM, et al Primary coloduodenal fistula in a patient with Crohn' disease. Dig Dis Sci 2007 Feb;50(2):239–50.
[25] Barisiae G, Krivokapiae Z, Adziae T, et al. Fecopneumothorax and colopleural fistula—uncommon complications of Crohn's disease. BMC Gastroenterol 2006;6:17.
[26] Poritz LS, Gagliano GA, McLeod RS, et al. Surgical management of entero and colocutaneous fistulae in Crohn's disease: 17 year's experience. Int J Colorectal Dis 2004;19(5): 481–5 [discussion: 486].
[27] Garcea G, Majid I, Sutton CD, et al. Diagnosis and management of colovesical fistulae: six-year experience of 90 consecutive cases. Colorectal Dis 2006;8(4):347–52.
[28] Bahadursingh AM, Longo WE. Colovaginal fistulas. Etiology and management. J Reprod Med 2003;48(7):489–95.
[29] Poritz LS, Rowe WA, Koltun WA. Remicade does not abolish the need for surgery in fistulizing Crohn's disease. Dis Colon Rectum 2002;45(6):771–5.
[30] Yamazaki Y, Ribeiro MB, Sachar DB, et al. Malignant colorectal strictures in Crohn's disease. Am J Gastroenterol 1991;86(7):882–5.
[31] Singh VV, Draganov P, Valentine J. Efficacy and safety of endoscopic balloon dilation of symptomatic upper and lower gastrointestinal Crohn's disease strictures. J Clin Gastroenterol 2005;39(4):284–90.

[32] Nomura E, Takagi S, Kikuchi T, et al. Efficacy and safety of endoscopic balloon dilation for Crohn's strictures. Dis Colon Rectum 2006;49(10 Suppl):S49–67.

[33] Scarpa M, Angriman I, Barollo M, et al. Role of stapled and hand-sewn anastomoses in recurrence of Crohn's disease. Hepatogastroenterology 2004;51(58):1053–7.

[34] Resegotti A, Astegiano M, Farina EC, et al. Side-to-side stapled anastomosis strongly reduces anastomotic leak rates in Crohn's disease surgery. Dis Colon Rectum 2005;48(3):464–8.

[35] Yamamoto T. Factors affecting recurrence after surgery for Crohn's disease. World J Gastroenterol 2005;11(26):3971–9.

[36] Munoz-Juarez M, Yamamoto T, Wolff BG, et al. Wide-lumen stapled anastomosis vs. conventional end-to-end anastomosis in the treatment of Crohn's disease. Dis Colon Rectum 2001;44(1):20–5 [discussion: 25–6].

[37] Hashemi M, Novell JR, Lewis AA. Side-to-side stapled anastomosis may delay recurrence in Crohn's disease. Dis Colon Rectum 1998;41(10):1293–6.

[38] Kostka R, Lukas M. Massive, life-threatening bleeding in Crohn's disease. Acta Chir Belg 2005;105(2):168–74.

[39] Belaiche J, Louis E, D'Haens G, et al. Acute lower gastrointestinal bleeding in Crohn's disease: characteristics of a unique series of 34 patients. Belgian IBD Research Group. Am J Gastroenterol 1999;94(8):2177–81.

[40] Pardi DS, Loftus EV Jr, Tremaine WJ, et al. Acute major gastrointestinal hemorrhage in inflammatory bowel disease. Gastrointest Endosc 1999;49(2):153–7.

[41] Veroux M, Angriman I, Ruffolo C, et al. Severe gastrointestinal bleeding in Crohn's disease. Ann Ital Chir 2003;74(2):213–5 [discussion: 216].

[42] Turnbull RB Jr, Weakley FL, Hawk WA, et al. Choice of operation for the toxic megacolon phase of nonspecific ulcerative colitis. Surg Clin North Am 1970;50(5):1151–69.

[43] Hyman NH, Cataldo P, Osler T. Urgent subtotal colectomy for severe inflammatory bowel disease. Dis Colon Rectum 2005;48(1):70–3.

[44] Ng RL, Davies AH, Grace RH, et al. Subcutaneous rectal stump closure after emergency subtotal colectomy. Br J Surg 1992;79(7):701–3.

[45] McKee RF, Keenan RA, Munro A. Colectomy for acute colitis: is it safe to close the rectal stump? Int J Colorectal Dis 1995;10(4):222–4.

[46] Wojdemann M, Wettergren A, Hartvigsen A, et al. Closure of rectal stump after colectomy for acute colitis. Int J Colorectal Dis 1995;10(4):197–9.

[47] Sirinek KR, Tetirick CE, Thomford NR, et al. Total proctocolectomy and ileostomy: procedure of choice for acute toxic megacolon. Arch Surg 1977;112(4):518–22.

[48] Ausch C, Madoff RD, Gnant M, et al. Aetiology and surgical management of toxic megacolon. Colorectal Dis 2006;8(3):195–201.

[49] Ribeiro MB, Greenstein AJ, Sachar DB, et al. Colorectal adenocarcinoma in Crohn's disease. Ann Surg 1996;223(2):186–93.

[50] Hamilton SR. Colorectal carcinoma in patients with Crohn's disease. Gastroenterology 1985;89(2):398–407.

[51] Greenstein AJ, Sachar DB, Smith H, et al. Patterns of neoplasia in Crohn's disease and ulcerative colitis. Cancer 1980;46(2):403–7.

[52] Friedman S. Cancer in Crohn's disease. Gastroenterol Clin North Am 2006;35(3):621–39.

[53] Choi PM, Zelig MP. Similarity of colorectal cancer in Crohn's disease and ulcerative colitis: implications for carcinogenesis and prevention. Gut 1994;35(7):950–4.

[54] Jess T, Loftus EV Jr, Velayos FS, et al. Risk of intestinal cancer in inflammatory bowel disease: a population-based study from Olmsted County, Minnesota. Gastroenterology 2006;130(4):1039–46.

[55] Maykel JA, Hagerman G, Mellgren AF, et al. Crohn's colitis: the incidence of dysplasia and adenocarcinoma in surgical patients. Dis Colon Rectum 2006;49(7):950–7.

[56] Ekbom A, Helmick C, Zack M, et al. Increased risk of large-bowel cancer in Crohn's disease with colonic involvement. Lancet 1990;336(8711):357–9.

[57] Mayer R, Wong WD, Rothenberger DA, et al. Colorectal cancer in inflammatory bowel disease: a continuing problem. Dis Colon Rectum 1999;42(3):343–7.
[58] Siegel CA, Sands BE. Risk factors for colorectal cancer in Crohn's colitis: a case-control study. Inflamm Bowel Dis 2006;12(6):491–6.
[59] Shanahan F. Review article: colitis-associated cancer—time for new strategies. Aliment Pharmacol Ther 2003;18(Suppl 2):6–9.
[60] Collins PD, Mpofu C, Watson AJ, et al. Strategies for detecting colon cancer and/or dysplasia in patients with inflammatory bowel disease. Cochrane Database Syst Rev 2006;2: CD000279.
[61] Eaden J. Review article: colorectal carcinoma and inflammatory bowel disease. Aliment Pharmacol Ther 2004;20(Suppl 4):24–30.
[62] Itzkowitz SH, Harpaz N. Diagnosis and management of dysplasia in patients with inflammatory bowel diseases. Gastroenterology 2004;126(6):1634–48.
[63] Greenson JK. Dysplasia in inflammatory bowel disease. Semin Diagn Pathol 2002;19(1): 31–7.
[64] Befrits R, Ljung T, Jaramillo E, et al. Low-grade dysplasia in extensive, long-standing inflammatory bowel disease: a follow-up study. Dis Colon Rectum 2002;45(5): 615–20.
[65] Jess T, Loftus EV Jr, Velayos FS, et al. Incidence and prognosis of colorectal dysplasia in inflammatory bowel disease: a population-based study from Olmsted County, Minnesota. Inflamm Bowel Dis 2006;12(8):669–76.
[66] Castellano TJ, Frank MS, Brandt LJ, et al. Metachronous carcinoma complicating Crohn's disease. Arch Intern Med 1981;141(8):1074–5.
[67] Cooper DJ, Weinstein MA, Korelitz BI. Complications of Crohn's disease predisposing to dysplasia and cancer of the intestinal tract: considerations of a surveillance program. J Clin Gastroenterol 1984;6(3):217–24.
[68] Andersson P, Olaison G, Hallbook O, et al. Segmental resection or subtotal colectomy in Crohn's colitis? Dis Colon Rectum 2002;45(1):47–53.
[69] Tekkis PP, Purkayastha S, Lanitis S, et al. A comparison of segmental vs subtotal/total colectomy for colonic Crohn's disease: a meta-analysis. Colorectal Dis 2006;8(2):82–90.
[70] Fichera A, McCormack R, Rubin MA, et al. Long-term outcome of surgically treated Crohn's colitis: a prospective study. Dis Colon Rectum 2005;48(5):963–9.
[71] Raab Y, Bergstrom R, Ejerblad S, et al. Factors influencing recurrence in Crohn's disease. An analysis of a consecutive series of 353 patients treated with primary surgery. Dis Colon Rectum 1996;39(8):918–25.
[72] Regimbeau JM, Panis Y, Pocard M, et al. Long-term results of ileal pouch-anal anastomosis for colorectal Crohn's disease. Dis Colon Rectum 2001;44(6):769–78.
[73] Hartley JE, Fazio VW, Remzi FH, et al. Analysis of the outcome of ileal pouch-anal anastomosis in patients with Crohn's disease. Dis Colon Rectum 2004;47(11):1808–15.
[74] Braveman JM, Schoetz DJ Jr, Marcello PW, et al. The fate of the ileal pouch in patients developing Crohn's disease. Dis Colon Rectum 2004;47(10):1613–9.
[75] Brown CJ, Maclean AR, Cohen Z, et al. Crohn's disease and indeterminate colitis and the ileal pouch-anal anastomosis: outcomes and patterns of failure. Dis Colon Rectum 2005; 48(8):1542–9.
[76] Reese GE, Lovegrove RE, Tilney HS, et al. The effect of Crohn's disease on outcomes after restorative proctocolectomy. Dis Colon Rectum 2007 Feb;50(2):239–50.
[77] Bissel AD. Localized chronic ulcerative ileitis. Ann Surg 1934;99:957–66.
[78] McKee RF, Keenan RA. Perianal Crohn's disease—is it all bad news? Dis Colon Rectum 1996;39(2):136–42.
[79] Solomon MJ. Fistulae and abscesses in symptomatic perianal Crohn's disease. Int J Colorectal Dis 1996;11(5):222–6.
[80] Homan WP, Tang C, Thorgjarnarson B. Anal lesions complicating Crohn disease. Arch Surg 1976;111(12):1333–5.

[81] Lew RJ, Ginsberg GG. The role of endoscopic ultrasound in inflammatory bowel disease. Gastrointest Endosc Clin N Am 2002;12(3):561–71.

[82] Laniado M, Makowiec F, Dammann F, et al. Perianal complications of Crohn disease: MR imaging findings. Eur Radiol 1997;7(7):1035–42.

[83] Bressler B, Sands BE. Review article: medical therapy for fistulizing Crohn's disease. Aliment Pharmacol Ther 2006;24(9):1283–93.

[84] Katz JA. Advances in the medical therapy of inflammatory bowel disease. Curr Opin Gastroenterol 2002;18(4):435–40.

[85] Ouraghi A, Nieuviarts S, Mougenel JL, et al. [Infliximab therapy for Crohn's disease anoperineal lesions]. Gastroenterol Clin Biol 2001;25(11):949–56 [in French].

[86] Sandborn WJ. Transcending conventional therapies: the role of biologic and other novel therapies. Inflamm Bowel Dis 2001;7(Suppl 1):S9–16.

[87] Buchmann P, Keighley MR, Allan RN, et al. Natural history of perianal Crohn's disease. Ten year follow-up: a plea for conservatism. Am J Surg 1980;140(5):642–4.

[88] Taylor BA, Williams GT, Hughes LE, et al. The histology of anal skin tags in Crohn's disease: an aid to confirmation of the diagnosis. Int J Colorectal Dis 1989;4(3):197–9.

[89] Basu A, Wexner SD. Perianal Crohn's disease. Curr Treat Options Gastroenterol 2002; 5(3):197–206.

[90] Wolkomir AF, Luchtefeld MA. Surgery for symptomatic hemorrhoids and anal fissures in Crohn's disease. Dis Colon Rectum 1993;36(6):545–7.

[91] Sangwan YP, Schoetz DJ Jr, Murray JJ, et al. Perianal Crohn's disease. Results of local surgical treatment. Dis Colon Rectum 1996;39(5):529–35.

[92] Makowiec F, Jehle EC, Becker HD, et al. Perianal abscess in Crohn's disease. Dis Colon Rectum 1997;40(4):443–50.

[93] Joo JS, Weiss EG, Nogueras JJ, et al. Endorectal advancement flap in perianal Crohn's disease. Am Surg 1998;64(2):147–50.

[94] Ellis CN, Clark S. Fibrin glue as an adjunct to flap repair of anal fistulas: a randomized, controlled study. Dis Colon Rectum 2006;49(11):1736–40.

[95] O'Connor L, Champagne BJ, Ferguson MA, et al. Efficacy of anal fistula plug in closure of Crohn's anorectal fistulas. Dis Colon Rectum 2006;49(10):1569–73.

[96] Hyder SA, Travis SP, Jewell DP, et al. Fistulating anal Crohn's disease: results of combined surgical and infliximab treatment. Dis Colon Rectum 2006;49(12):1837–41.

[97] Hull TL, Fazio VW. Surgical approaches to low anovaginal fistula in Crohn's disease. Am J Surg 1997;173(2):95–8.

[98] Sands BE, Blank MA, Patel K, et al. Long-term treatment of rectovaginal fistulas in Crohn's disease: response to infliximab in the ACCENT II Study. Clin Gastroenterol Hepatol 2004;2(10):912–20.

[99] Topstad DR, Panaccione R, Heine JA, et al. Combined seton placement, infliximab infusion, and maintenance immunosuppressives improve healing rate in fistulizing anorectal Crohn's disease: a single center experience. Dis Colon Rectum 2003;46(5): 577–83.

[100] Ardizzone S, Maconi G, Colombo E, et al. Perianal fistulae following infliximab treatment: clinical and endosonographic outcome. Inflamm Bowel Dis 2004;10(2):91–6.

[101] Bernard D, Morgan S, Tasse D. Selective surgical management of Crohn's disease of the anus. Can J Surg 1986;29(5):318–21.

[102] Fleshner PR, Schoetz DJ Jr, Roberts PL, et al. Anal fissure in Crohn's disease: a plea for aggressive management. Dis Colon Rectum 1995;38(11):1137–43.

[103] Linares L, Moreira LF, Andrews H, et al. Natural history and treatment of anorectal strictures complicating Crohn's disease. Br J Surg 1988;75(7):653–5.

[104] Galandiuk S, Kimberling J, Al-Mishlab TG, et al. Perianal Crohn disease: predictors of need for permanent diversion. Ann Surg 2005;241(5):796–801 [discussion: 801–2].

[105] Williamson ME, Hughes LE. Bowel diversion should be used with caution in stenosing anal Crohn's disease. Gut 1994;35(8):1139–40.

[106] Athanasiadis S, Oladeinde I, Kuprian A, et al. [Endorectal advancement flap-plasty vs. transperineal closure in surgical treatment of rectovaginal fistulas. A prospective long-term study of 88 patients]. Chirurg 1995;66(5):493–502 [in German].

[107] Ky A, Sohn N, Weinstein MA, et al. Carcinoma arising in anorectal fistulas of Crohn's disease. Dis Colon Rectum 1998;41(8):992–6.

[108] Chaikhouni A, Regueyra FI, Stevens JR. Adenocarcinoma in perineal fistulas of Crohn's disease. Dis Colon Rectum 1981;24(8):639–43.

[109] Nikias G, Eisner T, Katz S, et al. Crohn's disease and colorectal carcinoma: rectal cancer complicating longstanding active perianal disease. Am J Gastroenterol 1995;90(2):216–9.

[110] Sjodahl RI, Myrelid P, Soderholm JD. Anal and rectal cancer in Crohn's disease. Colorectal Dis 2003;5(5):490–5.

[111] Sweeney JL, Ritchie JK, Nicholls RJ. Anal fissure in Crohn's disease. Br J Surg 1988;75(1):56–7.

[112] Yamamoto T, Allan RN, Keighley MR. Effect of fecal diversion alone on perianal Crohn's disease. World J Surg 2000;24(10):1258–62 [discussion: 1262–3].

ELSEVIER
SAUNDERS

SURGICAL
CLINICS OF
NORTH AMERICA

Surg Clin N Am 87 (2007) 633–641

Elective and Emergent Operative Management of Ulcerative Colitis

Amanda M. Metcalf, MD

*Department of Surgery, Roy J. and Lucille A. Carver College of Medicine,
University of Iowa Hospitals and Clinics, 200 Hawkins Drive,
Iowa City, IA 52242, USA*

Approximately 25% of patients who have ulcerative colitis ultimately require colectomy for the management of their disease. The precise indication for surgical intervention plays an important role in the choice of surgical procedure chosen. Although most patients (and their surgeons) have the luxury of an elective resection, a small but significant number of patients require emergent therapy, the nature of which may well alter the possibility of subsequent restorative procedures.

Elective operative management of ulcerative colitis

Indications for surgical treatment

Intractable disease is the most common indication for elective operative management of ulcerative colitis. Intractable disease is considered to be present when medical therapy fails to adequately control symptoms or when symptoms are only controlled by therapy that carries an excessive long-term risk for morbidity (for example, high-dose corticosteroids). Growth failure in pediatric patients is considered to reflect intractable disease and should prompt consideration of surgical therapy [1]. Colectomy in patients who have intractable disease has been demonstrated to improve quality-of-life indices [2–4]. Non-adenomalike dysplasia-associated lesions (DALM), high-grade dysplasia, or low-grade dysplasia associated with stricture are also indications for elective colectomy [5]. This recommendation is strongest when two experienced gastrointestinal histopathologists have independently reviewed the specimens and are in diagnostic agreement [6]. Bernstein and colleagues [7] reported synchronous carcinoma at immediate colectomy in 43% of patients who had DALM, 42% of patients who had high-grade

E-mail address: amanda-metcalf@uiowa.edu

dysplasia, and 19% of patients who had low-grade dysplasia. There are issues regarding the distinction between DALM lesions and typical adenomas. DALM lesions have associated surrounding flat mucosa dysplasia, whereas typical adenomas do not. Some authors believe that if a lesion is surrounded by biopsy-proven normal mucosa, these lesions can be managed endoscopically without excessive carcinoma risk [8,9].

There is controversy concerning the management of patients who have low-grade dysplasia not associated with stricture. Bernstein and colleagues [7] demonstrated that patients who have low-grade dysplasia have a 16% to 29% incidence of progression to high-grade dysplasia, DALM, or cancer when followed endoscopically. There are reports suggesting that low-grade dysplasia may not be as ominous a finding, however. Befrits and colleagues [10] reported a group of 60 patients who had low-grade dysplasia followed for a mean period of 10 years, in whom only 18% progressed to high-grade dysplasia. This study has been criticized for not following standard histopathologic criteria, in that patients who had biopsies that were indefinite for dysplasia were included in the low-grade dysplasia group.

Stricture develops in 5% to 10% of patients who have ulcerative colitis, and up to 25% are malignant. Strictures that occur in patients who have longstanding colitis, are proximal to the splenic flexure, or are symptomatic have a higher risk for malignancy [11]. Although biopsy of strictures may be helpful, it is often unreliable in the diagnosis of dysplasia or malignancy [12,13], and therefore resection is reasonable.

This longitudinal risk for the development of carcinoma in patients who have ulcerative colitis may be mitigated by the use of 5-ASA medication in patients in clinical remission. There have been several reports that suggest a reduction in carcinoma with long-term use of these medications [14,15].

Surgical options

Proctocolectomy with ileostomy

Despite the popularity of restorative proctocolectomy with ileal pouch–anal anastomosis (IPAA), proctocolectomy with ileostomy remains the benchmark procedure against which others must be compared. It remains the procedure of choice in patients who have impaired sphincter function, significant comorbid conditions, or those who simply choose not to have a restorative procedure [5]. Complications are not uncommon and occur in up to 26%of patients [16]. These include small bowel obstruction, alterations in bladder and sexual function, infertility, failure of perineal wound healing, and stoma-related complications. Stoma-related complications are the most frequent.

Restorative proctocolectomy with ileal pouch–anal anastomosis

Proctocolectomy with IPAA has become the most common procedure performed for patients who have ulcerative colitis undergoing elective resection. It can be performed open or laparoscopically assisted. The benefits of a laparoscopic approach compared with an open approach seem to mimic those seen with less extensive resections (ie, decreased pain, decreased hospital stay, and improved cosmesis) [17]. Although it has been performed as a single-stage procedure in highly selected patients, it is most commonly performed in two stages with construction of a temporary loop ileostomy. Although there have been several configurations of pouches used (Fig. 1), none has clearcut advantage in functional results [5]. Overall, the J configuration is used most widely. Either a double-stapled technique or a mucosectomy with hand-sewn anastomosis can be used. Several studies have demonstrated no difference in functional results between the two techniques [18,19]. The double-stapled technique is technically easier, but is generally considered to be contraindicated if the procedure is being performed for dysplasia. Symptomatic inflammation in the retained mucosa and the potential development of dysplasia are long-term complications of the double-stapled technique. Long-term surveillance of any retained mucosa is recommended [5]. Age greater than 60 years, although not considered to be a contraindication, is associated with poorer functional results overall [20]. Patients who have a diagnosis of indeterminate colitis are candidates for this procedure. The incidence of pelvic sepsis and long-term pouch failure is higher in this group of patients, however [21]. Concomitant carcinoma is a relative contraindication to an immediate IPAA procedure; a subtotal colectomy with ileostomy with later conversion to an IPAA is usually more appropriate [5]. Overall, the IPAA has been demonstrated to be a safe, durable procedure with an acceptable morbidity (19% to 27%) and an extremely low mortality (0.2% to 0.4%) [22,23]. The quality of life following this procedure is near that of the normal population [24,25]. The risk for long-term pouch loss is 10% and is usually secondary to sepsis,

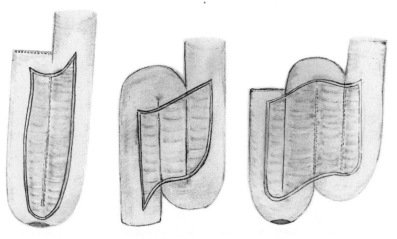

Fig. 1. J, S, and W configurations of ileal pouches.

which may be associated with the development of Crohn's disease [26]. The long-term risk for complications is significantly higher than after proctocolectomy with ileostomy (52% versus 26%) [16] and this relates primarily to pouchitis, the most frequent long-term complication of this procedure [27]. The diagnosis of pouchitis is often mainly on clinical grounds of diarrhea and associated deterioration of anorectal function. This complication occurs in up to 50% of patients postoperatively and is associated with extraintestinal manifestations of inflammatory bowel disease and sclerosing cholangitis [26]. It is most commonly believed to be an immunologic response to the altered bowel flora in the pouch and has been associated with sulfate-reducing bacteria [28,29]. Approximately 60% of patients have recurrent episodes; a minority of patients (5%–19%) develop refractory or chronic pouchitis that requires continuous therapy [30–32]. Treatment with metronidazole or ciprofloxacin alone or in combination is usually all that is needed. A minority of patients require more aggressive therapy with immunosuppressive agents, such as steroids or azathioprine [33]. Other treatment options include probiotics, budesonide enemas, short-chain fatty acid enemas, and even Remicade [33]. The development of ulcerations in the small bowel proximal to the pouch is considered to be suggestive of the development of Crohn's disease. Endoscopic biopsies usually demonstrate nonspecific inflammation.

Subtotal colectomy with ileostomy

Although this is not a common procedure for patients who require an elective resection, this may be an appropriate choice in some situations. One situation would be the unexpected finding of carcinoma at the time of surgery. If palliation is the only reasonable goal based on the findings at surgery, a procedure associated with the lowest risk for complications is a reasonable choice. If a serious attempt to convert to a pouch procedure in the future is anticipated, preservation of the presacral space and the ileocolic vessel by division of the mesentery adjacent to the cecum is extremely important. Several authors have advocated this approach with a delay of 12 months before attempted conversion to detect patients who have early recurrent cancer [34]. Pelvic irradiation following a pouch procedure is associated with a high risk for pouch loss and has a significantly deleterious effect on pouch function [35]. Although conversion to a restorative procedure following pelvic irradiation has not been performed frequently, it is certainly a theoretic possibility. Adjuvant therapy, whether chemotherapy or radiation therapy, is tolerated better with an end ileostomy compared with a high output loop ileostomy.

Proctocolectomy with Kock pouch construction (continent ileostomy)

Currently, this procedure is performed so infrequently that most surgical residents are unfamiliar with this option. Essentially, the distal ileum is intussuscepted into a pouch constructed of more proximal bowel to form a continent nipple valve (Fig. 2). This procedure is a reasonable alternative for patients who are not candidates for IPAA because of poor sphincter function, patients who are dissatisfied with an ileostomy, or patients who have a failed IPAA. Early complications occur in 25% and are most commonly related to sepsis. Late complications occur in at least 50% and include incontinence and obstruction because of nipple dysfunction [36]. These complications require valve revision. Patients who undergo a conversion to a Kock pouch have a significantly higher rate of long-term failure (46%) compared with those who had the procedure as a primary procedure (23%) [36]. Patients who have a functioning Kock pouch have a quality of life that is only slightly inferior to patients who have an IPAA [37]. Overall, the cumulative loss of small bowel if both an IPAA and a Kock pouch fail make conversion to a Kock pouch after a failed IPAA a procedure to be undertaken only after careful consideration.

Subtotal colectomy with ileoproctostomy

This option is reasonable only in highly selected patients who have minimal rectal involvement without anoperineal disease, as might be seen in patients who have indeterminate colitis [38–40]. It might be appropriate for a patient who has metastatic colon cancer who wishes to avoid a permanent stoma. Patients who have dysplasia or curative carcinoma should not have this procedure performed as a definitive procedure, however [41]. Although it is a safe procedure, the durability of this procedure is limited. Several studies have demonstrated a relatively high risk for failure, ranging between 12% and 50% with follow-up of more than 6 years [42,43]. An additional disadvantage is the need for long-term surveillance of the residual rectum.

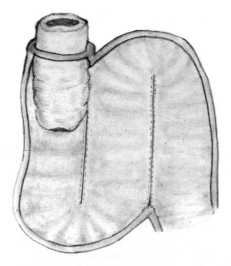

Fig. 2. Kock pouch demonstrating intussuscepted ileum forming nipple valve.

Emergent operative management

Indications for operative intervention

The indication for urgent or emergent surgical intervention includes patients who have fulminant colitis, toxic megacolon, or significant hemorrhage. Approximately 15% of patients who have ulcerative colitis present initially with severe colitis requiring hospitalization. Severe colitis as defined as more than 6 bloody stools per day, fever (temperature >37.5°C), tachycardia, anemia (hemoglobin <75% of normal), and elevated sedimentation rate. Fulminant colitis is defined as more than 10 bloody stools per day, fever and tachycardia as above, anemia requiring transfusion, elevated sedimentation rate, colonic distension by radiograph, and abdominal distension with tenderness [44,45]. Dilation of the transverse colon to greater than 6 cm defines a diagnosis of toxic megacolon and is an indication for emergent surgical intervention [5].

Some 20% to 30% of patients who have severe colitis require surgery [44,45]. Failure to respond adequately within 96 hours of initiation of medical treatment with high-dose corticosteroids, with or without intravenous cyclosporine, predicts a high risk for colectomy. In one study, patients who had more than eight stools per day or three to eight stools per day and an erythrocyte sedimentation rate 0.45 mg/mL after 3 days of therapy had an 85% chance of requiring colectomy during that hospitalization [46].

Perforation, either localized or free, is a serious complication of severe colitis and has a mortality rate between 27% and 57% [47,48]. Impending or actual perforation is suggested by continued or worsening colonic dilation, pneumatosis, localizing peritoneal signs, and the development of multisystem organ failure. As would be expected, the development of multisystem organ failure is extremely ominous. In one series 8 of 11 such patients died postoperatively [49].

Surgical options

Subtotal colectomy with ileostomy

Subtotal colectomy with ileostomy and Hartmann's pouch or mucous fistula is the appropriate choice of procedure for most patients requiring urgent or emergent colectomy. Mortality is extremely low in the absence of perforation [50,51]. Construction of a mucous fistula or transanal drainage of the Hartmann's pouch may decrease the incidence of pelvic sepsis [52,53]. Preservation of the entire length of the ileocolic vessel and nonviolation of the presacral space maximizes the chances for successful conversion to an IPAA procedure at a later date. Some authors have suggested that the optimal time interval to attempting conversion is 6 months because this interval seemed to result in a lower incidence of pelvic sepsis compared with that seen in patients who underwent earlier conversion [54].

Summary

Surgical therapy of ulcerative colitis is effective, safe, and provides an improved quality of life in those whose disease cannot be managed medically. It is life saving for patients who have dysplasia, cancer, or fulminant disease. In the elective setting, widespread acceptance of restorative proctocolectomy has made surgical therapy an attractive option in the overall management of ulcerative colitis. Enthusiasm for this procedure should be tempered by the acknowledgment of the significant incidence of pouchitis in the long term, however. Proctocolectomy with ileostomy remains a good surgical option for patients who are unsuitable for restorative procedures. The standard therapy for fulminant colitis or toxic megacolon remains subtotal colectomy with ileostomy. Patients undergoing subtotal colectomy are candidates for conversion to restorative procedures.

References

[1] Berger M, Gribetz D, Korelitz BI. Growth retardation in children with ulcerative colitis: the effect of medical and surgical therapy. Pediatrics 1975;55:459–67.

[2] McLeod RS, Churchill DN, Lock AM, et al. Quality of life of patients with ulcerative colitis preoperatively and postoperatively. Gastroenterology 1991;101:1307–13.

[3] McLeod RS, Baxter NN. Quality of life of patients with inflammatory bowel disease after surgery. World J Surg 1998;22:375–81.

[4] Muir AJ, Edwards LJ, Sanders LL, et al. A prospective evaluation of health-related quality of life after ileal pouch anal anastomosis for ulcerative colitis. Am J Gastroenterol 2001;96: 1480–5.

[5] Cohen JL, Strong SA, Hyman NH, et al. Practice parameters for the surgical treatment of ulcerative colitis. Dis Colon Rectum 2005;48:1997–2009.

[6] Dixon MF, Brown LJ, Gilmour HM, et al. Observer variation in the assessment of dysplasia in ulcerative colitis. Histopathology 1988;13:385–97.

[7] Bernstein CN, Shanahan F, Weinstein WM. Are we telling patients the truth about surveillance colonoscopy in ulcerative colitis? Lancet 1994;343:71–4.

[8] Rubin PH, Friedman S, Harpaz N, et al. Colonoscopic polypectomy in chronic colitis: conservative management after endoscopic management of dysplastic polyps. Gastroenterology 1999;117:1295–300.

[9] Odze RD, Farraye FA, Hecht JL, et al. Long-term follow-up after polypectomy treatment for adenoma-like dysplastic lesions in ulcerative colitis. Clin Gastroenterol Hepatol 2004; 2:534–41.

[10] Befrits R, Ljung T, Jaramillo E, et al. Low grade dysplasia in extensive, long-standing inflammatory bowel disease: a follow-up study. Dis Colon Rectum 2002;45:615–20.

[11] Gumaste V, Sachar DB, Greenstein AJ. Benign and malignant colorectal strictures in ulcerative colitis. Gut 1992;33:938–41.

[12] Lashner BA, Turner BC, Bostick DG, et al. Dysplasia and cancer complicating strictures in ulcerative colitis. Dig Dis Sci 1990;35:349–52.

[13] Reiser JR, Waye JD, Janowitz HD, et al. Adenocarcinoma in strictures of ulcerative colitis without antecedent dysplasia by colonoscopy. Am J Gastroenterol 1994;89:119–22.

[14] Moody GA, Jayanthi V, Probert CS, et al. Long-term therapy with sulphasalazine protects against colorectal cancer in ulcerative colitis; a retrospective study of colorectal cancer risk and compliance with treatment in Leicestershire. Eur J Gastroenterol Hepatol 1996;8: 1179–83.

[15] Eaden J, Abrams K, Ekbom A, et al. Colorectal cancer prevention in ulcerative colitis; a case-control study. Aliment Pharmacol Ther 2000;14:145–53.

[16] Camilleri-Brennan J, Munro A, Steele RJ. Does an ileoanal pouch offer a better quality of life than a permanent ileostomy for patients with ulcerative colitis? J Gastrointest Surg 2003;7:814–9.

[17] Larson DW, Cima RR, Dozois EJ, et al. Safety, feasibility, and short-term outcomes of laparoscopic ileal-pouch-anal anastomosis: a single institutional case-matched experience. Ann Surg 2006;243:667–72.

[18] Choen S, Tsunoda A, Nicholls RJ. Prospective randomized trial comparing anal function after hand-sewn ileoanal anastomosis with mucosectomy versus stapled ileoanal anastomosis without mucosectomy in restorative proctocolectomy. Br J Surg 1991;78:430–4.

[19] Reilly WT, Pemberton JH, Wolff BG, et al. Randomized prospective trial comparing ileal pouch-anal anastomosis performed by excising the anal mucosa to ileal pouch-anal anastomosis performed by preserving the anal mucosa. Ann Surg 1997;225:666–76.

[20] Ho KS, Chang CC, Baig MK, et al. Ileal pouch anal anastomosis for ulcerative colitis is feasible for septuagenarians. Colorectal Dis 2006;8:235–8.

[21] Tekkis PP, Heriot AG, Smith O, et al. Long-term outcomes of restorative proctocolectomy for Crohn's disease and indeterminate colitis. Colorectal Dis 2005;7:218–23.

[22] Fazio VW, Ziv Y, Church JM, et al. Ileal pouch-anal anastomosis complications and function in 1005 patients. Ann Surg 1995;222:120–7.

[23] Meagher AP, Farouk R, Dozois RR, et al. J ileal pouch-anal anastomosis for chronic ulcerative colitis: complications and long-term outcome in 1310 patients. Br J Surg 1998;85:800–3.

[24] Carmon E, Keidar A, Ravid A, et al. The correlation between quality of life and functional outcome in ulcerative colitis patients after proctocolectomy ileal pouch-anal anastomosis. Colorectal Dis 2003;5:228–32.

[25] Scarpa M, Angriman I, Ruffolo C, et al. Health-related quality of life after restorative proctocolectomy for ulcerative colitis: long-term results. World J Surg 2004;28:124–9.

[26] Penna C, Dozois R, Tremaine W, et al. Pouchitis after ileal pouch-anal anastomosis for ulcerative colitis occurs with increased frequency in patients with associated primary sclerosing cholangitis. Gut 1996;38:234–9.

[27] Lohmuller JL, Peberton JH, Dozois RR, et al. Pouchitis and extraintestinal manifestations of inflammatory bowel disease after ileal pouch-anal anastomosis. Ann Surg 1990;211: 622–7.

[28] Nasmyth DG, Godwin PG, Dixon MF, et al. Ileal ecology after pouch-anal anastomosis or ileostomy. A study of mucosal morphology, fecal bacteriology, fecal volatile fatty acids, and their interrelationship. Gastroenterology 1989;96:817–24.

[29] Duffy M, O'Mahony L, Coffey JC, et al. Sulfate-reducing bacteria colonize pouches formed for ulcerative colitis but not for adenomatous polyposis. Dis Colon Rectum 2002;45:384–8.

[30] Mowschenson PM, Critchlow JF, Peppercorn MA. Ileoanal pouch operation: long-term outcome with or without diverting ileostomy. Arch Surg 2000;135:463–5.

[31] Hurst RD, Chung TP, Rubin M, et al. The implications of acute pouchitis on the long-term functional results after restorative proctocolectomy. Inflamm Bowel Dis 1998;4:280–4.

[32] Madiba TE, Bartolo DC. Pouchitis following restorative proctocolectomy for ulcerative colitis: incidence and therapeutic outcome. J R Coll Surg Edinb 2001;46:334–7.

[33] Shen B, Lashner BA. Pouchitis: a spectrum of diseases. Curr Gastroenterol Rep 2005;7: 404–11.

[34] Stelzner M, Fonkalsrud EW. The endorectal ileal pullthrough procedure in patients with ulcerative colitis and familial polyposis with carcinoma. Surg Gynecol Obstet 1989;169: 187–94.

[35] Wiltz O, Hashmi HF, Schoetz DJ Jr, et al. Carcinoma and the ileal pouch-anal anastomosis. Dis Colon Rectum 1991;34:805–9.

[36] Fazio VW, Church JM. Complications and function of the continent ileostomy at the Cleveland Clinic. World J Surg 1988;12:148–54.

[37] Litle VR, Barbour S, Schrock TR, et al. The continent ileostomy: long-term durability and patient satisfaction. J Gastrointest Surg 1999;3:625–32.

[38] Parc R, Legrand M, Frileux P, et al. Comparitive clinical results of ileal-pouch anal anasto-mosis and ileorectal anastomosis in ulcerative colitis. Hepatogastroenterology 1989;36:235–9.

[39] Khubchandani IT, Kontostolis SB. Outcome of ileorectal anastomosis in an inflammatory bowel disease surgery experience of three decades. Arch Surg 1994;129:866–9.

[40] Pastore RL, Wolff BG, Hodge D. Total abdominal colectomy and ileorectal anastomosis for inflammatory bowel disease. Dis Colon Rectum 1977;40:1455–64.

[41] Kvist N, Jacobsen O, Kvist HK, et al. Malignancy in ulcerative colitis. Scand J Gastroenterol 1989;24:497–506.

[42] Saito Y, Sawada T, Tsuno N, et al. Total colectomy and ileorectal anastomosis in ulcerative colitis. J Gastroenterol 1995;30(Suppl 8):131–4.

[43] Leijonmarck CE, Lofberg R, Ost A, et al. Long-term results of ileorectal anastomosis in ulcerative colitis in Stockholm County. Dis Colon Rectum 1990;33:195–200.

[44] Hanauer SB. Inflammatory bowel disease. N Engl J Med 1996;334:841–8.

[45] Katz JA. Medical and surgical management of severe colitis. Semin Gastrointest Dis 2000;11:18–32.

[46] Present DH. Toxic megacolon. Med Clin North Am 1993;77:1129–48.

[47] Greenstein AJ, Barth JA, Sachar DB, et al. Free colonic perforation without dilation in ulcerative colitis. Am J Surg 1986;152:272–5.

[48] Heppell J, Farkouh E, Dube S, et al. Toxic megacolon. An analysis of 70 cases. Dis Colon Rectum 1986;29:789–92.

[49] Caprilli R, Latella G, Vernia P, et al. Multiple organ dysfunction in ulcerative colitis. Am J Gastroenterol 2000;95:1258–62.

[50] Travis SP, Farrant JM, Ricketts C, et al. Predicting outcome in severe ulcerative colitis. Gut 1996;38:905–10.

[51] Hyman NH, Cataldo P, Osler T. Urgent subtotal colectomy for severe inflammatory bowel disease. Dis Colon Rectum 2005;48:70–3.

[52] Carter FM, McLeod RS, Cohen Z. Subtotal colectomy for ulcerative colitis: complications related to the rectal remnant. Dis Colon Rectum 1991;34:1005–9.

[53] Karch LA, Bauer JJ, Gorfine SR, et al. Subtotal colectomy with Hartmann's pouch for inflammatory bowel disease. Dis Colon Rectum 1995;38:635–9.

[54] Dinnewitzer AJ, Wexner SD, Baig MK, et al. Timing of restorative proctocolectomy following subtotal colectomy in patients with inflammatory bowel disease. Colorectal Dis 2006;8:278–82.

ELSEVIER
SAUNDERS

SURGICAL
CLINICS OF
NORTH AMERICA

Surg Clin N Am 87 (2007) 643–658

Inflammatory Bowel Disease in the Pediatric Patient

Todd Ponsky, MD[a], Anna Hindle, MD[b],
Anthony Sandler, MD[a],*

[a]Children's National Medical Center, 111 Michigan Ave., NW, Washington,
DC 20010-2970, USA
[b]George Washington University, 901 23rd St. NW, Washington, DC 20037, USA

Inflammatory bowel disease (IBD) is a general term used to describe two chronic bowel disorders, Crohn's disease (CD) and ulcerative colitis (UC), both of which are characterized by autoimmune-related inflammation of the intestines. UC is limited to the colonic mucosa, whereas CD can involve any part of the intestinal tract from the mouth to the anus. The true etiology of UC and CD is still unknown, although extensive research has identified some genetic and environmental factors [1–3]. This article discusses current clinical concepts of both diseases in the pediatric population.

Ulcerative colitis

Epidemiology and pathophysiology

The incidence of UC is approximately 2.2 per 100,000, and does not appear to be increasing, unlike CD, which is steadily rising [2,4,5]. There does not appear to be gender predominance for UC. Both UC and CD demonstrate a bimodal age distribution pattern in the second or third decade of life and then again in the sixth decade of life [2,4]. Thirty percent of patients who have IBD are diagnosed during childhood. Although our understanding of the etiology of UC is improving with the introduction of multi-institutional databases and registries, the true cause of UC continues to evade us. Close examination of the epidemiology of UC suggests a combination of genetic and environmental factors. Several recent studies

---

* Corresponding author.
    E-mail address: asandler@cnmc.org (A. Sandler).

0039-6109/07/$ - see front matter © 2007 Elsevier Inc. All rights reserved.
doi:10.1016/j.suc.2007.03.002   *surgical.theclinics.com*

demonstrate a genetic component: there is a 44.4% concordance rate of IBD among monozygotic twins compared with 3.8% concordance among dizygotic twins [6]. Family history is shown to be a significant risk factor for IBD [7], and it is suggested that the incidence of UC is higher in Ashkenazi Jews [8]. Recently, several genetic markers are found to be associated with IBD, such as the nucleotide-binding oligomerization domain containing 2 (NOD2) leucine-rich repeat variants for CD, and a genome wide association study identifying interleukin 23 (IL23R) as an inflammatory gene for both UC and CD [9,10].

Besides a genetic predisposition for UC, environmental factors also appear to play an important role [3]. There appears to be a higher incidence of IBD in children who have improved hygiene in infancy [11–13].

The natural history of UC in children is different from that of adults. Specifically, there is a higher probability of proximal extension and pancolitis in children. Kugathasan and colleagues [14] reported a 90% incidence of pancolitis in newly diagnosed children who have UC, compared with 37% in newly diagnosed adults [14,15]. Furthermore, the chance of disease progression from left-sided disease proximally is greater in children when compared with adults [2,16].

Workup/diagnosis

The diagnosis of UC can be elusive because the presenting signs and symptoms are so variable. Although the most common presenting symptoms of UC are abdominal pain and diarrhea, some children present with hematochezia, arthralgias, lethargy, weight loss, anorexia, growth and sexual delay, or iron deficiency [2,17,18]. Following a thorough history and physical, the workup for UC should begin with routine blood work, looking for anemia, leukocytosis, electrolyte abnormalities from extensive diarrhea, and low albumin from chronic disease state. Elevated liver enzymes and bilirubin may suggest biliary disease, possibly from sclerosing cholangitis. Stool should be analyzed and cultured for *Salmonella, Shigella, Campylobacter*, and *Yersinia*, and stool assays performed for *Clostridium difficile* and *Entamoeba histolytica*. Abdominal plain films can show evidence of toxic megacolon or visceral perforation. An upper gastrointestinal series with small bowel follow-through may help identify small bowel disease and enteric fistulas that will suggest CD and rule-out the diagnosis of UC. A contrast enema can demonstrate findings consistent with UC, such as mucosal ulcerations, psuedopolyps, and loss of haustral markings giving a "lead pipe" appearance. The ultimate diagnostic test for UC is colonoscopy with biopsies. Patients who have UC will have friable, ulcerative mucosa with pseudopolyp formation in the rectum with possible proximal extension. Small bowel involvement suggests a diagnosis of CD, because UC is limited to the colon. In 10% to 15% of patients, the diagnosis of UC cannot be differentiated from CD [18]. Recently, the use of serologic markers has drastically increased our ability to diagnose IBD, and even to differentiate between UC and Crohn's disease with a 92% to 100% sensitivity [19].

Medical therapy

Once the diagnosis of UC is established, patients are started on medical therapy, based upon the severity of their disease. The strategies of medical therapy can be categorized into remission induction and remission maintenance.

Remission induction therapy

Remission induction therapy is targeted at treating the acute flare-up. The general strategy for medical therapy is to start treatment with 5-aminosalicilic acid (5-ASA) alone, and add additional medications if there is no response. The limiting factor in the benefit of 5-ASA is the poor compliance with this medication. The large number of pills necessary for the child to consume to achieve an adequate response has led to only 40% compliance [20]. Approximately one third of patients will not be successfully treated with 5-ASA, and require the addition of corticosteroids to the treatment regimen. Fifty-four percent of patients treated with oral prednisone will have complete remission [21]. Although steroid therapy is effective, it is not without complications. Prolonged use of high-dose steroids may lead to Cushing's syndrome, which consists of moon facies, buffalo hump, acne, and weight gain. High-dose steroid therapy may also lead to poor wound healing and infection.

The use of cyclosporine has gained popularity in UC remission induction therapy. Lichtiger and colleagues [22] demonstrated that cyclosporine, an immunomodulator, is a viable therapeutic option for severe UC that is refractory to corticosteroids. Although efficacious, there are serious side effects of cyclosporine, which include renal insufficiency, *Pneumocystis carinii* infections, seizures, tremor, gingival hyperplasia, and hypertension [23,24]. Despite the risk of complications from cyclosporine, it remains a safe viable option for acute therapy [25].

Remission maintenance therapy

Remission maintenance therapy is directed at prevention of recurrent flare-ups. Fewer than 10% of children who have UC will be sustained on medical therapy without a relapse [26]. The mainstay of medical maintenance therapy for UC is 5-ASA. This is the tried and true therapy for IBD, and has a dose-response up to 4.8 g/d [24,27]. 5-ASA has been shown to maintain remission. Kane and colleagues [28] demonstrated that patients who were compliant with taking 5-ASA had a lower risk of relapse than the noncompliant patients.

Another option for maintenance therapy is 6-mercaptopurine (6-MP), an immunomodulator. 6-MP takes several months to achieve efficacy, and for that reason it is not useful in the treatment of an acute flare-up, but is an effective therapy in remission maintenance. Only 11% of patients who are started on 6-MP failed to achieve remission [29]. In fact, 6-MP may be effective as a monotherapy for UC remission maintenance, and may obviate the need for 5-ASA compounds [30]. As with all other immunomodulators, 6-MP may have significant side effects. Specifically, leucopenia with associated infections, hepatotoxicity, and pancreatitis may develop [24,31]. Despite the risk of complications from 6-MP, it remains a safe viable option for remission maintenance therapy [31,32].

Other therapies

Other newer medical therapies are also shown to be effective or may show promise in the treatment of UC. Tacrolimus (FK506), a calcineurin inhibitor, is used for treatment of acute flare-ups in children who have steroid-refractory disease. Although almost 70% responded initially, fewer than 50% achieved long-term remission [33].

The use of biologic agents such as the tumor necrosis factor (TNF)-alpha antibody infliximab has revolutionized medical therapy for CD, but the results with UC are not as promising. Several studies have shown mixed results with infliximab targeting of TNF-alpha [34–37], and more convincing studies are needed before it can be recommended in the routine treatment of UC.

Surgical therapy

Fortunately, a curative option exists for UC in a total proctocolectomy. A total proctocolectomy, however, carries significant morbidity, including bleeding, infection, nerve injury, and the potential for a permanent ileostomy. Timing of surgery for children is perhaps one of the most widely debated topics in the treatment of UC. Four groups of patients can be defined when considering indications for surgical therapy.

There is no controversy in the need for surgical therapy in patients who have acute complications of their disease such as toxic megacolon, persistent bleeding, hemorrhage, or hollow viscus perforation.

Patients who have UC and who may benefit from a total colectomy are those children who fail to enter into remission after several weeks of medical therapy. These children become significantly at risk not only from the side effects of high-dose steroids and other immunomodulators, but also from the complications of the disease itself.

Another group of patients who should also benefit from surgery are those who have chronic disease and continue to go in and out of remission. These patients often find themselves on frequent high doses of steroids. Children on chronic steroids are at risk of significant growth retardation and delayed sexual maturation.

Perhaps the most difficult and controversial issue in the treatment of UC is the role and timing of surgical therapy in the child who has medically controlled chronic disease. Prolonged use of periodic steroids may lead to growth delay, wound healing impairment, and poor nutrition. Sher and colleagues [38] reported a 65% complication rate from steroids compared with a 15% complication rate from a restorative proctocolectomy. Those patients undergoing prolonged medical care had more blood transfusions, weight loss, and significantly higher medical costs compared with the surgically treated group. Even patients who may have symptomatic control with medical therapy are at risk for colonic mucosal aneuploidy and neoplasia [26,39]. Furthermore, after 10 years of disease, UC carries a 10% to 20% risk of colon cancer per decade [40].

Although surgical therapy is curative, it is not without risk. Most studies quote a 20% risk of complication for both the open and laparoscopic approach [41,42]. The complications typically include anastomotic leak, pelvic abscess, peptic ulcer, dehydration, and anastomotic stricture [42]. Therefore, most gastroenterologists advocate surveillance endoscopy in the medically controlled patient [18]. Annual colonoscopic surveillance with random biopsies is shown to be an effective alternative to colectomy [43–46]. Magnifying chromoendoscopy and dye spraying are newer techniques that improve the accuracy in the detection of dysplasia or neoplasia in surveillance endoscopy in children who have UC [43,47]. Patients who are found to have dysplasia, neoplasia, or adenomatous polyps on colonoscopy should undergo a proctocolectomy.

The surgical options include total proctocolectomy with ileostomy or restorative proctocolectomy. Although most patients will choose a restorative proctocolectomy because it offers stool continence, some prefer a permanent end ileostomy. In fact, patients who choose an ileostomy have equal quality of life satisfaction without the morbidity of the pelvic pouch [48,49].

Restorative proctocolectomy is the most common operation performed. The usual method of restorative proctocolectomy is an endorectal ileal pull-through. There are many variations to this procedure. The classic three-stage procedure consists of first performing a total abdominal colectomy with loop ileostomy, then returning in about 6 weeks to perform a rectal mucosectomy with ileal pull-through, and finally returning a third time to reverse the ileostomy. The three-stage procedure is advocated because it delays the ileo-anal anastomosis until the patient is off of steroid therapy.

Many advocate the two-stage procedure, which combines the total abdominal colectomy, rectal mucosectomy, ileal pull through, and ileostomy at the first operation, followed by eventual ileostomy takedown. Nicholls and colleagues [50] report that the three-stage operation offers no advantage except in patients in whom "urgent surgery is required for the complications of ulcerative colitis, when malignancy or Crohn's disease cannot be ruled out, and when a patient who has active colitis has a combination of a low hemoglobin value (male less than 13.5 g/dL, female less than 11.5 g/dL), a low serum albumin level (less than 40 g/L), and is taking oral steroids."

Variations also exist in the method of pulling down the ileum to the anus. Some prefer to create an ileal pouch reservoir, whereas others prefer a straight ileal pull-through. The advantage of creating a pouch is that it creates a reservoir for stool and decreases the stool frequency, allowing for continence; however, this technique, which involves looping the ileum upon itself and creating a side-to-side entero-enterostomy, decreases the length of the ileum and may create tension on the ileo-anal anastomosis.

The data are mixed when comparing the results of pouch pull-through versus straight pull-through. Most studies suggest improved functional outcome with a pouch [51,52], but others show no difference [53]. There are multiple variations to the pouch creation, including the classic single loop J-pouch or the multiple loop pouch (S- or W-pouch). Some have also described a straight pull-through technique with multiple myotomies, which had equal functional outcome as the pouch [54,55].

Finally, laparoscopy has made its way into the realm of colorectal surgery, and is the preferred method of many for colectomy. In the hands of an experienced laparoscopic surgeon, the laparoscopic approach does not increase the chance of operative morbidity [41]. In fact, the laparoscopic approach may offer earlier return of intestinal function and decreased length of hospital stay [42].

The diagnostic workup and treatment of UC is advancing. Serum assays for UC such as interleukin (IL)-6 and IL-8 are becoming increasingly more accurate [56] and the use of newer imaging techniques such as MRI in the diagnosis of UC is evolving [57–60]. Newer medical therapies are being developed, such as CDP-571, an anti-tumor necrosis factor (TNF) drug that may show promise in the treatment of UC [61]. Finally, advances in minimally invasive surgery may make the surgical treatment of UC less morbid and still provide outcomes that are compatible with a satisfactory standard of daily living.

Crohn's disease

Epidemiology and pathophysiology

CD is a chronic inflammatory condition that can affect the entire bowel. The disease may manifest itself by the formation of intestinal fistulas, strictures, ulceration, or perforation secondary to inflammation of the bowel wall. Typical lesions in CD are ulcerating, granulomatous, transmural lesions [62]. The pathogenesis of the disease is multifactorial, and there seem to be environmental, genetic, and immunological causes that overlap each other and contribute to the development of CD [63].

Epidemiologic trends exist in patients who have CD suggesting that there is an environmental component to the development of the disease. There is a higher incidence of the disease in developed countries and in urban areas. There is also an increase in the rates of disease in areas with improved sanitation. The hypothesis is proposed that improved hygiene alters innate immunity by changing the bacteria to which a person is exposed, thus combining the environmental and immunologic causes. Finally, smoking is another environmental risk factor that may predispose individuals to developing CD, but is probably of less importance in the pediatric population [63].

The development of CD is thought to be a dysregulation of the immune system that is naturally present in the intestine. The bowel is constantly exposed to a heavy load of intraluminal bacteria, and the immune cells of the bowel have the task of maintaining immune homeostasis while preventing systemic infection from the intraluminal bacteria [64]. There is a physical barrier to intraluminal bacteria through tight junctions of the epithelial cells and the production of mucus. The antigen presenting cells within the bowel wall are key components of the immune system in their ability to sample the contents of bacteria in the bowel and regulate immunity. An inability to maintain an appropriate physical barrier (ie, failure to maintain tight junc-tions) or an inappropriate (biased) immune response to intraluminal bacteria may result in activation of the inflammatory response that contributes to the pathologic findings of CD.

There is a familial predisposition to CD that led scientists to study the genetics of patients who have CD [65]. Mutations in the nuclear oligomerization domain 2 (NOD2) gene on chromosome 16 were found to be associated with a higher incidence of CD [9,66]. The NOD2 gene, also known as caspase activation and recruitment domain 15 (CARD 15), is involved with mediation of the immune response in the bowel [62,63,67]. NOD2/CARD15 is a cytoplasmic protein that recognizes certain aspects of the bacterial cell wall and regulates the immune response to these bacteria [64]. The protein is present in macrophages, dendritic cells, and Paneth cells. Upregulation is shown to produce an increase in TNF alpha that contributes to the activation of cytokines and diffuse inflammation [62]. NOD2/CARD15 may help to allow controlled activation of the immune system, and a defect in this system produces the uncontrolled inflammation that is present in CD.

There are several other loci that may confer an increased risk for CD. These include IBD 5, 3, and 6 on chromosomes 5, 6, and 19 respectively [67]. The isolation of multiple genes in patients who have CD demonstrates the heterogeneity that exists among Crohn's patients. Most patients who have CD represent sporadic cases, which supports the conclusion that the cause for the disease is multifactorial, and that there are potentially further genes to be discovered [63]. There is an attempt to correlate the genetics of Crohn's with the expected course of the disease [68]. The genetic factors that are suggested to have an influence in the development of CD all seem to play a role in the immunoregulatory system of the bowel.

Genetics, the environment, and immunology are all intertwined in the development of the chronic mucosal inflammation that leads to the development of CD. A better understanding of these factors may help in determining the cause of the disease and in direct development of therapeutic options.

Workup and diagnosis

Patients who have CD frequently present with complaints of abdominal pain, diarrhea, and weight loss. In children, these symptoms may or may not all be present, and it may be very difficult to make the diagnosis of CD. For example, children may simply present with lethargy and mild abdominal pain, or commonly, a delay in growth. Because of the variety of manifestations of CD, especially in children, there may be a delay in the diagnosis of the disease [69].

The majority of patients who have CD have diarrhea [69]. Children may also present with extra-intestinal manifestations of CD that include arthropathies, weight loss, oral or anal inflammation, granulomatosis, or erythema nodosum [69,70]. Pediatric patients may present with growth failure alone [71].

In the pediatric population, physicians must have a high degree of suspicion for IBD. Making the diagnosis of CD is a multidisciplinary endeavor, and there is no single test that can definitively diagnose CD [70]. Because CD involves diffuse inflammation of the gastrointestinal tract, some serum markers of inflammation can help support the diagnosis. C-reactive protein is an acute phase protein with a short half-life that is a marker for acute inflammation; an elevated c-reactive protein is commonly seen in CD [72]. Other markers of inflammation include erythrocyte sedimentation rate, white blood cell count, platelet count, and fecal leukocyte analysis. All of the above are nonspecific markers of inflammation, and there is no one laboratory test to diagnose CD.

Because CD may affect any part of the gastrointestinal tract, it is important to study the length of the intestinal tract to aid in a diagnosis. CD typically appears as a patchy, segmental inflammatory process. Endoscopy may illustrate involvement of the upper gastrointestinal tract; the presence of apthous ulcers or granulomas is diagnostic. Colonoscopy into the terminal ileum with multiple biopsies allows determination of the extent of disease and obtains a tissue diagnosis [70]. Histologic examination may reveal segmental disease with transmural lymphoid aggregates or granulomas. There may also be evidence of fissures, sinuses, or fistulas [73].

The most common area of involvement is the terminal ileum and right colon, with up to half of the patients also having gastroduodenal involvement. Most patients who have CD have ileocecal involvement [69]. Other modalities to assess the extent of bowel involved include capsule endoscopy, small bowel barium studies, MRI, ultrasound, or technetium-labeled scintigraphy to detect inflammation [70].

Medical treatment

Many treatments are used in pediatric patients who have CD; unfortunately, much of the pediatric management is based on adult management, and has not been extensively tested in children. Management must be multidisciplinary, because there are nutritional and psychological issues involved in the treatment of CD [70]. Because growth failure is a common presentation for the pediatric Crohn's patient, nutrition must be addressed with all Crohn's patients. When treating CD using medical therapies, it is important to distinguish between the treatment of active disease and maintenance of remission. With active disease there is the further separation of mild-to-moderate disease versus severe disease [74].

Active disease

With mild-to-moderate active disease, steroids are the first line of therapy to attempt to induce remission in the adult population, although there is an effort to avoid steroids in children. Oral prednisone or budesonide may be used and then weaned as the patient enters remission [70]. Budesonide is a controlled-release steroid, and is used for patients who have involvement of the terminal ileum and right colon [74]. In an effort to mitigate the potential side effects of steroids on the pediatric patient's growth, vitamin D and Calcium should be given with the steroids. Intravenous steroids should be used for patients who have severe pancolitis [70].

In adults, 5-aminosalicylates (sulphasalazine, mesalasine, and the like) may be used as a monotherapy for active disease, but children usually have a more severe form of the disease and are usually treated with 5-aminosalicylates as an adjunct to steroids. In an effort to avoid steroids in children, exclusive enteral nutrition (EEN) has recently been used to induce remission. EEN is a solution of whole protein given as the sole source for nutrition for 6 to 8 weeks; food is then re-introduced slowly [70]. The aminosalycylates may be used in conjunction with EEN.

Some patients will not respond to the above therapies, and other methods of immunosuppression must be considered. Infliximab is a monoclonal antibody against TNF-alpha that may be used for active intestinal disease or for fistulizing anal disease. It is an intravenous therapy that often must be repeated [70,74]. Other second-line therapies include methotrexate, cyclosporine, and tacrolimus.

Disease in remission

Once remission has been achieved, 6-mercaptopurine can be effective as maintenance therapy to reduce the incidence of relapse and to wean patients off the steroids. Children must be closely followed because 6-mercaptopurine may cause bone marrow suppression or pancreatitis [70].

Many studies have examined the utility of using antibiotics in patients who have CD. Broad-spectrum antibiotics should be used in patients who have fulminant CD or in toxic patients who have fever. Some benefit has also been found with long-term metronidazole in patients who have chronic perianal disease [70].

Surgical therapy

There is no surgical cure for CD. In fact, the rate of recurrence after bowel resection requiring a second operation is 24% [75,76]. Despite this fact, approximately 58% to 92% of patients who have CD will require surgery, depending on the location of the disease [77].

The indications for surgical therapy in patients who have CD are failure of medical therapy or complications of the disease. Medical therapy can be considered a failure not only if the disease persists, but also if there is non-compliance or if unacceptable complications of immunosuppression occur, such as failure to thrive or delayed puberty. Complications of the disease include hemorrhage, perforation, symptomatic fistula formation, abscess, or bowel obstruction.

Stricture

The majority of patients who require surgical therapy for CD have an isolated stricture in the terminal ileum. These patients often undergo an ileocecectomy. Although gross inflammation at the resection margin does increase the chance of recurrence, use of frozen sections to achieve microscopic disease-free margins does not improve recurrence rates [78–80]. Therefore, resection should include all gross disease, but wide resection margins are not advocated.

Although the standard therapy for small bowel stricture has been segmental resection, strictureplasty has gained popularity in patients who have multiple strictures to preserve bowel length. Some even advocate strictureplasty in patients who have single-segment disease. Sampietro and colleagues [81] reported that strictureplasty may yield equal if not better outcomes than resection. These patients did not have a higher recurrence rate than patients who undergo resection.

Laparoscopy in the treatment of CD has been adapted by many surgeons in the last decade. Recent reports suggest that laparoscopic bowel resection in adolescents may lead to a shorter length of stay and decreased postoperative narcotic use [82–84]. Although not exclusively studied in children, other studies have suggested improved postoperative pulmonary function, reduction in duration of postoperative ileus, decrease in hospital costs, and a decrease in surgical morbidity [85–87].

Hemorrhage

Uncontrollable bleeding from inflamed small bowel poses a challenge to the surgeon, because localization of the bleeding site can be difficult. In patients who have an isolated segment of disease, the decision of which segment to resect may be straightforward; however, in patients who have skip lesions, identification of the bleeding segment may be difficult. Preoperative localization is critical. Although push enteroscopy and barium enteroclysis have been the standard localization techniques for small bowel bleeding, capsule endoscopy has recently become recognized as the most sensitive diagnostic and localization technique [88]. If the site of bleeding is not obvious at exploration, intraoperative enteroscopy may aid in identifying the bleeding segment. In combination with preoperative localization by capsule endoscopy, laparoscopic resection has been successfully used [89].

Intra-abdominal abscess

There are three general treatment options for intra-abdominal or pelvic abscesses in CD: medical therapy, percutaneous drainage, or surgical drainage. Although abscess drainage has shown superior results to medical therapy, approximately 50% of patients can be successfully treated with medical therapy alone [90]; however, patients who are drained earlier have a better outcome, so a decision to drain should be made early. Equal outcomes are reported between percutaneous versus surgical drainage. Most of these studies agree, however, that abdominal abscesses with associated fistulas are more successfully treated with surgical drainage [91–93]. A staged approach is occasionally indicated, in which a drainage procedure is performed at presentation of the intra-abdominal abscess, following which resection is performed for either persistent symptomatic disease or for entero-cutaneous fistula formation.

Perianal disease

The management of perianal disease in CD is challenging. Almost 40% of patients who have CD have perianal disease [94]. Perianal disease consists of fistulas and abscesses, both of which have a high recurrence rate following treatment. Fistulas are typically managed initially with medical therapy consisting of antibiotics, steroids, and 5-ASA. More recently, anti-TNF antibody, (infliximab), has shown promise as a primary or adjunct therapy for perianal fistulas in CD. Many studies show promising results with infliximab, especially when combined with surgical therapy [95–98]; however, most studies have demonstrated that infliximab has not supplanted surgical therapy [94,99]. Surgical therapy for perianal fistulas includes abscess drainage and or fistulotomy.

Perirectal abscesses should be drained surgically if there is no response to antibiotics. Most abscesses have an associated fistula. The management of the associated fistula depends on the depth of invasion through the sphincter muscles. If a simple fistulotomy would involve cutting greater than 30% of the sphincter complex, a seton should be placed. Otherwise, abscess drainage with fistulotomy is appropriate. The fistula tract should be debrided to reduce the chance of recurrence, although management of perirectal fistulae can be a chronically vexing problem.

References

[1] Cohen M, Seldman E, Winter H, et al. Controversies in pediatric inflammatory bowel disease. Inflamm Bowel Dis 1998;4:203–27.

[2] Mamula P, Markowitz JE, Baldassano RN. Inflammatory bowel disease in early childhood and adolescence: special considerations. Gastroenterol Clin North Am 2003;32(3):967–95.

[3] Fiocchi C. Inflammatory bowel disease: etiology and pathogenesis. Gastroenterology 1998;(115):182–205.

[4] Logan R. Inflammatory bowel disease incidence: up, down or unchanged? Gut 1998;42: 309–11.

[5] Yang E, Johnson S, Ziegler M. Inflammatory bowel disease and intestinal cancer. In: Ashcraft K, Holcomb G, Murphy J, editors. Pediatric surgery. Philadelphia: Elsevier Saunders; 2005.

[6] Tysk C, Lindberg E, Jarnerot G, et al. Ulcerative colitis and Crohn's disease in an unselected population of monozygotic and dizygotic twins. A study of heritability and the influence of smoking. Gut 1988;29:990–6, p. 558–76.

[7] Gilat T, Hacohen D, Lilos P, et al. Childhood factors in ulcerative colitis and Crohn's disease: an international cooperative study. Scand J Gastroenterol 1987;22:1009–24.

[8] Roth M, Petersen G, McElree C, et al. Geographic origins of Jewish patients with inflammatory bowel disease. Gastroenterology 1989;97:900–4.

[9] Hugot J, Chamaillard M, Zouali H, et al. Association of NOD2 leucine-rich repeat variants with susceptibility to Crohn's disease. Nature 2001;411(6837):599–603.

[10] Duerr RH, Taylor KD, Brant SR, et al. A genome-wide association study identifies IL23R as an inflammatory bowel disease gene. Science 2006;314(5804):1461–3.

[11] Bernstein CN, Rawsthorne P, Cheang M, et al. A population-based case control study of potential risk factors for IBD. Am J Gastroenterol 2006;101(5):993–1002.

[12] Danese S, Sans M, Fiocchi C. Inflammatory bowel disease: the role of environmental factors. Autoimmun Rev 2004;3(5):394–400.

[13] Koutroubakis I, Manousos ON, Meuwissen SG, et al. Environmental risk factors in inflammatory bowel disease. Hepatogastroenterology 1996;43(8):381–93.

[14] Kugathasan S, Judd R, Khan F, et al. Epidemiologic and clinical characteristics of newly diagnosed inflammatory bowel disease in children in the state of Wisconsin: results of a prospective state wide population based study. J Pediatr Gastroenterol Nutr 2002;35:A421.

[15] Farmer R, Easley K, Rankin G. Clinical patterns, natural history, and progression of ulcerative colitis. A long-term follow-up of 1116 patients. Dig Dis Sci 1993;38:1137–46.

[16] Mir-Madjlessi S, Michener W, Farmer R. Course and prognosis of idiopathic ulcerative proctosigmoiditis in young patients. J Pediatr Gastroenterol Nutr 1986;5:571–5.

[17] Baldassano R, Piccoli D. Inflammatory bowel disease in pediatric and adolescent patients. Gastroenterol Clin North Am 1999;28:445–58.

[18] Fish D, Kugathasan S. Inflammatory bowel disease. Adolesc Med Clin 2004;15(1):67–90.

[19] Ruemmele FM, Targan SR, Levy G, et al. Diagnostic accuracy of serological assays in pediatric inflammatory bowel disease. Gastroenterology 1998;115(4):822–9.

[20] Kane SV, Cohen RD, Aikens JE, et al. Prevalence of nonadherence with maintenance mesalamine in quiescent ulcerative colitis. Am J Gastroenterol 2001;96(10):2929–33.

[21] Faubion WA Jr, Loftus EV Jr, Harmsen WS, et al. The natural history of corticosteroid therapy for inflammatory bowel disease: a population-based study. Gastroenterology 2001; 121(2):255–60.

[22] Lichtiger S, Present DH, Kornbluth A, et al. Cyclosporine in severe ulcerative colitis refractory to steroid therapy. N Engl J Med 1994;330(26):1841–5.

[23] Jani N, Regueiro MD. Medical therapy for ulcerative colitis. Gastroenterol Clin North Am 2002;31(1):147–66.

[24] Friedman S. General principles of medical therapy of inflammatory bowel disease. Gastroenterol Clin North Am 2004;33(2):191–208, viii.

[25] Garcia-Lopez S, Gomollon-Garcia F, Perez-Gisbert J. Cyclosporine in the treatment of severe attack of ulcerative colitis: a systematic review. Gastroenterol Hepatol 2005;28(10): 607–14.

[26] Buchmiller-Crair T. Ulcerative colitis. In: Oldham K, et al, editors. Principles and practice of pediatric surgery. Philadelphia: Lippincott, Williams & Wilkins; 2005. p. 1365–80.

[27] Hanauer SB. New lessons: classic treatments, expanding options in ulcerative colitis. Colorectal Dis 2006;8(Suppl 1):20–4.

[28] Kane S, Huo D, Aikens J, Hanauer S. Medication nonadherence and the outcomes of patients with quiescent ulcerative colitis. Am J Med 2003;114(1):39–43.

[29] George J, Present DH, Pou R, et al. The long-term outcome of ulcerative colitis treated with 6-mercaptopurine. Am J Gastroenterol 1996;91(9):1711–4.

[30] Mantzaris GJ, Sfakianakis M, Archavlis E, et al. A prospective randomized observer-blind 2-year trial of azathioprine monotherapy versus azathioprine and olsalazine for the maintenance of remission of steroid-dependent ulcerative colitis. Am J Gastroenterol 2004;99(6): 1122–8.

[31] Sandborn WJ. Azathioprine: state of the art in inflammatory bowel disease. Scand J Gastroenterol Suppl 1998;225:92–9.

[32] Hibi T, Naganuma M, Kitahora T, et al. Low-dose azathioprine is effective and safe for maintenance of remission in patients with ulcerative colitis. J Gastroenterol 2003;38(8): 740–6.

[33] Bousvaros A, Kirschner BS, Werlin SL, et al. Oral tacrolimus treatment of severe colitis in children. J Pediatr 2000;137(6):794–9.

[34] Sands BE, Tremaine WJ, Sandborn WJ, et al. Infliximab in the treatment of severe, steroid-refractory ulcerative colitis: a pilot study. Inflamm Bowel Dis 2001;7(2):83–8.

[35] Kaser A, Mairinger T, Vogel W, et al. Infliximab in severe steroid-refractory ulcerative colitis: a pilot study. Wien Klin Wochenschr 2001;113(23–24):930–3.

[36] Chey WY, Hussain A, Ryan C, et al. Infliximab for refractory ulcerative colitis. Am J Gastroenterol 2001;96(8):2373–81.

[37] Chang JC, Cohen RD. Medical management of severe ulcerative colitis. Gastroenterol Clin North Am 2004;33(2):235–50, viii.

[38] Sher ME, Weiss EG, Nogueras JJ, et al. Morbidity of medical therapy for ulcerative colitis: what are we really saving? Int J Colorectal Dis 1996;11(6):287–93.

[39] Befrits R, Hammarberg C, Rubio C, et al. DNA aneuploidy and histologic dysplasia in long-standing ulcerative colitis. A 10-year follow-up study. Dis Colon Rectum 1994;37(4):313–9 [discussion: 319–20].

[40] Devroede GJ, Taylor WF, Sauer WG, et al. Cancer risk and life expectancy of children with ulcerative colitis. N Engl J Med 1971;285(1):17–21.

[41] McNevin MS, Bax T, MacFarlane M, et al. Outcomes of a laparoscopic approach for total abdominal colectomy and proctocolectomy. Am J Surg 2006;191(5):673–6.

[42] Marcello PW, Milsom JW, Wong SK, et al. Laparoscopic restorative proctocolectomy: case-matched comparative study with open restorative proctocolectomy. Dis Colon Rectum 2000;43(5):604–8.

[43] Bernstein CN. Neoplasia in inflammatory bowel disease: surveillance and management strategies. Curr Gastroenterol Rep 2006;8(6):513–8.

[44] Chambers WH, Warren BF, Jewell DP, et al. Cancer surveillance in ulcerative colitis. Br J Surg 2005;92(8):928–36.

[45] Khorrami Mashhadi S, Trapero M, Gisbert JP, et al. A pilot study on the endoscopic surveillance of colorectal dysplasia and cancer in long-standing ulcerative colitis. Rev Esp Enferm Dig 2005;97(1):16–23.

[46] Rutter MD, Saunders BP, Wilkinson KH, et al. Cancer surveillance in longstanding ulcerative colitis: endoscopic appearances help predict cancer risk. Gut 2004;53(12):1813–6.

[47] Kiesslich R, Neurath MF. Chromoendoscopy and other novel imaging techniques. Gastroenterol Clin North Am 2006;35(3):605–19.

[48] Jimmo B, Hyman NH. Is ileal pouch-anal anastomosis really the procedure of choice for patients with ulcerative colitis? Dis Colon Rectum 1998;41(1):41–5.

[49] Lichtenstein GR, Cohen R, Yamashita B, et al. Quality of life after proctocolectomy with ileoanal anastomosis for patients with ulcerative colitis. J Clin Gastroenterol 2006;40(8): 669–77.

[50] Nicholls RJ, Holt SD, Lubowski DZ. Restorative proctocolectomy with ileal reservoir. Comparison of two-stage vs. three-stage procedures and analysis of factors that might affect outcome. Dis Colon Rectum 1989;32(4):323–6.

[51] Rintala RJ, Lindahl H. Restorative proctocolectomy for ulcerative colitis in children—is the J-pouch better than straight pull-through? J Pediatr Surg 1996;31(4):530–3.

[52] Taylor BM, Beart RW Jr, Dozois RR, et al. Straight ileoanal anastomosis v ileal pouch— anal anastomosis after colectomy and mucosal proctectomy. Arch Surg 1983;118(6): 696–701.

[53] Stoller DK, Coran AG, Drongowski RA, et al. Physiologic assessment of the four commonly performed endorectal pullthroughs. Ann Surg 1987;206(5):586–94.

[54] Tonelli F, Batignani G, Ficari F, et al. Straight ileoanal anastomosis with multiple ileal myotomies as an alternative to pelvic pouch. Int J Colorectal Dis 1997;12(5):261–6.

[55] Landi E, Landa L, Fianchini A, et al. Straight ileo-anal anastomosis with myectomy as an alternative to ileal pouch-anal anastomosis in restorative proctocolectomy. Int J Colorectal Dis 1994;9(1):45–9.

[56] Umehara Y, Kudo M, Nakaoka R, et al. Serum proinflammatory cytokines and adhesion molecules in ulcerative colitis. Hepatogastroenterology 2006;53(72):879–82.

[57] Ambrosini R, Barchiesi A, Di Mizio V, et al. Inflammatory chronic disease of the colon: how to image. Eur J Radiol 2006;61(3):442–8.

[58] Haykir R, Karakose S, Karabacakoglu A, et al. Three-dimensional MR and axial CT colonography versus conventional colonoscopy for detection of colon pathologies. World J Gastroenterol 2006;12(15):2345–50.

[59] Mackalski BA, Bernstein CN. New diagnostic imaging tools for inflammatory bowel disease. Gut 2006;55(5):733–41.

[60] Leighton JA, Loftus EV Jr. Evolving diagnostic modalities in inflammatory bowel disease. Curr Gastroenterol Rep 2005;7(6):467–74.

[61] Su C, Salzberg BA, Lewis JD, et al. Efficacy of anti-tumor necrosis factor therapy in patients with ulcerative colitis. Am J Gastroenterol 2002;97(10):2577–84.

[62] Sanders DS. Mucosal integrity and barrier function in the pathogenesis of early lesions in Crohn's disease. J Clin Pathol 2005;58(6):568–72.

[63] Hanauer SB. Inflammatory bowel disease: epidemiology, pathogenesis, and therapeutic opportunities. Inflamm Bowel Dis 2006;12(Suppl 1):S3–9.

[64] Abraham C, Cho JH. Functional consequences of NOD2 (CARD15) mutations. Inflamm Bowel Dis 2006;12(7):641–50.

[65] Curran ME, Lau KF, Hampe J, et al. Genetic analysis of inflammatory bowel disease in a large European cohort supports linkage to chromosomes 12 and 16. Gastroenterology 1998;115(5):1066–71.

[66] Hampe J, Grebe J, Nikolaus S, et al. Association of NOD2 (CARD 15) genotype with clinical course of Crohn's disease: a cohort study. Lancet 2002;359(9318):1661–5.

[67] Newman B, Siminovitch KA. Recent advances in the genetics of inflammatory bowel disease. Curr Opin Gastroenterol 2005;21(4):401–7.

[68] Hampe J, Cuthbert A, Croucher PJ, et al. Association between insertion mutation in NOD2 gene and Crohn's disease in German and British populations. Lancet 2001;357(9272): 1925–8.

[69] Sawczenko A, Sandhu BK. Presenting features of inflammatory bowel disease in Great Britain and Ireland. Arch Dis Child 2003;88(11):995–1000.

[70] Beattie RM, Croft NM, Fell JM, et al. Inflammatory bowel disease. Arch Dis Child 2006; 91(5):426–32.

[71] Caprilli R, Gassull MA, Escher JC, et al. European evidence based consensus on the diagnosis and management of Crohn's disease: special situations. Gut 2006;55(Suppl 1):i36–58.

[72] Vermeire S, Van Assche G, Rutgeerts P. Laboratory markers in IBD: useful, magic, or unnecessary toys? Gut 2006;55(3):426–31.

[73] Yantiss RK, Odze RD. Diagnostic difficulties in inflammatory bowel disease pathology. Histopathology 2006;48(2):116–32.

[74] Egan LJ, Sandborn WJ. Advances in the treatment of Crohn's disease. Gastroenterology 2004;126(6):1574–81.

[75] Lowney JK, Dietz DW, Birnbaum EH, et al. Is there any difference in recurrence rates in laparoscopic ileocolic resection for Crohn's disease compared with conventional surgery? A long-term, follow-up study. Dis Colon Rectum 2006;49(1):58–63.

[76] Fichera A, McCormack R, Rubin MA, et al. Long-term outcome of surgically treated Crohn's colitis: a prospective study. Dis Colon Rectum 2005;48(5):963–9.

[77] Farmer RG, Whelan G, Fazio VW. Long-term follow-up of patients with Crohn's disease. Relationship between the clinical pattern and prognosis. Gastroenterology 1985;88(6):1818–25.

[78] Kotanagi H, Kramer K, Fazio VW, et al. Do microscopic abnormalities at resection margins correlate with increased anastomotic recurrence in Crohn's disease? Retrospective analysis of 100 cases. Dis Colon Rectum 1991;34(10):909–16.

[79] Heimann TM, Greenstein AJ, Lewis B, et al. Prediction of early symptomatic recurrence after intestinal resection in Crohn's disease. Ann Surg 1993;218(3):294–8 [discussion: 298–9].

[80] Pennington L, Hamilton SR, Bayless TM, et al. Surgical management of Crohn's disease. Influence of disease at margin of resection. Ann Surg 1980;192(3):311–8.

[81] Sampietro GM, Cristaldi M, Maconi G, et al. A prospective, longitudinal study of nonconventional strictureplasty in Crohn's disease. J Am Coll Surg 2004;199(1):8–20 [discussion: 20–2].

[82] Diamond IR, Langer JC. Laparoscopic-assisted versus open ileocolic resection for adolescent Crohn disease. J Pediatr Gastroenterol Nutr 2001;33(5):543–7.

[83] von Allmen D, Markowitz JE, York A, et al. Laparoscopic-assisted bowel resection offers advantages over open surgery for treatment of segmental Crohn's disease in children. J Pediatr Surg 2003;38(6):963–5.

[84] Bonnard A, Fouquet V, Berrebi D, et al. Crohn's disease in children. Preliminary experience with a laparoscopic approach. Eur J Pediatr Surg 2006;16(2):90–3.

[85] Bemelman WA, Slors JF, Dunker MS, et al. Laparoscopic-assisted vs. open ileocolic resection for Crohn's disease. A comparative study. Surg Endosc 2000;14(8):721–5.

[86] Young-Fadok TM, HallLong K, McConnell EJ, et al. Advantages of laparoscopic resection for ileocolic Crohn's disease. Improved outcomes and reduced costs. Surg Endosc 2001; 15(5):450–4.

[87] Milsom JW, Hammerhofer KA, Bohm B, et al. Prospective, randomized trial comparing laparoscopic vs. conventional surgery for refractory ileocolic Crohn's disease. Dis Colon Rectum 2001;44(1):1–8 [discussion: 8–9].

[88] Triester SL, Leighton JA, Leontiadis GI, et al. A meta-analysis of the yield of capsule endoscopy compared to other diagnostic modalities in patients with non-stricturing small bowel Crohn's disease. Am J Gastroenterol 2006;101(5):954–64.

[89] Kim J, Kim YS, Chun HJ, et al. Laparoscopy-assisted exploration of obscure gastrointestinal bleeding after capsule endoscopy: the Korean experience. J Laparoendosc Adv Surg Tech A 2005;15(4):365–73.

[90] Garcia JC, Persky SE, Bonis PA, et al. Abscesses in Crohn's disease: outcome of medical versus surgical treatment. J Clin Gastroenterol 2001;32(5):409–12.

[91] Ayuk P, Williams N, Scott NA, et al. Management of intra-abdominal abscesses in Crohn's disease. Ann R Coll Surg Engl 1996;78(1):5–10.

[92] Gutierrez A, Lee H, Sands BE. Outcome of surgical versus percutaneous drainage of abdominal and pelvic abscesses in Crohn's disease. Am J Gastroenterol 2006;101(10):2283–9.

[93] Sahai A, Belair M, Gianfelice D, et al. Percutaneous drainage of intra-abdominal abscesses in Crohn's disease: short and long-term outcome. Am J Gastroenterol 1997;92(2):275–8.

[94] Danelli P, Bartolucci C, Sampietro GM, et al. [Surgical options in the treatment of perianal Crohn's disease]. Ann Ital Chir 2003;74(6):635–40.

[95] Hyder SA, Travis SP, Jewell DP, et al. Fistulating anal Crohn's disease: results of combined surgical and infliximab treatment. Dis Colon Rectum 2006;49(12):1837–41.

[96] Asteria CR, Ficari F, Bagnoli S, et al. Treatment of perianal fistulas in Crohn's disease by local injection of antibody to TNF-alpha accounts for a favourable clinical response in selected cases: a pilot study. Scand J Gastroenterol 2006;41(9):1064–72.

[97] Regueiro M, Mardini H. Treatment of perianal fistulizing Crohn's disease with infliximab alone or as an adjunct to exam under anesthesia with seton placement. Inflamm Bowel Dis 2003;9(2):98–103.

[98] Osterman MT, Lichtenstein GR. Infliximab in fistulizing Crohn's disease. Gastroenterol Clin North Am 2006;35(4):795–820.

[99] Poritz LS, Rowe WA, Koltun WA. Remicade does not abolish the need for surgery in fistulizing Crohn's disease. Dis Colon Rectum 2002;45(6):771–5.

SURGICAL
CLINICS OF
NORTH AMERICA

ELSEVIER
SAUNDERS

Surg Clin N Am 87 (2007) 659–672

Associated Neoplastic Disease in Inflammatory Bowel Disease

Juan C. Cendan, MD, Kevin E. Behrns, MD*

*Department of Surgery, Division of General and GI Surgery, University of Florida,
1600 SW Archer Road, P.O. Box 100286, Gainesville, FL 32610, USA*

Since 1925 when Crohn and Rosenberg [1] discovered colon cancer in a patient who had ulcerative colitis (UC), the development of intestinal carcinoma in the setting of inflammatory bowel disease (IBD) has been recognized as an unsavory outcome of chronic inflammation of the bowel. Similar to sporadic colon cancer, which is associated with a well-known adenoma-to-carcinoma sequence, intestinal cancer developing in the setting of inflammatory bowel disease arises through an inflammation-to-dysplasia-to carcinoma sequence that can be longitudinally assessed in this patient population [2]. Because this patient population can be followed endoscopically over time, numerous studies have recently documented the clinical and morphologic features of malignant transformation in this closely-followed group of patients [3,4]. This article highlights the recent findings of these population-based studies with specific attention to surgical concepts and frames these data in the context of surgical approaches to cancer arising in inflammatory disease. Specifically, the authors address the pathobiology of malignant transformation, the management of colorectal cancer in inflammatory bowel disease, the development of dysplasia in UC, surveillance of patients who have IBD, chemoprevention of cancer, and special features of surgical oncologic management.

Chronic inflammatory states and cancer

Virchow hypothesized in 1863 that malignant neoplasms occurred at sites of chronic inflammation. There are numerous clinical conditions that provide support for that observation. For example, the North American

---

* Corresponding author.
  E-mail address: kevin.behrns@surgery.ufl.edu (K.E. Behrns).

0039-6109/07/$ - see front matter © 2007 Elsevier Inc. All rights reserved.
doi:10.1016/j.suc.2007.03.010 *surgical.theclinics.com*

Pima Indians have an elevated risk for gallbladder cancer, which directly correlates with the increased prevalence of cholecystitis, cholelithiasis, and obesity in this population. The cumulative risk for gallbladder cancer in patients who have cholecystitis after 20 years is about 1%, representing a threefold increase in risk compared with those who do not have a history of cholecystitis. Furthermore, the risk for gallbladder cancer increases with size and duration of gallstones and calcification in the mucosal epithelium (porcelain gallbladder).

Similarly, chronic inflammation from *Helicobacter pylori* infection increases the risk for gastric cancer. *H pylori* has been identified as a major cause of atrophic gastritis, mucosal ulcers of the stomach and duodenum, and, most importantly, a twofold relative risk for gastric adenocarcinoma [5]. This Gram-negative bacterium colonizes the luminal surface of the stomach and survives the acid environment by penetrating the mucous layer.

As a final example, the risk for cancer among individuals who have Barrett esophagus seems to be also elevated [6]. Most studies report a relative risk for esophageal cancer that is 40 to 125 times higher in patients who have Barrett's esophagus than that of the general population. Estimates of the absolute risk for esophageal adenocarcinoma in the setting of Barrett's esophagus vary from 0% to almost 3% per patient-year. A meta-analysis of these data suggests that a reasonable estimate of absolute risk is approximately 0.5% per patient-year [7].

The cytokine milieu in these inflammatory-cancer conditions revealed seems to be altered. In Barrett's esophagus, specifically, there is a relative increase in the T-helper type II cytokines, interleukin-4 and -10, in the affected mucosa compared with normal esophagus [8]. In the case of gastric cancer and *H pylori*, metaplasia and neoplastic transformation occur alongside an inflammatory reaction by producing chemotactic factors that attract neutrophils, mononuclear cells, and proinflammatory cytokines [5].

Pathobiology of intestinal cancer in inflammatory bowel disease

The development of carcinoma is a potential outcome of chronic inflammation of multiple alimentary tract organs, including the gut [9], esophagus [10], liver [11], and pancreas [12]. The underlying molecular and cellular events that govern this malignant transformation therefore likely have common features. Several studies have demonstrated that chronic inflammation increases intracellular reactive oxygen species, which lead to alterations in cellular signaling with up-regulation of signaling pathways that promote cellular proliferation and, potentially, aberrant growth [9–12]. The progression from chronic inflammation to dysplasia with the ultimate development of intestinal carcinoma is a well-recognized cellular transition in IBD [2]. In IBD, nearly all (>90%) cancers arise through this sequence of events, and therefore the recognition of dysplasia is a critical observation in the management of these patients [2].

Dysplasia in inflammatory bowel disease

Dysplasia arising in IBD may be grossly undetectable or endoscopically visible as flat lesions or as mass lesions called dysplasia-associated lesion or mass (DALM) [13]. Dysplasia in flat lesions is often undetectable because it arises in normal-appearing mucosa, and thus the diagnosis of dysplasia in this setting depends on biopsy specimens. The current recommendations for biopsy specimens suggest that two to four biopsies are obtained every 10 cm in the bowel [13]. Rigorous biopsy programs have identified that 33 biopsy specimens result in detection of 90% of dysplastic lesions with 64 biopsies required for a 95% probability of detecting dysplasia [14]. The recent introduction of chromoendoscopy (methylene blue-aided) has also been shown to increase by 300% the detection of dysplastic lesions that are not grossly visible endoscopically [15].

Generally, the histopathology of dysplasia in IBD includes regenerative features in chronic inflammation followed by a transition to morphologic features that are negative for dysplasia, indefinite for dysplasia, and subsequently progress to low-grade and finally high-grade dysplasia. It is important to recognize, however, that not all carcinomas arise from direct progression through this sequence and that some carcinomas arise out of lesions with few histologic characteristics of even low-grade dysplasia [13]. In addition, the histologic diagnosis of the various forms of dysplasia is difficult, and agreement of dysplastic findings in biopsy specimens may vary significantly among pathologists. As a result, additional histologic immunostains, such as alpha-methylacyl-CoA racemase, which is evident in 96% and 80% of low- and high-grade dysplastic lesions, respectively, may significantly enhance the diagnosis of dysplasia in IBD [16].

The significance of undetectable or endoscopically visible dysplasia in IBD is controversial. The bulk of evidence suggests that the finding of low-grade dysplasia leads to progression to high-grade dysplasia or carcinoma. The probability of finding high-grade dysplasia or carcinoma after an initial diagnosis of low-grade dysplasia is 16% to 29% [17]. Furthermore, other investigators have found that the likelihood of progressing from low-grade dysplasia to high-grade dysplasia or cancer is 54% at 5 years [18]. Similarly, other studies have demonstrated that this high rate of progression is plausible given that Mount Sinai and the Mayo Clinic reported rates of progression of 53% and 33%, respectively [19,20]. Although these results strongly argue that the identification of low-grade dysplasia is an indication for colectomy, two studies have reported progression rates of 0% from Sweden [21] and 10% from the United Kingdom [22]. In addition, DALM and polypoid lesions are not necessarily associated with the development of cancer, and two studies have shown that these lesions can be followed for up to 4 years without malignant transformation [23,24]. Because the preponderance of evidence suggests that the finding of low-grade dysplasia is associated with progression to high-grade dysplasia or carcinoma, colectomy is strongly encouraged for these early lesions that should be cured by surgical resection.

Intestinal cancer in inflammatory bowel disease

Ulcerative colitis

The cherished dogma that colorectal cancer is a nearly inevitable result of long-standing UC has recently been challenged. In the early 1970s, some reports suggested that 60% of patients would develop colorectal cancer over a duration of 40 years [25]. More recent evidence suggest that the risk is much lower, however, and in fact some studies suggest that the overall survival of patients who have UC is improved compared with the general population [26,27].

A recent meta-analysis by Eaden et al [3] provides absolute risk data from more than 54,000 patients that were published in 116 different studies (Table 1). Although this large number of patients provides a "big-picture"–type analysis, the types and quality of the publications included in this meta-analysis vary markedly, and thus the results should be interpreted with caution. Nonetheless, they found that the prevalence of colorectal cancer in UC was 3.7% and the incidence was 0.3%, or one cancer in every 333 patients. The cumulative probability (likelihood of cancer developing over time) was 8.3% at 20 years and 18.4% at 30 years. Several other contemporary publications noted a lower annual incidence ranging from 0.06% to 0.16% [28–32]. These data suggest that the overall incidence of colorectal cancer is

Table 1
Comparison of dysplasia and colorectal cancer risk in patients who have inflammatory bowel diseases

Disease	Author	Relative risk and 95% CI
Ulcerative colitis	Winther et al 2004 [31]	1.05 (0.6–1.8)
	Jess et al 2006 [29]	1.1 (0.4–2.4)
	Palli et al 2000 [28]	1.79 (0.9–3.3)
	Bernstein et al 2001 [30]–in rectal involvement	1.9 (1.0–3.4)
	Bernstein et al 2001 [30]–in colonic involvement	2.75 (1.9–4.0)
Crohn's	Gyde et al 1980 [49]	23.8 in Crohn's colitis 4.3 in general Crohn's population
	Greenstein et al 1981 [52]	6.9
	Ekbom et al 1990 [50]	5.6 (2.1–12.2) in Crohn's colitis 3.2 (0.7–9.2) in ileitis population
	Canavan et al 2006 [54] (meta-analysis)	2.5 (1.3–4.7) in all Crohn's population 4.5 (1.3–14.9) in Crohn's colitis population

decreased as compared with decades earlier. The reasons for a decreased risk are not readily apparent but may include factors such as improved surveillance for colorectal cancer, aggressive and earlier medical treatment of UC, chemoprevention of colorectal cancer in UC, and an aggressive surgical approach to patients who have UC.

Although the overall risk for developing colorectal cancer in UC may be decreasing, several risk factors are associated with the development of carcinoma (Table 2). These risk factors include the duration of IBD, the extent of inflammation, the severity of inflammation, the presence of primary sclerosing cholangitis, a family history of colorectal cancer, age at the time of diagnosis, and backwash ileitis [33]. The association of colorectal cancer with the duration of disease has been demonstrated in multiple studies, and some evidence suggests that duration of the disease beyond 30 years results in a significant increase in the risk for colorectal cancer [34]. This finding has prompted the argument for more frequent colonoscopic surveillance, but other studies have not documented a marked increased in risk past 30 years [35]. The extent of IBD is a well-known cancer risk factor

Table 2
Risk factors for dysplasia and colorectal cancer in patients who have ulcerative colitis

Strength of evidence	Factor	Observed effect
Established	Duration of disease	Annual incidence of CRC increases from 0.1%–0.2% in 1st decade of UC to 1.2%–1.3% in 3rd decade of UC
	Extent of disease	Proctitis alone increases CRC risk slightly, left colon disease increases CRC risk 2.8-fold, and pancolitis increases risk 14-fold
Highly suggestive	Sclerosing cholangitis	At 20 years, CRC in 31% of patients who have UC + PSC; CRC in 5% of patients who have UC-PSC
	Family history of sporadic CRC	Twice the risk for patients without a family history of sporadic CRC
	Severity of disease	Histologic and gross markers of inflammation correlate with increase CRC risk. Exact risk not as clear
	Young age at presentation	Younger age at UC diagnosis increases risk for dysplasia and CRC. Exact risk not as clear

Abbreviations: CRC, colorectal cancer; PSC, primary sclerosing cholangitis.

for IBD patients who have pancolitis, and is associated with a cancer risk 14 times higher than expected, whereas left-sided colitis increases the risk 2.8 times and proctitis alone carries a risk of 0.7 [4]. A recent study by Rutter and colleagues [36] found that endoscopic and histologic scoring of the severity of UC was associated with an odds ratio of 4.7 for the development of colorectal cancer. Somewhat surprisingly, the mere presence of primary sclerosing cholangitis leads to an increased risk for colorectal cancer in UC. A Swedish study demonstrated that at 20 years 31% of patients who had IBD and primary sclerosing cholangitis developed cancer, whereas only 5% of patients who had UC alone developed neoplasia [37]. The mechanisms underlying the increased risk for colorectal cancer in patients who have primary sclerosing cholangitis are unknown. Additional risk factors include a family history of sporadic colon cancer, which is associated with a fourfold increased risk for colorectal cancer in IBD [38]. Young age at the onset of UC is also an independent risk factor for cancer development, although a specific discriminatory age has not been identified [33]. Finally, the presence of backwash ileitis may be associated with an increased risk for colorectal cancer. A single study showed that the presence of terminal ileal inflammation was associated with colorectal cancer in 29% of patients who had pancolitis, but only 9% of patients who had pancolitis without ileitis developed cancer [39].

Total proctocolectomy and restorative J-pouch

Given the totality of risk factors for UC developing into colorectal cancer, should the surgeon perform a hand-sewn or double-stapled technique in the performance of total proctocolectomy with J-pouch reconstruction? The surgeon is called on to perform a total colectomy with J-pouch reconstruction for the definitive treatment of UC. One issue that presents itself is the need for removal of the transitional zone because this may pose a future rectal cancer risk. The observation of this phenomenon is particularly well documented in patients who have familial adenomatous polyposis syndrome (FAP). Patients who have FAP who undergo total proctocolectomy with J-pouch reconstruction can develop polyps in the anastomotic region. In these patients a double-stapled technique (technically leaving the transition zone) leads to polyps in the transition zone more frequently (21 of 76) than in patients who have a hand-sewn (technically removing the transition zone) anastomosis (6 of 42) [40]. This difference translates to a 7-year risk for developing polyps at the anastomosis in these patients of 31% in double-stapled and 10% in hand-sewn reconstructions, respectively [41].

In patients who have UC, transition zone dysplasia develops in 8 of 178 postoperative patients between 4 and 123 months (mean 9 months) after surgery with careful follow-up. No association has been found with regard to gender, age, preoperative disease duration, or extent of colitis. There is a correlation between the development of dysplasia in the transition zone if the original specimen had dysplasia or colorectal cancer, however. No patient developed cancer in this study [42]; however, there are several case reports of transition zone–related cancers in the UC patients [43]. Taken together, FAP patients being at risk for developing polyps in the transition zone and patients who have UC developing dysplasia/colorectal cancer in the transition zone has led some authors to support complete mucosectomy in cases of UC with ileal pouch anal anastomosis (IPAA) reconstruction. Even with complete mucosectomy some cases of primary ileal cancer in the pouch are now documented in the literature. These are cases in which the cancer developed not in the transition zone, but within the J-pouch, suggesting an inflammatory process [44,45]. These findings support the need for continued vigilance of the pouch and transition zone even when a complete mucosectomy and hand-sewn reconstruction are performed.

Pouch function is frequently cited as equally critical and there are arguments for a functional advantage to the double-stapled technique. Several studies have documented that the double-stapled technique is safer with fewer leaks reported [46]. In fact, studies support that the double-stapled technique is safer and more anatomically functional [47]. A recent meta-analysis has failed to document a functional or manometrically evident advantage to one technique over the other, however [48]. The surgeon needs to discuss all of these issues with the patient to determine the best surgical option.

Crohn's disease

Colorectal cancer

Like patients who have UC, patients who have Crohn's disease (CD) are at increased risk for developing intestinal cancer either in the large or small bowel. In addition, some data suggest that these patients are at risk for lymphomas, leukemias, and carcinoid tumors. Patients who have CD most at risk are those who have colitis, whereas patients who have disease limited to the ileum probably have a low risk for intestinal cancer.

Hospital and population-based data indicate that patients who have Crohn's colitis have a standardized incidence or relative risk that ranges from 0.8 to 23.8, but most studies suggest that the risk is about five times greater than those patient in whom CD is not limited to the colon [29, 49–53]. A recent meta-analysis [54] also suggests that the relative risk for colorectal cancer in CD is 4.5 and further supports the concept that patients who have Crohn's colitis are at a substantially increased risk for developing colorectal cancer.

Patients who have CD undergoing surgery occasionally have dysplasia (2.3%) or even colorectal cancer (2.7%) in the specimen. These findings are not always evident in preoperative screening. Colorectal cancer and dysplasia are found more frequently in patients of advanced age (38 versus 30 years old), in cases of longer clinical duration (16 versus 10 years duration), and in cases of extensive involvement of the colon (90% extensive versus 59% limited extent) [55].

The risk factors for the development of colorectal cancer in CD are similar to those for patients who have UC [56]. These factors include young age at the onset of CD, the extent of disease, the duration of disease, and dysplasia in CD colitis. Other risk factors, however, are unique to patients who have CD and include the presence of colonic strictures, bypassed intestinal segments, and fistulas with cancer. These distinct risk factors, with special consideration to the surgical management, are discussed later. A table comparing the development of CRC and dysplasia between UC and Crohn's follows (see Table 1).

Prior intestinal bypass in Crohn's disease

Patients who have prior intestinal bypasses may be at risk for colorectal cancer. Although this operation is not performed frequently, patients who have had a prior segmental bypass for CD have an increased colorectal cancer risk. In theory, this is because of ongoing inflammation in an area that may not benefit from orally ingested medications. Practically, the situation is aggravated by the inaccessibility of bypassed segments using routine endoscopic techniques. Patients who have long-standing bypass segments may require CT enterography, or revision/takedown of bypassed segments [56].

Risk for cancer in strictures related to Crohn's disease

Patients who have CD-related strictures of the colon are at risk for colorectal cancer. Strictures of the colon develop in 4% to 16% of patients who have Crohn's colitis. Colonoscopy in this setting can be challenging because the stricture is difficult to traverse. Pediatric colonoscopes can improve the technical ability to complete the study. The risk for developing colorectal cancer is 10 times greater in strictured areas, as compared with areas without stricture. A review by Yamakazi identified 10 colorectal cancers related to strictures in a group of 980 patients who had 132 strictures [57]. In this light, 6.8% of patients who had stricture developed colorectal cancer compared with 0.7% of patients who did not have stricture.

Current evaluation of strictures in Crohn's disease

It has been standard practice to use small bowel follow-through in combination with CT scans to plan surgery in Crohn's disease with stricture. Currently we are combining standard radiographs with positron emission tomography (PET) or CT enterography. Starting 75 minutes before the scan the patient drinks intralumen bowel contrast (Volumen). Just before scan, 1 mg of IV glucagon is administered to paralyze the bowel for scanning. A bolus injection of intravenous contrast (such as Omnipaque350) is used and thin-section scans are obtained of the abdomen and pelvis. A single-phase (portal venous) acquisition is then used. The patient is administered 12.9 mCi of F-18 FDG and a combined PET/CT study of the abdomen and pelvis is performed to observe for sites of active inflammation. Fig. 1 shows an example of a patient who has terminal ileal stricture.

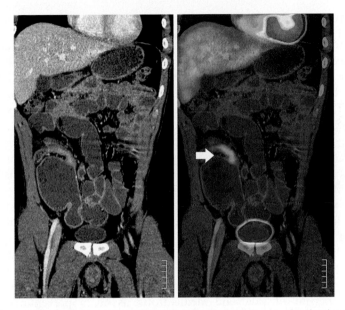

Fig. 1. Computerized tomography enterography of a Crohn's disease–related stricture with an associated area of active inflammation in the terminal ileum. The use of fluorodeoxyglucose (2-fluoro-2-deoxy-D-glucose) more commonly referred to as FDG (*green; arrow*) may assist with the diagnosis of active inflammation. A comparison of the CT and PET images allows precise definition of the location of the active inflammation highlighted by active uptake of F-18 FDG. (*Courtesy of* Walt Drane, MD, Gainesville, Florida.)

Small intestinal adenocarcinoma

Despite the rarity of adenocarcinoma of the small bowel, patients who have CD are at a substantially increased risk for developing this disease. Several studies document the large increased risk, but it is important to keep in mind that even though the risk is substantial the actual number of patients who have small bowel adenocarcinoma in CD is low. The adjusted incidence ratios for the risk for small intestinal adenocarcinoma range from 0 to 66.7, but the actual number of observed cases ranges from 0 to 5 [29,30,51,58–61]. Although the risk is high, the frequency of encountering small bowel carcinoma in CD is uncommon. Identifying risk factors for the development of small intestinal adenocarcinoma in CD is difficult because of the rarity of the disease. Potential risk factors include jejunal inflammation, chronic ileal inflammation, treatment with 6-mercaptopurine, and exposure to halogenated aromatic compounds [56].

In addition, some studies suggest that the risk for development of extra-intestinal cancers and carcinoids in CD is increased [56]. Lymphomas and leukemias are cited as malignancies that arise more frequently than in the general population. Although the data are not strong, close observation for lymphomas and leukemia is warranted because of the increasing use of immunomodulatory medical therapy for CD.

Chemoprevention

Chemoprevention to prevent the development of colorectal cancer in IBD has received significant attention in the last decade. Numerous medical therapies are used to stem the recurrence or halt the progression of IBD, and some of these therapies may be effective in reducing the risk for colorectal cancer. The agents that have been examined as antineoplastic medications include 5-aminosalicylates, nonsteroidal anti-inflammatory drugs, corticosteroids, immunomodulators, ursodeoxycholic acid, folate, calcium, and statins. Of these drugs, nonsteroidal anti-inflammatory drugs, immunomodulators, calcium, and statins have not been shown to decrease the risk significantly either because they are ineffective or because data are too sparse to warrant widespread use. Corticosteroids are associated with decreased risk, and the long-term toxicity of the medication outweighs the beneficial outcomes of chemoprevention.

Salicylate derivatives have been the best studied chemopreventative medications because they are generally well tolerated and not associated with significant toxicity. Several cohort and cross-sectional studies have examined the benefit of salicylate medications as chemopreventative agents over several years, but the most tightly controlled trial by Eaden and colleagues [62] demonstrated that patients who had UC who took regular 5-ASA medications for 5 to 10 years reduced the risk for colorectal cancer by 75%.

Patients who have UC and primary sclerosing cholangitis are at significantly increased risk for developing colorectal cancer, and this finding has prompted studies to determine the effectiveness of ursodeoxycholic acid (UCDA) for chemoprevention. Because the combination of these two diseases is uncommon, the studies performed include small numbers of patients. Two of three studies, however, demonstrated a protective effect of UDCA for the development of dysplasia or cancer [63].

Because patients who have IBD typically have low folate concentrations because of poor nutritional status and enhanced intestinal loss by way of inflamed bowel, supplementation with folate has been examined as a chemopreventative medication. Furthermore, previous studies have demonstrated that low folate concentrations are associated with the development of sporadic colorectal cancer. Of six trials performed, one has found that folate administration is associated with a decreased risk for dysplasia or cancer [63]. Although only a single study achieved statistical significance, many of the other reports showed trends that support the use of folate as a chemopreventative agent.

In addition to the above-mentioned chemopreventative agents, the use of infliximab, although costly, will undoubtedly be examined in the future as a chemopreventative medication. Other agents that may be worthy of examination include COX-2 inhibitors, antioxidants, thiazolidinediones, and short-chain fatty acids.

Surveillance for colorectal cancer in inflammatory bowel disease

A Cochrane Database review of strategies for detection of dysplasia and colorectal cancer in patients who have IBD failed to identify a clear benefit for surveillance in this patient group. Patients who had extensive colitis who underwent routine colonic surveillance did not have a survival advantage. There was evidence that cancers tended to be detected at an earlier stage in those patients who underwent routine surveillance. The authors reviewed indirect evidence that surveillance decreases the risk for death and an acceptable cost likely because of a lead-time bias improvement [64]. It is because of the lead-time issue that authors continue to implore surveillance [65].

References

[1] Crohn BB, Rosenberg H. The sigmoidoscopic picture of chronic ulcerative colitis. Am J Med Sci 1925;170:220–7.
[2] Itzkowitz SH, Harpaz N. Diagnosis and management of dysplasia in patients with inflammatory bowel diseases. Gastroenterology 2004;126(6):1634–48.
[3] Eaden JA, Abrams KR, Mayberry JF. The risk of colorectal cancer in ulcerative colitis: a meta-analysis. Gut 2001;48(4):526–35.
[4] Ekbom A, Helmick C, Zack M, et al. Ulcerative colitis and colorectal cancer. A population-based study. N Engl J Med 1990;323(18):1228–33.
[5] Schottenfeld D, Beebe-Dimmer J. Chronic inflammation: a common and important factor in the pathogenesis of neoplasia. CA Cancer J Clin 2006;56(2):69–83.
[6] Shaheen N, Ransohoff DF. Gastroesophageal reflux, Barrett esophagus, and esophageal cancer: clinical applications. JAMA 2002;287(15):1982–6.
[7] Shaheen NJ, Crosby MA, Bozymski EM, et al. Is there publication bias in the reporting of cancer risk in Barrett's esophagus? Gastroenterology 2000;119(2):333–8.
[8] Slehria S, Sharma P. Barrett esophagus. Curr Opin Gastroenterol 2003;19(4):387–93.
[9] Hwang JT, Kim YM, Surh YJ, et al. Selenium regulates cyclooxygenase-2 and extracellular signal-regulated kinase signaling pathways by activating AMP-activated protein kinase in colon cancer cells. Cancer Res 2006;66(20):10057–63.
[10] Farhadi A, Fields J, Banan A, et al. Reactive oxygen species: are they involved in the pathogenesis of GERD, Barrett's esophagus, and the latter's progression toward esophageal cancer? Am J Gastroenterol 2002;97(1):22–6.
[11] Black D, Bird MA, Samson CM, et al. Primary cirrhotic hepatocytes resist TGFbeta-induced apoptosis through a ROS-dependent mechanism. J Hepatol 2004;40(6):942–51.
[12] Weydert C, Roling B, Liu J, et al. Suppression of the malignant phenotype in human pancreatic cancer cells by the overexpression of manganese superoxide dismutase. Mol Cancer Ther 2003;2(4):361–9.
[13] Odze RD. Pathology of dysplasia and cancer in inflammatory bowel disease. Gastroenterol Clin North Am 2006;35(3):533–52.
[14] Rubin CE, Haggitt RC, Burmer GC, et al. DNA aneuploidy in colonic biopsies predicts future development of dysplasia in ulcerative colitis. Gastroenterology 1992;103(5):1611–20.
[15] Kiesslich R, Fritsch J, Holtmann M, et al. Methylene blue-aided chromoendoscopy for the detection of intraepithelial neoplasia and colon cancer in ulcerative colitis. Gastroenterology 2003;124(4):880–8.
[16] Dorer R, Odze RD. AMACR immunostaining is useful in detecting dysplastic epithelium in Barrett's esophagus, ulcerative colitis, and Crohn's disease. Am J Surg Pathol 2006;30(7):871–7.

[17] Bernstein CN, Shanahan F, Weinstein WM. Are we telling patients the truth about surveillance colonoscopy in ulcerative colitis? Lancet 1994;343(8889):71–4.

[18] Connell WR, Lennard-Jones JE, Williams CB, et al. Factors affecting the outcome of endoscopic surveillance for cancer in ulcerative colitis. Gastroenterology 1994;107(4):934–44.

[19] Ullman T, Croog V, Harpaz N, et al. Progression of flat low-grade dysplasia to advanced neoplasia in patients with ulcerative colitis. Gastroenterology 2003;125(5):1311–9.

[20] Ullman TA, Loftus EV Jr, Kakar S, et al. The fate of low grade dysplasia in ulcerative colitis. Am J Gastroenterol 2002;97(4):922–7.

[21] Befrits R, Ljung T, Jaramillo E, et al. Low-grade dysplasia in extensive, long-standing inflammatory bowel disease: a follow-up study. Dis Colon Rectum 2002;45(5):615–20.

[22] Lim CH, Dixon MF, Vail A, et al. Ten year follow up of ulcerative colitis patients with and without low grade dysplasia. Gut 2003;52(8):1127–32.

[23] Rubin PH, Friedman S, Harpaz N, et al. Colonoscopic polypectomy in chronic colitis: conservative management after endoscopic resection of dysplastic polyps. Gastroenterology 1999;117(6):1295–300.

[24] Engelsgjerd M, Farraye FA, Odze RD. Polypectomy may be adequate treatment for adenoma-like dysplastic lesions in chronic ulcerative colitis. Gastroenterology 1999;117(6):1288–94.

[25] Devroede GJ, Taylor WF, Sauer WG, et al. Cancer risk and life expectancy of children with ulcerative colitis. N Engl J Med 1971;285(1):17–21.

[26] Masala G, Bagnoli S, Ceroti M, et al. Divergent patterns of total and cancer mortality in ulcerative colitis and Crohn's disease patients: the Florence IBD study 1978–2001. Gut 2004; 53(9):1309–13.

[27] Jess T, Loftus EV Jr, Harmsen WS, et al. Survival and cause specific mortality in patients with inflammatory bowel disease: a long term outcome study in Olmsted County, Minnesota, 1940–2004. Gut 2006;55(9):1248–54.

[28] Palli D, Trallori G, Bagnoli S, et al. Hodgkin's disease risk is increased in patients with ulcerative colitis. Gastroenterology 2000;119(3):647–53.

[29] Jess T, Loftus EV Jr, Velayos FS, et al. Risk of intestinal cancer in inflammatory bowel disease: a population-based study from Olmsted County, Minnesota. Gastroenterology 2006; 130(4):1039–46.

[30] Bernstein CN, Blanchard JF, Kliewer E, et al. Cancer risk in patients with inflammatory bowel disease: a population-based study. Cancer 2001;91(4):854–62.

[31] Winther KV, Jess T, Langholz E, et al. Long-term risk of cancer in ulcerative colitis: a population-based cohort study from Copenhagen County. Clin Gastroenterol Hepatol 2004; 2(12):1088–95.

[32] Lakatos L, Mester G, Erdelyi Z, et al. Risk factors for ulcerative colitis-associated colorectal cancer in a Hungarian cohort of patients with ulcerative colitis: results of a population-based study. Inflamm Bowel Dis 2006;12(3):205–11.

[33] Loftus EV Jr. Epidemiology and risk factors for colorectal dysplasia and cancer in ulcerative colitis. Gastroenterol Clin North Am 2006;35(3):517–31.

[34] Itzkowitz SH, Present DH. Consensus conference: colorectal cancer screening and surveillance in inflammatory bowel disease. Inflamm Bowel Dis 2005;11(3):314–21.

[35] Rutter MD, Saunders BP, Wilkinson KH, et al. Thirty-year analysis of a colonoscopic surveillance program for neoplasia in ulcerative colitis. Gastroenterology 2006;130(4):1030–8.

[36] Rutter MD, Saunders BP, Wilkinson KH, et al. Cancer surveillance in longstanding ulcerative colitis: endoscopic appearances help predict cancer risk. Gut 2004;53(12):1813–6.

[37] Broome U, Lofberg R, Veress B, et al. Primary sclerosing cholangitis and ulcerative colitis: evidence for increased neoplastic potential. Hepatology 1995;22(5):1404–8.

[38] Velayos FS, Loftus EV Jr, Jess T, et al. Predictive and protective factors associated with colorectal cancer in ulcerative colitis: a case-control study. Gastroenterology 2006;130(7): 1941–9.

[39] Heuschen UA, Hinz U, Allemeyer EH, et al. Backwash ileitis is strongly associated with colorectal carcinoma in ulcerative colitis. Gastroenterology 2001;120(4):841–7.

[40] Remzi FH, Church JM, Bast J, et al. Mucosectomy vs. stapled ileal pouch-anal anastomosis in patients with familial adenomatous polyposis: functional outcome and neoplasia control. Dis Colon Rectum 2001;44(11):1590–6.

[41] van DP, Vasen HF, Bertario L, et al. Cumulative risk of developing polyps or malignancy at the ileal pouch-anal anastomosis in patients with familial adenomatous polyposis. J Gastrointest Surg 1999;3(3):325–30.

[42] Remzi FH, Dietz DW, Unal E, et al. Combined use of preoperative provocative angiography and highly selective methylene blue injection to localize an occult small-bowel bleeding site in a patient with Crohn's disease: report of a case. Dis Colon Rectum 2003;46(2):260–3.

[43] Rotholtz NA, Pikarsky AJ, Singh JJ, et al. Adenocarcinoma arising from along the rectal stump after double-stapled ileorectal J-pouch in a patient with ulcerative colitis: the need to perform a distal anastomosis. Report of a case. Dis Colon Rectum 2001;44(8): 1214–7.

[44] Knupper N, Straub E, Terpe HJ, et al. Adenocarcinoma of the ileoanal pouch for ulcerative colitis-a complication of severe chronic atrophic pouchitis? Int J Colorectal Dis 2006;21(5): 478–82.

[45] Hassan C, Zullo A, Speziale G, et al. Adenocarcinoma of the ileoanal pouch anastomosis: an emerging complication? Int J Colorectal Dis 2003;18(3):276–8.

[46] Ziv Y, Fazio VW, Church JM, et al. Stapled ileal pouch anal anastomoses are safer than handsewn anastomoses in patients with ulcerative colitis. Am J Surg 1996;171(3):320–3.

[47] Reilly WT, Pemberton JH, Wolff BG, et al. Randomized prospective trial comparing ileal pouch-anal anastomosis performed by excising the anal mucosa to ileal pouch-anal anastomosis performed by preserving the anal mucosa. Ann Surg 1997;225(6):666–76.

[48] Schluender SJ, Mei L, Yang H, et al. Can a meta-analysis answer the question: is mucosectomy and handsewn or double-stapled anastomosis better in ileal pouch-anal anastomosis? Am J Surg 2006;72(10):912–6.

[49] Gyde SN, Prior P, Macartney JC, et al. Malignancy in Crohn's disease. Gut 1980;21(12): 1024–9.

[50] Ekbom A, Helmick C, Zack M, et al. Increased risk of large-bowel cancer in Crohn's disease with colonic involvement. Lancet 1990;336(8711):357–9.

[51] Jess T, Winther KV, Munkholm P, et al. Intestinal and extra-intestinal cancer in Crohn's disease: follow-up of a population-based cohort in Copenhagen County, Denmark. Aliment Pharmacol Ther 2004;19(3):287–93.

[52] Greenstein AJ, Sachar DB, Smith H, et al. A comparison of cancer risk in Crohn's disease and ulcerative colitis. Cancer 1981;48(12):2742–5.

[53] Gillen CD, Andrews HA, Prior P, et al. Crohn's disease and colorectal cancer. Gut 1994; 35(5):651–5.

[54] Canavan C, Abrams KR, Mayberry J. Meta-analysis: colorectal and small bowel cancer risk in patients with Crohn's disease. Aliment Pharmacol Ther 2006;23(8):1097–104.

[55] Maykel JA, Hagerman G, Mellgren AF, et al. Crohn's colitis: the incidence of dysplasia and adenocarcinoma in surgical patients. Dis Colon Rectum 2006;49(7):950–7.

[56] Friedman S. Cancer in Crohn's disease. Gastroenterol Clin North Am 2006;35(3):621–39.

[57] Yamazaki Y, Ribeiro MB, Sachar DB, et al. Malignant colorectal strictures in Crohn's disease. Am J Gastroenterol 1991;86(7):882–5.

[58] Fireman Z, Grossman A, Lilos P, et al. Intestinal cancer in patients with Crohn's disease. A population study in central Israel. Scand J Gastroenterol 1989;24(3):346–50.

[59] Mellemkjaer L, Johansen C, Gridley G, et al. Crohn's disease and cancer risk (Denmark). Cancer Causes Control 2000;11(2):145–50.

[60] Palascak-Juif V, Bouvier AM, Cosnes J, et al. Small bowel adenocarcinoma in patients with Crohn's disease compared with small bowel adenocarcinoma de novo. Inflamm Bowel Dis 2005;11(9):828–32.

[61] Persson PG, Karlen P, Bernell O, et al. Crohn's disease and cancer: a population-based cohort study. Gastroenterology 1994;107(6):1675–9.

[62] Eaden J, Abrams K, Ekbom A, et al. Colorectal cancer prevention in ulcerative colitis: a case-control study. Aliment Pharmacol Ther 2000;14(2):145–53.

[63] Chan EP, Lichtenstein GR. Chemoprevention: risk reduction with medical therapy of inflammatory bowel disease. Gastroenterol Clin North Am 2006;35(3):675–712.

[64] Collins PD, Mpofu C, Watson AJ, et al. Strategies for detecting colon cancer and/or dysplasia in patients with inflammatory bowel disease. Cochrane Database Syst Rev 2006;(2): CD000279.

[65] Siegel CA, Sands BE. Risk factors for colorectal cancer in Crohn's colitis: a case-control study. Inflamm Bowel Dis 2006;12(6):491–6.

SURGICAL
CLINICS OF
NORTH AMERICA

ELSEVIER
SAUNDERS

Surg Clin N Am 87 (2007) 673–680

Extra-Intestinal Manifestations of Crohn's Disease

Kimberly Ephgrave, MD, FACS

Department of Surgery, University of Iowa Hospitals and Clinics, 200 Hawkins Drive,
Iowa City IA, 52242, USA

Crohn's disease is associated with inflammatory processes affecting organ systems outside the gastrointestinal tract, which are collectively known as the extra-intestinal manifestations (EIM) of inflammatory bowel disease (IBD). The prevalence of these processes varies according to how EIM are defined, and whether asymptomatic lesions are included. Classically, the 1979 National Cooperative Crohn's Disease Study of 569 patients found that 24% had true EIM [1], and that perianal disease was present in the majority. The prevalence of perianal disease varied from 58% for patients who had disease confined to the small bowel, to 76% for Crohn's disease patients who had ileocolitis.

The lowest recent estimate of extra-intestinal manifestations of IBD comes from a population database study reporting that only 6.2% of patients who had IBD carried any of the classic extra-intestinal diagnoses. The most prevalent extra-intestinal manifestations of IBD in this database study were musculoskeletal. For Crohn's disease, this was most commonly ankylosing spondylitis, at 2.7% of the total patients, or over one third of those Crohn's patients who had any extra-intestinal diagnosis [2]. Recent reports from China [3] and Hungary [4] suggest that at least 20% of Crohn's disease patients are diagnosed with extra-intestinal manifestations. Active screening for EIM produces much higher estimates of prevalence. For instance, screening IBD patients with plain films (and CT follow-up when indicated) produced a. 9.9% incidence for ankylosing spondylitis, and fully 45.7% for all forms of spondyloarthropathy [5].

The three organ systems most commonly associated with EIM of Crohn's disease are musculoskeletal, ocular, and mucocutaneous [6]. More recently described are associations of Crohn's disease with pulmonary disease, psychological syndromes, osteoporosis, and thromboembolism [7]. The diseases

E-mail address: kimberly-ephgrave@uiowa.edu

0039-6109/07/$ - see front matter © 2007 Published by Elsevier Inc.
doi:10.1016/j.suc.2007.03.003   *surgical.theclinics.com*

that recently have been recognized to occur more frequently than expected in Crohn's disease patients include a very wide range of pathologic conditions, such as dental caries [8], atherosclerosis (documented in intimal media thickness of the common carotid artery) [9], various malignancies [10], and abnormal Pap smears in females who have Crohn's disease [11]. These myriad associations with Crohn's disease are tantalizing because they may provide clues about the etiology of inflammatory bowel disease in general, and Crohn's disease in particular. No one mechanistic explanation has yet emerged, though, to explain the bowel findings and the associated extraintestinal manifestations of IBD [12].

For clinicians with responsibility for Crohn's disease patients, it is useful to maintain a focus on those inflammatory processes that seem most closely linked etiologically with Crohn's disease, such as the inflammatory joint, skin, and ocular processes, and those which are found frequently as complications of the nutritional derangements and the corticosteroid treatments for Crohn's disease, such as osteoporosis. Ulcerative colitis (UC) is of course also associated with EIM, and in comparison with Crohn's disease is more frequently associated with primary sclerosing cholangitis. Primary sclerosing cholangitis is rarely associated with Crohn's disease, but is nevertheless important, because it may require liver transplantation and contribute to mortality. UC and Crohn's disease have a similar incidence of ocular manifestations, but Crohn's disease is more frequently associated with both peripheral and axial joint inflammation [2].

Ocular manifestations of Crohn's disease

The ocular manifestations of inflammatory bowel disease are myriad (blurred vision, tearing, burning and itching, pain, photophobia, hyperemia, and decreased visual acuity), but because they occur in 10% or fewer of cases, may be overlooked. Recent authors recommend ophthalmologic examinations for all inflammatory bowel disease patients, because the consequences can be as severe as blindness [13] or corneal perforation [14]. Eye findings can be the first sign of inflammatory bowel disease; screening in a uveitis clinic for the prevalence of a family history of inflammatory bowel disease showed 3 to 15 times the expected incidence of family members who had already received an IBD diagnosis [15]. Even in patients who have known IBD, ocular flares do not always indicate active bowel disease [7].

The more common ocular manifestations of IBD are episcleritis, or hyperemia without pain or visual deficits, and uveitis, which is associated with both pain and visual disturbance. The uveitis requires urgent treatment with steroids, which if untreated may lead to blindness. Case reports demonstrate utility for cyclosporine A and infliximab in steroid-refractory cases [6]. Additionally, treatment with infliximab for ankylosing spondylitis was associated with a prophylactic ocular benefit, reducing uveitis flares from 15.6 to 6.9 per 100 patient years [16].

Musculoskeletal manifestations of Crohn's disease

Musculoskeletal manifestations are the most common extra-intestinal diagnoses associated with Crohn's disease, with approximately 22% incidence of joint inflammation in comparison with 11% for ulcerative colitis patients [4]. The musculoskeletal diseases associated with Crohn's disease include peripheral joint inflammation, axial arthritis, and osteoporosis. The peripheral joint inflammation tends to track the bowel disease, and can respond to medical or surgical treatment of the bowel disease. In contrast, the axial disease, such as sacroiliitis or psoriatic arthritis, does not seem to remit with treatment of the bowel disease [7].

First-line treatment of the arthropathy associated with inflammatory bowel disease remains acetaminophen, with steroids and methotrexate the traditional second-line treatments [6]. One early trial of Crohn's disease patients specifically noted improvement in two patients who had axial arthropathy, as well as in three who had peripheral arthropathy after anti-tumor necrosis factor (TNF) antibody infusions [17]. Whether anti-TNF antibody infusions will prove to be cost-effective to use as first- or second-line treatment for Crohn's arthropathy in the future remains to be seen.

From the point of view of rheumatologists, at least 5% to 10% of their ankylosing spondylitis patients have Crohn's disease. Moreover, the incidence of subclinical gut inflammation is much higher when screened with endoscopy or gut histology [18]. Treatment of ankylosing spondylitis with nonsteroidal anti-inflammatory agents is thus problematic, because it may cause a flare of IBD or subclinical gut inflammation, and anti-TNF agents may thus become a preferred treatment for active ankylosing spondylitis.

Osteoporosis or decreased bone mineral density and fracture rates are both increased in patients who have inflammatory bowel disease [19,20]. Steroid use is definitely associated with decreased bone mineral density [21,22]; however, because more Crohn's disease patients than ulcerative colitis patients are hypocalcemic and bowel resection is one of the significant predictors for decreased bone density, it appears that Crohn's disease patients have a nutritional contribution, in addition to a direct steroid effect, that makes them particularly prone to decreased bone mineral density.

Fracture risk appears to be highly elevated in IBD patients, even beyond what would be expected from their decreased bone mineral density [19]. No specific osteomalacia or disordered bone formation has been described, however. Circulating levels of osteoprotegerin have been found to be elevated in IBD patients, and the inflamed intestinal tissue secretes this molecule, which may play a role. Levels of osteoprotegerin are inversely associated with bone marrow density; however, in animal models of inflammatory bowel disease, treatment with exogenous osteoprotegerin reversed osteopenia, suggesting that it is not likely to be the cause of osteoporosis observed in patients who have inflammatory bowel disease [19].

At the present time, management of osteoporosis in Crohn's disease patients should be similar to management of all other patients who have decreased bone mineral density, including modification of other risk factors with weight-bearing exercise, calcium and vitamin D supplementation, correction of hormone deficiencies, and smoking cessation. Additionally, the biphosphonates risedronate and alendronate have been shown to reduce fracture risk in patients who have osteoporosis induced by steroids, which would apply to most surgical patients who have Crohn's disease [20]. The anti-TNF agents are not known to induce osteoporosis, and in fact seem to increase bone mineral density, but no data are yet available to determine whether this translates into a clinical benefit [6].

Mucocutaneous manifestations of Crohn's disease

Dermatologic problems commonly associated with Crohn's disease include the erythema nodusum and pyoderma gangrenosum lesions most commonly found near the tibia on the lower extremities, and aphthous ulcerations of mucous membranes. Both erythema nodusum and pyoderma gangrenosum are reported to occur in up to 20% of Crohn's disease patients; however, the erythema nodusum is a more benign lesion that tends to regress with regression of active bowel disease, whereas the painful ulcerations of pyoderma gangrenosum may warrant specific treatment with corticosteroids, cyclosporine, or tacrolimus [6].

The association of papulo-pustular lesions of skin, aphthous ulcerations of mucosae, and arthritis composes Behcet's disease, which has also long been known to have an association with IBD and can appear in advance of the bowel symptoms of Crohn's disease [23].

Although erythema nodusum and pyoderma gangrenosum are most commonly found on the lower extremities, Crohn's disease with granulomas and multinucleated giant cells can appear as skin disease essentially anywhere, with morbid consequences [24]. Metastatic cutaneous Crohn's disease [25] and pyoderma gangrenosum [26] have both been reported to respond to anti-TNF therapy.

Psoriasis, characterized by thick, red, scaly skin plaques, is another chronic inflammatory condition that is relatively common as an extra-intestinal manifestation of Crohn's disease. As is seen with the relationship between Crohn's disease and ankylosing spondylitis, the presence of psoriasis also confers an elevated risk for later development of IBD [27]. Corticosteroids and anti-metabolites are both effective for psoriasis as well as Crohn's disease. Additionally, anti-TNF therapy was recently tested in 249 patients who had severe psoriasis, with 75% improvement noted in the majority of actively treated patients compared with fewer than 10% of those receiving placebo [28].

Pulmonary associations with Crohn's disease

Pulmonary disease associated with inflammatory bowel disease has only recently been recognized. The prevalence may be fairly high, however, because screening with a self-administered questionnaire and peak expiratory flow rate revealed that over half of Crohn's and UC patients had respiratory symptoms. The most common underlying disorder was asthma [29]; however, a large study of over 500,000 young Israeli military personnel inducted from 1980 to 2003 revealed a reverse association from that of most other inflammatory processes with IBD—that asthmatic personnel were less likely to also have other autoimmune diseases, including inflammatory bowel disease [30].

Two relatively uncommon pulmonary conditions, bronchiolitis [31] and bronchiectasis [32], have recently been linked to inflammatory bowel disease. Bronchiolitis refers to inflammation and scarring affecting small conducting airways, and is essentially a nonspecific finding. Bronchiectasis is classically considered to be a consequence of chronic infections, which could be a complication of chronic immune-suppressive therapy; however, in a recent series of 10 patients who had both inflammatory bowel disease and bronchiectasis, 8 had a clinical flare following surgery. The study authors postulated that the flares of bronchiectasis after surgery for inflammatory bowel disease might stem from the withdrawal of medical therapy that had been suppressing the pulmonary inflammation. In this small series of IBD and bronchiectasis patients, half had Crohn's disease and half had ulcerative colitis, suggesting similar incidence of bronchiectasis in both forms of inflammatory bowel disease [32].

Psychological symptoms and Crohn's disease

Both anxiety and depression are associated with many chronic diseases, including inflammatory bowel disease [33]. This is true for pediatric as well as adult patients. For children who have inflammatory bowel disease, the patterns of depressions and anxiety are increased compared with healthy children, and seem to be similar to those seen with other pediatric chronic diseases [34]. Although these symptoms may be a complication of treatment or a natural consequence of the morbidity of the disease, it is also possible that inflammatory bowel disease patients are particularly susceptible because of direct effects of their disease on the central nervous system. Data from a mouse model of inflammatory bowel disease demonstrated that animals exhibited anxiety-like behaviors very early in the process. The behavioral changes were unlikely to reflect a response to inflammation or pain, because they occurred before detectable colonic inflammation [35].

Mental health professionals have noted the link between inflammatory bowel disease and depression, and questioned whether adequate control of the depression might have a beneficial impact on the somatic complaints associated with inflammatory bowel disease [33]. Twelve studies regarding the effects of anti-depressant therapy on inflammatory bowel disease were reported, none of which were randomized. The majority of studies found benefit for both psychological and somatic symptoms of inflammatory bowel disease from treatment with serotonin uptake inhibitors, but amitriptyline only impacted the psychological symptoms; however, the design of the reports limits the conclusions that can be drawn.

According to two large Canadian surveys, the true prevalence of depression in inflammatory bowel disease appears to be triple that of the normal population, at about 15% [36]. Fewer than half of these patients were actively treated for depression, but 47% recalled having suicidal ideation at some point. Factors that were associated with depression included female sex, being without a partner, being young, having greater pain, and having functional limitations. Screening for depression and treatment when appropriate may thus be an important way clinicians can decrease patient suffering from inflammatory bowel disease.

Beyond the anxiety and depression, which can often accompany any significant chronic somatic disease, clinicians have questioned whether inflammatory bowel disease might be associated with increased rates of psychosis; however, examination of British epidemiologic data suggests that schizophrenia may actually be less commonly diagnosed in patients who have inflammatory bowel disease than in the normal population [37]. The odds ratio for Crohn's disease versus controls was 0.74 (95% Confidence Interval: 0.44–1.3).

Crohn's disease and quality of life

Recently, clinicians have become more aware of the importance of quality of life for patients who have chronic diseases. Inflammatory bowel disease patients may have impairment of both physical and mental health, so both the physical and mental components summary scores were recently analyzed in 314 patients treated in Philadelphia [38]. For the physical component, low quality of life was associated most strongly with the activity of their inflammatory bowel disease, followed by the degree of arthritis, heart disease, age, anemia, and back/shoulder pain. For the mental health-related quality of life, the primary component was again inflammatory bowel disease activity, followed by depression/anxiety. Taking this study with the Canadian studies on the prevalence of depression [36] suggests that control of inflammatory bowel disease itself, along with control of painful EIM, are the most effective ways to improve the quality of life for patients who have Crohn's disease.

Summary

Extra-intestinal manifestations occur in at least 25% of Crohn's disease patients, and can be an important source of morbidity. Some of the EIM, such as erythema nodusum and peripheral arthropathy, will wax and wane in keeping with the inflammation in the bowel. The more severe cutaneous ulcerations, uveitis, and axial arthropathy may precede the bowel disease or persist after it subsides. Screening may be appropriate for eye disease to prevent complications, including permanent visual impairment, and for osteoporosis, because prophylactic measures may prevent fractures.

Medical management for extra-intestinal diseases is generally similar to effective medical treatment for Crohn's disease, with corticosteroids the mainstay. As in other chronic diseases, pain and psychological conditions such as depression are associated with IBD, and their control can be of benefit for patients' quality of life. Recent small studies with anti-TNF agents are promising for activity against most of the EIM of Crohn's disease, and may permit more steroid-sparing control of disease in the future.

References

[1] Rankin GB, Watts HD, Melnyk CS, Kelley ML Jr. National Cooperative Crohn's Disease Study: extraintestinal manifestations and perianal complications. Gastroenterology 1979;77: 914–20.

[2] Bernstein CN, Blanchard JF, Rawsthorne P, et al. The prevalence of extra-intestinal diseases in inflammatory bowel disease: a population-based study. Am J Gastroenterol 2001;96: 1116–22.

[3] Jiang L, Xia B, Li J, et al. Retrospective survey of 452 patients with inflammatory bowel disease in Wuhan City, central China. Inflamm Bowel Dis 2006;12:212–7.

[4] Lakotos L, Pandur T, David G, et al. Association of extraintestinal manifestations of inflammatory bowel disease in a province of western Hungary with disease phenotype: results of a 25 year follow-up study. World J Gastroenterol 2003;9:2300–7.

[5] Turkcaper N, Toruner M, Soykan I, et al. The prevalence of extraintestinal manifestations and HLA association in patients with inflammatory bowel disease. Rheumatol Int 2006;26: 663–8.

[6] Barrie A, Plevy S. Treatment of immune-mediated extraintestinal manifestations of inflammatory bowel disease with infliximab. Gastroenterol Clin North Am 2006;35:883–93.

[7] Rothfuss KS, Stange EF, Herrlinger KR. Extraintestinal manifestations and complications in inflammatory bowel diseases. World J Gastroenterol 2006;12:4819–31.

[8] Grossner-Schreiber B, Fetter T, Hedderich J, et al. Prevalence of dental caries and periodontal disease in patients with inflammatory bowel disease: a case-control study. J Clin Periodontol 2006;33:478–84.

[9] Papa A, Danese G, Urgesi R, et al. Early atherosclerosis in patients with inflammatory bowel disease. Eur Rev Med Pharmacol Sci 2006;10:7–11.

[10] Stange EF. Review article: the effect of aminosalicylates and immunomodulation on cancer risk in inflammatory bowel disease. Aliment Pharmacol Ther 2006;24(Suppl 3):64–7.

[11] Bhatia J, Bratcher J, Korelitz B, et al. Abnormalities of the uterine cervix in women with inflammatory bowel disease. World J Gastroenterol 2006;12:6167–71.

[12] Danese S, Fiocchi C. Etiopathogenesis of inflammatory bowel diseases. World J Gastroenterol 2006;12:4807–12.

[13] Mintz R, Feller ER, Bahr RL, et al. Ocular manifestations of inflammatory bowel disease. Inflammatory Bowel Diseases 2004;10:135–9.

[14] Tan MH, Chen SD, Rubinstein A, et al. Corneal perforation due to severe peripheral ulcerative keratitis in Crohn disease. Cornea 2006;25:628–30.

[15] Lin P, Tessler HH, Goldstein DA. Family history of inflammatory bowel disease in patients with idiopathic ocular inflammation. Am J Ophthalmol 2006;141:1097–104.

[16] Braun J, Baraliakos X, Listing J, et al. Decreased incidence of anterior uveitis in patients with ankylosing spondylitis treated with the anti-tumor necrosis factor agents infliximab and etanercept. Arthritis Rheum 2005;52:2447–51.

[17] Van den Bosch F, Kruithof E, De Vos M, et al. Crohn's disease associated with spondyloarthropathy: effect of TNF-alpha blockade with infliximab on articular symptoms. Lancet 2000;356:821–2.

[18] Rudwaleit M, Baeten D. Ankylosing spondylitis and bowel disease. Best Pract Res Clin Rheumatol 2006;20:451–71.

[19] Bernstein CN. Inflammatory bowel diseases as secondary causes of osteoporosis. Curr Osteoporos Rep 2006;4:116–23.

[20] Katz S. Osteoporosis in patients with inflammatory bowel disease: risk factors, prevention, and treatment. Rev Gastroenterol Disord 2006;6:63–71.

[21] Frei P, Fried M, Hungerbuhler Ve, et al. Analysis of risk factors for low bone mineral density in inflammatory bowel disease. Digestion 2006;73:40–6.

[22] Zali M, Bahari A, Firouzi F, et al. Bone mineral density in Iranian patients with inflammatory bowel disease. Int J Colorectal Dis 2006;21:758–66.

[23] Akay N, Boyvat A, Heper AO, et al. Behcet's disease-like presentation of bullous pyoderma gangrenosum associated with Crohn's disease. Clin Exp Dermatol 2006;31:384–6.

[24] Goyal A. Metastatic cutaneous Crohn's disease of the nipple. Dis Colon Rectum 2006;49: 132–4.

[25] Konrad A, Seibold F. Response of cutaneous Crohn's disease to infliximab and methotrexate. Dig Liver Dis 2003;35:351–6.

[26] Brooklyn TN, Dunnill GS, Shetty A, et al. Infliximab for the treatment of pyoderma gangrenosum: a randomised, double-blind placebo-controlled trial. Gut 2006;55:505–9.

[27] Bernstein CN, Wajda A, Blanchard JF. The clustering of other chronic inflammatory diseases in inflammatory bowel disease: a population-based study. Gastroenterology 2005; 129:827–36.

[28] Gottlieb AB, Evans R, Li S, et al. Infliximab induction therapy for patients with severe plaque-type psoriasis: a randomized, double-blind, placebo-controlled trial. J Am Acad Dermatol 2004;51:534–42.

[29] Sivagnamam P, Coutsoumpas A, Forbes A. Respiratory symptoms in patients with inflammatory bowel disease and the impact of dietary salicylates. Dig Liver Dis 2006; [Epub ahead of print].

[30] Tirosh A, Mandel D, Mimouni FB, et al. Autoimmune diseases in asthma. Ann Intern Med 2006;144:877–83.

[31] Visscher DW, Myers JL. Bronchiolitis: the pathologist's perspective. Proc Am Thorac Soc 2006;3:41–7.

[32] Kelly MG, Frizelle FA, Thornley PT, et al. Inflammatory bowel disease and the lung: is there a link between surgery and bronchiectasis? Int J Colorectal Dis 2006;21:754–7.

[33] Mikocka-Walus AA, Turnbull DA, Moulding NT, et al. Anti-depressants and inflammatory bowel disease: a systematic review. Clin Pract Epidemol Ment Health 2006;2:24.

[34] Mackner LM, Crandall WV, Szigethy EM. Psychosocial functioning in pediatric inflammatory bowel disease. Inflamm Bowel Dis 2006;12:239–44.

[35] Lyte M, Li W, Opitz N, et al. Induction of anxiety-like behavior in mice during the initial stages of infection with the agent of murine colonic hyperplasia *Citrobacter rodentium.* Physiol Behav 2006;89:350–7.

[36] Fuller-Thomson E, Sulman J. Depression and inflammatory bowel disease: findings from two nationally representative Canadian surveys. Inflamm Bowel Dis 2006;12:697–707.

[37] West J, Logan RF, Hubbard RB, et al. Risk of schizophrenia in people with celiac disease, ulcerative colitis and Crohn's disease: a general population-based study. Aliment Pharmacol Ther 2006;23:71–4.

[38] Pizzi LT, Weston CM, Goldfarb NI, et al. Impact of chronic conditions on quality of life in patients with inflammatory bowel disease. Inflamm Bowel Dis 2006;12:47–52.

ELSEVIER
SAUNDERS

SURGICAL
CLINICS OF
NORTH AMERICA

Surg Clin N Am 87 (2007) 681–696

Immunologic and Molecular Mechanisms in Inflammatory Bowel Disease

M. Nedim Ince, MD, David E. Elliott, MD, PhD*

*Division of Gastroenterology and Hepatology, Department of Internal Medicine,
University of Iowa, Carver College of Medicine,
4611 JCP, 200 Hawkins Drive, Iowa City, IA 52242, USA*

Human idiopathic inflammatory bowel disease (IBD) consists of two diseases, ulcerative colitis (UC) and Crohn's disease (CD). Chronic, relapsing intestinal inflammation is a common feature of both disorders, and is believed to result from a dysregulated, aberrant immune response to intestinal flora. Under normal conditions, the human colon is colonized by a dense bacterial load, against which a nonpathogenic and highly regulated immune response is generated. This ever-present but limited immune response permits rapid reaction to pathogens while ensuring survival of commensal bacteria that provide the individual with nutrients and vitamins. Additionally, bacteria-derived mediators deliver survival signals to intestinal epithelium that are important for self-renewal [1]. Immunological homeostasis in the gut is disturbed in IBD.

The disturbed immune response in IBD is believed to be directed against the commensal flora, and it is determined by genetic as well as environmental factors. Genomic analysis of IBD kindreds suggests that changes in genes coding for proteins that sense bacterial structures, cytokines, adhesion molecules, or proteins involved in cytokine signaling confer risk for the disease [2]. Often, an environmental factor, such as nonsteroidal anti-inflammatory drug (NSAID) use [3] or cytomegalovirus (CMV) infection [4], triggers colitis that does not resolve. In this article, the authors focus on normal intestinal immune regulation and its loss in IBD, with particular emphasis on genetic and environmental factors, and how they may modify disease activity. First, we introduce the cellular elements of the intestine and how they maintain immunological homeostasis.

---

* Corresponding author.
E-mail address: david-elliott@uiowa.edu (D.E. Elliott).

Cellular constituents of the intestinal immune system

The intestinal immune system consists of the lining epithelium, intraepithelial lymphocytes, and lamina propria cells that include T and B lymphocytes, monocytes, macrophages, dendritic cells, and polymorphonuclear leukocytes (Fig. 1). At certain locations within the gastrointestinal tract, some of these cellular elements organize into lymphoid structures named gut-associated lymphoid tissue (GALT). These GALTs include the appendix and Peyer's patches, densely organized lymphoid follicles of the small intestine. The cells constituting the lamina propria or Peyer's patches are in continuous exchange with other lymphoid compartments found in blood, lymph nodes, or spleen.

The intestinal immune responses are divided into innate and adaptive (acquired) immunity. Innate immune responses operate without previous exposure to pathogens, but their specificity is limited to shared microbial structures. Innate immune capacity includes the barrier function of the intestinal mucosa that prevents bacterial translocation, and the acid pH of the stomach that inhibits bacterial overgrowth. Phagocytic cells (eg, neutrophils and macrophages) and antibacterial proteins (eg, complement and

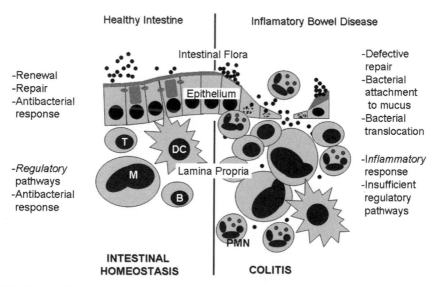

Fig. 1. Intestinal responses to gut flora during homeostasis (healthy intestine) and IBD. Immune regulation dominates the healthy intestine. Intestinal flora stimulate epithelial renewal, repair, and antibacterial responses. Macrophages and dendritic cells have a noninflammatory phenotype. Similarly, T cells and B cells are involved in immunologic homeostasis. IBD is characterized by epithelial damage (abnormal mucus production, defective repair). An acute and chronic inflammatory infiltrate driven by intestinal flora expands the lamina propria. Cells migrating to lamina propria include B cells (*B*), T cells (*T*), macrophages (*M*), dendritic cells (*DC*) and polymorphonuclear leukocytes (*PMN*). Lamina propria cells produce inflammatory cytokines. Immune regulation fails to dampen this inflammatory response.

defensins) also participate in innate responses against bacteria. Acquired (adaptive) responses are pathogen-specific, and are usually generated in circumstances in which the innate immune system is unable to circumvent a pathogen challenge. Activation of the acquired immune system after exposure to a pathogen usually takes days, and the specific response against this pathogen is made possible by the large repertoire of receptors within the B and T cell population. Survival of some responsive T and B cells after the pathogen is eradicated (memory cells) enables fast responses in subsequent infections with the same pathogen.

Antigen-specific adaptive responses are able to differentiate the host's own antigenic determinant's "self" from pathogen-related antigen's "nonself." Auto-antibodies directed against host proteins are produced in IBD, suggesting that self–non-self discrimination may be disturbed; however, the pathologic significance of auto-antibodies in IBD is not known. No specific microbial pathogen has been identified to cause IBD. The disease is believed to be driven by intestinal flora, because it responds to antibiotics [5], or diversion of fecal stream [6]. The epithelium and cellular constituents of the lamina propria take part in responses against the bacterial flora during colitis.

The gastrointestinal epithelium is a simple columnar cell layer, with tight junctions between cells preventing transfer of luminal antigens into deeper layers of the intestine. Epithelial lining has a high turnover rate, with signals delivered by luminal flora contributing to epithelial regeneration [7]. Although the intestinal epithelial cells can respond to commensal bacteria [8,9], the exact role of the epithelium and its contribution to colitis remains to be established. Epithelial integrity is disturbed in IBD, and mice who have deficient epithelial barrier function develop colitis [10]. NSAIDs may aggravate the disease. Permeability of the intestinal epithelium to bacterial flora is increased by administering aspirin to patients who have CD [11]. Paneth cells of the small intestine and colon are specialized elements of the epithelium that make antibacterial defensins and lectins [12,13]. Expression of specific defensins may be decreased in mucosa of IBD patients [14].

Antigen-presenting cells such as dendritic cells and macrophages are constituents of the lamina propria. Dendritic cells can extend their processes between the epithelial cells to sample bacteria [15], and during their interaction with the epithelium they may be conditioned to stimulate T cells toward a "non-inflammatory response" in order to preserve intestinal homeostasis [15,16]. Macrophages are major producers of inflammatory cytokines, such as interleukin (IL)6, IL12, and tumor necrosis factor (TNF)α, and therefore are regarded as effector cells of colitis. Lamina propira macrophages of uninflamed mucosa have a noninflammatory phenotype, and do not respond to bacteria-derived mediators by inflammatory cytokine production [17]. Immune regulatory cytokines IL10 and tumor growth factor (TGF)β may play a role in the induction and maintenance of this noninflammatory phenotype.

B lymphocytes and plasma cells make immunoglobulins against pathogens, but also can generate autoantibodies against the host's own proteins. Although autoantibodies, such as perinuclear anti-neutrophil cytoplasmic antibodies (p-ANCA), are produced in UC [18], their contribution to IBD pathogenesis is unknown. A few mouse models have demonstrated the importance of B cells in colitis [19]. In all these models, B cells regulate inflammation and suppress colitis, rather than taking part in immune pathology by antibody production. These observations suggest that B cells may help regulate inflammation in the gut.

CD and UC are viewed as T-cell–driven disease processes [20]. T cells develop in the thymus, where they first undergo receptor rearrangement. After rearrangement, each thymic T cell expresses one unique and specific T-cell receptor that allows this cell to respond to a limited number of unique antigens. To become peripheral T lymphocytes, thymic T cells undergo negative selection, in which potentially self-reactive T cells are eliminated to prevent immune pathology or autoimmune disorders. Lymphocytes that pass negative selection can become peripheral T cells, which respond to specific antigens. The enormous diversity of receptors represented on the surface of the peripheral T cell population enables adaptive responses to a broad range of pathogens. Occasionally, some T cells escape negative selection and can respond to self-antigens. Combating this are thymically selected T lymphocytes that develop into regulatory T cells (Treg). These Treg inhibit other effector T cell responses and prevent immune pathology. Peripheral immune regulatory pathways may be defective in IBD (Fig. 2).

Peripheral T cells express an antigen-specific T-cell receptor complex (TcR; CD3), and are grouped based on CD4 or CD8 protein expression on their surface. CD8+ T cells recognize protein antigens that are processed in the cytosol of cells and presented to CD8+ T cells after being attached to a major histocompatibility Class I (MHC Class I) molecule. The MHC molecules in people are called human leukocyte antigens (HLA). MHC-TcR interaction is important in CD8+ T lymphocyte-mediated surveillance and destruction of virus-infected or tumor cells. The importance of CD8+ T cells in colitis is not clear-cut, although in certain models intestinal CD8+ T cells may contribute to the control of inflammation [21].

Proteins processed in endosomes of antigen presenting cells (dendritic cells, macrophages, or B cells) are attached to MHC Class II proteins and presented to CD4+ T cells. CD4+ T cells, also called Thelper (Th) cells, are grouped as Th1, Th2, or Th17 effector lymphocytes based on their cytokine production profiles (see Fig. 2). Differentiation of these T cells requires specific transcription factors, which are T-bet for Th1 [22], GATA3 for Th2 [23], and RORγt for Th17 cells [24]. Different T-cell subsets are associated with specific cytokine production. Cytokines are important mediators of the immune response, and mucosal cytokine production patterns define the pathway of inflammation (see Fig. 2). Effector functions of T cells are counter-regulated by other T-cell subtypes. These include IL10-producing

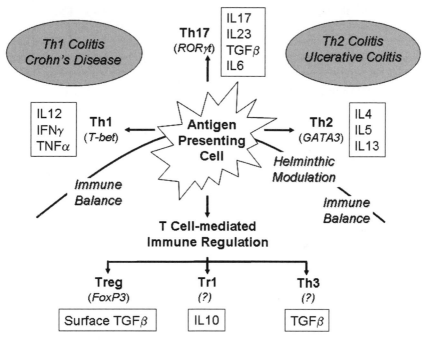

Fig. 2. Intestinal immune pathways. CD4 T cell differentiation includes four different paths. Differentiation starts after antigenic stimulation of T cells by antigen-presenting cells. Each of these paths is characterized by expression of T-cell-lineage–specific transcription factor and cytokines. They are T-bet for Th1, GATA3 for Th2, RORγt for Th17, and FoxP3 for Treg. According to mucosal cytokine patterns, Crohn's disease is a Th1 colitis, and ulcerative colitis has similarities to Th2 colitis. Enhanced expression of IL17 in intestinal mucosa of IBD patients has been documented. Treg, TGFβ-, or IL10-dominated environments exhibit immune balance. Helminth infection is associated with mucosal Th2 and regulatory responses.

Tr1, TGFβ-producing Th3, and thymus-derived CD4+ CD25+ Tregs that inhibit effector T lymphocyte responses by cell-to-cell contact. Generation of CD4+ CD25+ Tregs requires the transcription factor, FoxP3 [25]. Based on data from adoptive T-cell transfers in mice [26] and the effects of depletion or functional inhibition of T cells on IBD in patients [20], T cells are major conductors of intestinal immune responses. Besides CD4+ T cells, intraepithelial γδ T cells or natural killer T (NKT) cells that respond to lipid antigens may play a role in intestinal immune regulation, as shown by different animal models of colitis [27].

Intestinal immune responses in inflammatory bowel disease patients

Cells of the immune system that expand the lamina propria in IBD patients display disease-specific cellular responses to in vitro stimulation (see Fig. 2). CD is characterized by a Th1-type mucosal immune response with increased IFNγ, TNFα, and IL12, and with concomitant decrease in

IL4 generation. By contrast, UC is often designated as a Th2 response because of increased IL5 and IL13 secretion, although the prototypic Th2 cytokine IL4 secretion is not increased in mucosal T cells of UC patients [28]. Enhanced IL17 expression in intestinal mucosa has been reported in both diseases (see Fig. 2) [29,30].

These IBD immune responses may target intestinal flora. In uninflamed intestine, the commensal flora stimulate epithelial repair to preserve barrier function. During colitis, the epithelium becomes permeable, allowing bacterial translocation [31], amplifying the chronic inflammation [32]. Immune pathology is also contributed by dysfunctional immune regulation. For example, there may be an inadequate TGFβ signaling in intestinal leukocyte subsets of IBD patients [33,34], so that the immunoregulatory cytokine TGFβ fails to curtail effector T-cell responses. Therefore, IBD is regarded as a disease of impaired epithelial barrier function and excessive immune response, driven by commensal flora, T cells, and cytokines in the setting of insufficient immune regulation. These elements of inflammation have been addressed in animal models of colitis.

Lessons learned from animal models

Animal models are important tools of IBD research, because the characteristics of inflammation simulate human disease. Most of these models show some recurring themes. First, colitis responds to antibiotics or is not generated in bacteria-free or gnotobiotic (limited bacteria) environments, demonstrating the involvement of bacteria. Second, animals whose epithelial barrier is disturbed develop intestinal inflammation [10,11,27], showing the importance of epithelial integrity. Third, colitis is driven by T-cell–generated cytokines, indicating the central importance of T cells in intestinal inflammation. Fourth, interference with immune regulatory mechanisms worsens colitis, attesting to the critical role of self-regulation in the immune system.

In mice or rats, rectal infusion of trinitrobenzene sulfonic acid (TNBS) causes mucosal injury and results in excessive mucosal Th1 responses [35]. One of these T cell cytokines is TNFα, and previous studies have shown that TNFα-deficient animals are protected from TNBS colitis, whereas TNFα over-expressing mice have higher susceptibility [36]. Further evidence for the importance of Th1 cytokines in this model came from studies in which IL12-blocking antibodies interfered with inflammation after TNBS-mediated mucosal damage [37]. IL12 is produced by monocytes, macrophages, or dendritic cells, and stimulates T cells to generate Th1 cytokines such as IFNγ or TNFα. Subsequent experience in clinical practice attested to the importance of blocking TNFα in CD patients, in whom mucosal inflammation is driven by Th1 cytokines [3]. Furthermore, blocking the p40 subunit of IL12 has been shown to reduce the inflammation in CD [38]. The same IL12p40 protein also constitutes one subunit of IL23, which stimulates IL17-mediated inflammatory processes. Recently, the relevance of IL17 circuit has been validated in TNBS colitis, as blockage of IL17 signaling by overexpression of an IL-17R IgG1 fusion protein significantly attenuated colonic inflammation [39]. Although induction or maintenance of Th17 cells requires IL6, TGFβ, and IL23 [40,41], in TNBS colitis, IL12, rather than IL23, may be the critical cytokine driving the inflammation [42].

In a few chemically induced colitis models, inflammation is driven by Th2 cytokines or results from defective immune regulation. Oxazolone administration results in injury to the epithelium, and is characterized by enhanced mucosal IL4 and IL5, and decreased IFNγ responses. IL4 is important in oxazolone colitis because blocking IL4 with antibodies treats the disease [43]. Mucosal injury could also be generated by NSAIDs in mice [44], similar to NSAID-associated disease flares in IBD patients. IL10 appears to protect from colitis after TNBS or NSAID-induced injury [44,45], suggesting defective immune regulation is a characteristic of colitis, and that absence of immune regulation may underlie the disease process. Augmented TGFβ circuits similarly protect from TNBS injury [46].

Mucosa protection is in part achieved by immune regulatory cytokines such as IL10 and TGFβ. IL10 knock-out (IL10$^{-/-}$) mice develop spontaneous colitis [47,48]. To identify cellular elements that produce IL10 to protect mucosa from colitis, T cell-enriched lamina propria lymphocytes from IL10$^{-/-}$ mice were transferred into T- and B-cell–deficient, recombinase-activating gene knock-out (RAG$^{-/-}$) recipients [49]. Although RAG$^{-/-}$ mice do not develop inflammation spontaneously or after T-cell transfer from wild type (WT) animals, they developed colitis following T- and not B- cell transfer from IL10$^{-/-}$ donors. These experiments suggested that mucosal injury in IL10$^{-/-}$ mice was mediated by IL10-defective T cells.

TGFβ is another important immune regulator in the intestine. Mice that lack TGFβ develop severe inflammation [48]. Although all constituents of the intestine could produce TGFβ, recent evidence suggests that T-cell TGFβ production is crucial to prevent colitis [50]. Similar to TGFβ$^{-/-}$ animals [48,50], mice with T-cell–targeted TGFβ signaling defects develop intestinal inflammation [51,52], suggesting that T cell regulation by TGFβ is important. Indeed, TGFβ inhibits Th1, Th2 differentiation, and also impairs CD8 T-cell function. TGFβ signaling involves phosphorylation of intracellular Smad proteins, and TGFβ signaling defects have been characterized in mice that develop colitis and in IBD patients [34,46].

Further importance of T cells in colitis was shown by adoptive transfer experiments using specific T-cell subsets. Peripheral T cells may be grouped as naïve (no previous antigen experience), memory (previous antigen experience), or effector (activated by antigen) lymphocytes. These subgroups may be identified and experimentally selected by cell surface markers, such as CD45Rb expression level. Transfer of total peripheral T cells from normal WT animals into immunodeficient scid mice did not cause intestinal inflammation, whereas administration of naïve CD4 T cells, enriched in CD45Rb^{high} fraction, into immunodeficient *scid* mice resulted in colitis. Colitis in this transfer model was triggered by bacteria and did not occur in germ-free conditions [26]. Co-transfer of CD45Rb^{low} cells with CD45Rb^{high} fraction prevented intestinal inflammation. This experiment has shown the importance of peripheral regulatory mechanisms to prevent immune pathology, and indicated that CD45Rb^{high} T cells contain a cellular subset that can cause colitis. CD45Rb^{low} T cells contain a group of cells that inhibit immune pathology. Additional data have shown that this regulation involves TGFβ [53] and IL10 [54] production. Attempts to characterize the regulatory cellular elements within the CD45Rb^{low} T cells have revealed CD4+ CD25+ thymus-derived, *FoxP3*-expressing natural Treg [26]. Further experiments have shown resolution of colitis after transfer of CD+CD25+ Tregs. The exact mechanism of immune suppression by Tregs is not known, and may involve cell-to-cell contact, IL10, TGFβ, or inhibitory molecule (e.g. CTLA4) expression [26,55]. Tregs or T cells with regulatory properties can be generated in the periphery, and they even may be induced to express FoxP3. Whether IL10-producing Tr1 or TGFβ-producing Th3 cells constitute different T cell subsets from thymus-derived natural Tregs is not entirely clear (see Fig. 2).

T-cell migration to the intestine during colitis requires expression of certain cell surface adhesion molecules. The α4β1 and α4β7 integrins are two of these adhesion molecules expressed on T lymphocytes and other white blood cell subsets. Although spontaneous colitis was blocked in an animal model using anti-α4 integrin antibodies [56] and initial clinical trials using a similar approach showed some clinical benefit, α4 integrin blockage can be complicated by progressive multifocal leukoencephalopathy (PML) [57]. Integrin blockade may have clinical role if targeting a more narrow subset of these adhesion molecules permits reduction in inflammation without impeding surveillance for neurotropic agents.

Animal models of colitis with similarities to human disease help us dissect intestinal inflammatory pathways and design novel therapeutics, such as anti-TNFα antibodies. Additional insight into IBD pathogenesis has come from studies that identify genetic changes in IBD patients.

Genetic changes associated with inflammatory bowel disease

First-degree relatives of people who have IBD are at greater risk for the disease than the general population. The concordance rate for CD is as high as 50% to 60% among monozygotic twins [58,59]. A lesser but significant genetic association was found in UC, where 6% to 18% of monozygotic twins were affected. To identify genes that confer risk for IBD, genomewide studies using microsatellite markers have been performed. These studies have found several chromosomal locations designated as IBD susceptibility loci in human genome. Each of them was given a number.

One of these regions is located on chromosome 16 and named *IBD1* [60]. This region contains the gene encoding the protein caspase activation and recruitment domain 15 (CARD15), also designated as nuclear oligomerization domain 2 (NOD2). Cloning and functional characterization has shown that CARD15/NOD2 is an intracellular receptor recognizing bacterial muramyldipeptide (MDP). CARD15/NOD2 alleles predisposing to IBD are found in heterozygous form in up to 30% of CD patients and in up to 15% of people who do not have IBD [61]. Homozygous or compound heterozygous CARD15/NOD2 alleles are detected in 3% to 15% of CD patients, and in up to 1% of disease-free controls. CARD15/NOD2 mutations are neither sufficient nor necessary for disease, but they do confer risk for CD. CARD15/NOD2 variants do not increase risk of UC.

CARD15/NOD2 is expressed by Paneth cells, specialized epithelial elements of intestinal crypts involved in production of antibacterial peptides, such as lysozyme or defensins [62,63]. Therefore, CARD15/NOD2 mutations may affect Paneth-cell–mediated antibacterial defense in the gut. CARD15/NOD2 is also expressed in macrophages and dendritic cells, and activates NF-κB, a transcription factor important in inflammation. NF-κB activity is enhanced in the intestine of CD patients. Because NF-κB stimulates the production of proinflammatory cytokines such as TNFα and IL6, the effects of native and CD-associated mutant CARD15/NOD2 proteins on NF-κB activity has been studied. CARD15/NOD2 knock-out mice displayed severe defects of NF-κB activity, and were unable to clear bacterial challenge, supporting the hypothesis that CARD15/NOD2 is involved in antibacterial host defense [64]. Expression of CD-associated mutant CARD15/NOD2 proteins in cells by transient transfection showed diminished NF-κB activation [65]. These studies suggest that CARD15/NOD2 variants have impaired capability to activate NF-κB, impairing bacterial defense and leading to chronic unresolved inflammation; however, another study in mice used a CD-associated truncated CARD15/NOD2 protein knocked into the murine genomic CARD15/NOD2 locus, and showed enhanced NF-κB activity in the intestine, with increased production of proinflammatory cytokines [66]. Currently it is unclear whether CARD15/NOD2 variations discovered in CD patients are gain-of-function or loss-of-function mutations.

Expression of variant CARD15/NOD2 protein is associated with small intestinal CD. Several studies have linked CARD15/NOD2 mutations to fistulizing or fibrostenosing phenotype, suggesting deeper inflammation and more severe disease course in patients who have dysfunctional CARD15/NOD2 protein [67,68]. Whether this is the result of preferential small intestinal involvement in CARD15/NOD2-positive CD, or CARD15/NOD2 mutation predisposes to fibrostenosing phenotype independent of disease location remains to be established.

IBD3 locus on chromosome 6p is located in proximity to the coding region of polymorphic HLA or MHC genes. This locus carries a very high gene density, and studies have indicated the association of several classical and nonclassical MHC alleles with IBD susceptibility [69]. The link between HLA gene polymorphism and IBD is not well-established. Interestingly, this region also contains the coding DNA sequence for the proinflammatory cytokine TNFα, whose importance in IBD pathogenesis is established [70].

IBD5 on chromosome 5q designates another susceptibility locus, and is close to several cytokine genes, such as IL3, IL4, IL5, and IL13. Individuals carrying the microsatellite marker associated with disease susceptibility in *IBD5* locus may have more severe disease course requiring surgery, but the exact cytokine genes or mutations linked to this region remain to be established [61]. *IBD5* also contains the coding sequences for organic cation transporter 1 (OCTN1) and organic cation transporter 2 (OCTN2). Functional variants of these transporters have been linked to CD susceptibility [71]. How genetic changes that affect these transporter proteins lead to intestinal inflammation is unknown, but intestinal epithelial cell injury is believed to result from interference with epithelial transporter function. Single nucleotide polymorphisms have been found in another epithelial cell transporter gene not part of the *IBD5* locus. This cell membrane protein is encoded by the ATP-binding cassette, subfamily B, member 1 (ABCB1) also named the multidrug resistance 1 (MDR1) gene, which is located on chromosome 7q. ABCB1/MDR1 transporter raised particular attention when mice deficient for this protein were found to develop spontaneous intestinal inflammation [72]. Genetic studies linked ABCB1/MDR1 polymorphism and IBD [73]. ABCB1/MDR1 is probably involved in expulsion of cellular toxins. With dysfunctional ABCB1/MDR1 protein expression, the epithelial cell may be predisposed to injury by intracellular accumulation of damaging products.

Other genome-wide studies have identified additional loci (*IBD2, 4, 6, 8, 9*) [61]. The gene products for these regions that confer disease risk remain to be identified. In addition, these loci may predispose to disease in certain populations but not others. Similar genetic studies have identified polymorphisms in previously named genes, and therefore not given an IBD locus number.

Interleukin 23 recently gained attention as an important cytokine mediator of colitis in mice [74–76], and a recent study found that a variant IL23 receptor (IL23R) gene allele on chromosome 1p31 is protective against CD [77]. IL23 helps to maintain proinflammatory Th17 cells [24,74–76]. Perhaps the protective IL23R variant has inefficient signaling that reduces Th17 activity. IL23 is protein heterodimer that consists of IL23p19 and IL12p40. Anti-IL12p40 antibody treatment may induce remission in CD patients [38].

Toll-like receptors (TLR) are major sensors of bacteria in the eukaryotic host, and are important in stimulating inflammatory cytokine responses, including IL12 or IL23 secretion [78,79]. So far, ten TLR are defined in humans. Among these receptors, TLR2 recognizes gram-positive bacterial peptidoglycan (PGN), TLR4 gram-negative bacterial lipopolysaccharide

(LPS), and TLR9 unmethylated CpG motifs of bacterial DNA. Studies have found association between TLR4 or TLR9 polymorphism and human IBD [80–82]. TLR4 alleles associated with UC or CD show impaired NF-κB activation after LPS stimulation, suggesting that a loss-of-function allele is related to human IBD. These data raised the interesting question of how loss of LPS signaling can trigger colitis. Animal studies suggest that a major function of TLR4 signaling in the intestine is to stimulate tissue repair in response to injury [7,83,84]. In certain conditions, intestinal T cells also produce TGFβ in response to LPS, which may help immune regulation [85]. The association between TLR9 polymorphism and CD has been reported [82]. Consistent with that observation, probiotic bacteria may be beneficial in human IBD-related pouchitis [86], and in mice they may exert their immune regulatory functions by means of stimulating TLR9 [87,88]. TLR1, TLR2, and TLR6 polymorphism could also contribute to IBD pathogenesis [89]. TLR2 signaling may play a role in regulatory responses [90].

Bacterial flagellin is a dominant antigen in IBD, and it binds to TLR5. Many bacterial species express flagellin. In mice, flagellin-reactive T cells were able to transfer disease to recipient animals by adoptive transfer [91]. A recent study found a dominant negative TLR5 polymorphism (a loss-of-function allele) protects from CD, further suggesting that innate responses to flagellin have a role in stimulating pathologic intestinal inflammation [92].

Characterization of genetic changes in IBD is currently at its early stage of development. Further characterization of these genetic changes will help us better understand how host responses malfunction in IBD.

Environmental factors

Although patients who have IBD may have genetic predisposition, the concordance rate even in genetically identical monozygotic twins is only 50% for CD. This indicates that environmental factors are important in the pathogenesis of IBD. NSAID use, CMV infection, and pseudomembranous colitis by *Clostridium difficile* are among common environmental factors that may precipitate colitis that develops into IBD.

Besides being a common precipitant of IBD flares [3], NSAIDs also cause ulcers in the terminal ileum that are difficult to differentiate from CD [93]. NSAIDs inhibit the enzyme cyclooxygenase (Cox), and thereby prevent accumulation of prostaglandins in the mucosa, which are important for epithelial renewal. Unlike wild type mice, IL10$^{-/-}$ mice are prone to severe NSAID injury [44]. This suggests that NSAID-mediated mucosal damage may precipitate colitis when the regulatory pathways are deficient.

There are also environmental factors that may protect from IBD. The hygiene hypothesis suggests that exposure to infections such as helminths during childhood may prevent pathologic immune reactivity in later years [94]. Helminth colonization alters the host immune reactivity to antigens unrelated to the parasite [95]. It also induces the secretion of immune regulatory cytokines, IL10, and TGFβ [94]. Two clinical trials have shown benefits in UC and CD patients [96,97]. In mice, the mechanism of helminthic immune modulation involves induction of intestinal T-cell regulatory responses [85,98] in which adoptive transfer of T cells from worm-colonized mice to colitic recipients was associated with downregulation of inflammation.

Summary

Molecular and immunologic mechanisms underlying inflammation in IBD are still largely unknown. Recent studies have helped us better characterize genetic and environmental factors associated with colitis. Discoveries of genetic variants such as CARD15/NOD2 or IL23R have confirmed previous observations that IBD is a bacteria- and cytokine-driven pathologic immune response. Data from animal models and patients have demonstrated that certain T cell subsets (Th1, Th2, or Th17) are important in executing the inflammatory cascade. Insufficient regulatory cell activity or modulatory cytokine production results in unrestrained inflammation. These recent advances have been applied to clinical practice where biologic agents that block inflammatory cytokines (anti-TNFα antibodies) have been used successfully to treat IBD.

Biologic therapy in IBD was a major breakthrough but with major disadvantages. Biologic agents are expensive, and are associated with potential severe side effects and infectious complications. Recent advances have also identified mucosal regulatory pathways that include natural Tregs, TGFβ, or IL10-producing T cells. Although results of initial trials with IL10 were discouraging [20] (likely because of the very short half-life of the cytokine), agents that stimulate mucosal regulatory T cells and mucosal IL10 production appear to be beneficial in recent clinical trials. Future research will help us better characterize mucosal regulatory pathways and facilitate the development of less expensive, safer medications to treat this chronic and often devastating illness.

References

[1] Clevers H. At the crossroads of inflammation and cancer. Cell 2004;118:671–4.
[2] Bamias G, Nyce MR, De La Rue SA, et al. New concepts in the pathophysiology of inflammatory bowel disease. Ann Intern Med 2005;143:895–904.
[3] Podolsky DK. Inflammatory bowel disease. N Engl J Med 2002;347:417–29.
[4] Hommes DW, Sterringa G, van Deventer SJ, et al. The pathogenicity of cytomegalovirus in inflammatory bowel disease: a systematic review and evidence-based recommendations for future research. Inflamm Bowel Dis 2004;10:245–50.
[5] Sartor RB. Therapeutic manipulation of the enteric microflora in inflammatory bowel diseases: antibiotics, probiotics, and prebiotics. Gastroenterology 2004;126:1620–33.

[6] Rutgeerts P, Goboes K, Peeters M, et al. Effect of faecal stream diversion on recurrence of Crohn's disease in the neoterminal ileum. Lancet 1991;338:771–4.

[7] Rakoff-Nahoum S, Paglino J, Eslami-Varzaneh F, et al. Recognition of commensal microflora by toll-like receptors is required for intestinal homeostasis. Cell 2004;118:229–41.

[8] Cario E, Podolsky DK. Differential alteration in intestinal epithelial cell expression of toll-like receptor 3 (TLR3) and TLR4 in inflammatory bowel disease. Infect Immun 2000;68: 7010–7.

[9] Cario E, Rosenberg IM, Brandwein SL, et al. Lipopolysaccharide activates distinct signaling pathways in intestinal epithelial cell lines expressing Toll-like receptors. J Immunol 2000;164: 966–72.

[10] Hermiston ML, Gordon JI. Inflammatory bowel disease and adenomas in mice expressing a dominant negative N-cadherin. Science 1995;270:1203–7.

[11] Cobrin GM, Abreu MT. Defects in mucosal immunity leading to Crohn's disease. Immunol Rev 2005;206:277–95.

[12] Salzman NH, Ghosh D, Huttner KM, et al. Protection against enteric salmonellosis in transgenic mice expressing a human intestinal defensin. Nature 2003;422:522–6.

[13] Cash HL, Whitham CV, Behrendt CL, et al. Symbiotic bacteria direct expression of an intestinal bactericidal lectin. Science 2006;313:1126–30.

[14] Wehkamp J, Salzman NH, Porter E, et al. Reduced Paneth cell alpha-defensins in ileal Crohn's disease. Proc Natl Acad Sci U S A 2005;102:18129–34.

[15] Rescigno M, Urbano M, Valzasina B, et al. Dendritic cells express tight junction proteins and penetrate gut epithelial monolayers to sample bacteria. Nat Immunol 2001;2:361–7.

[16] Rimoldi M, Chieppa M, Salucci V, et al. Intestinal immune homeostasis is regulated by the crosstalk between epithelial cells and dendritic cells. Nat Immunol 2005;6:507–14.

[17] Smith PD, Ochsenbauer-Jambor C, Smythies LE. Intestinal macrophages: unique effector cells of the innate immune system. Immunol Rev 2005;206:149–59.

[18] Joossens S, Reinisch W, Vermeire S, et al. The value of serologic markers in indeterminate colitis: a prospective follow-up study. Gastroenterology 2002;122:1242–7.

[19] Mizoguchi A, Bhan AK. A case for regulatory B cells. J Immunol 2006;176:705–10.

[20] Korzenik JR, Podolsky DK. Evolving knowledge and therapy of inflammatory bowel disease. Nat Rev Drug Discov 2006;5:197–209.

[21] Metwali A, Setiawan T, Blum AM, et al. Induction of CD8+ regulatory T cells in the intestine by Heligmosomoides polygyrus infection. Am J Physiol Gastrointest Liver Physiol 2006; 291:G253–9.

[22] Szabo SJ, Kim ST, Costa GL, et al. A novel transcription factor, T-bet, directs Th1 lineage commitment. Cell 2000;100:655–69.

[23] Zheng W, Flavell RA. The transcription factor GATA-3 is necessary and sufficient for Th2 cytokine gene expression in CD4 T cells. Cell 1997;89:587–96.

[24] Ivanov II, McKenzie BS, Zhou L, et al. The orphan nuclear receptor RORgammat directs the differentiation program of proinflammatory IL-17+ T helper cells. Cell 2006; 126:1121–33.

[25] Williams LM, Rudensky AY. Maintenance of the Foxp3-dependent developmental program in mature regulatory T cells requires continued expression of Foxp3. Nat Immunol 2007;8:277–84.

[26] Izcue A, Coombes JL, Powrie F. Regulatory T cells suppress systemic and mucosal immune activation to control intestinal inflammation. Immunol Rev 2006;212:256–71.

[27] Strober W, Fuss IJ, Blumberg RS. The immunology of mucosal models of inflammation. Annu Rev Immunol 2002;20:495–549.

[28] Bouma G, Strober W. The immunological and genetic basis of inflammatory bowel disease. Nat Rev Immunol 2003;3:521–33.

[29] Nielsen OH, Kirman I, Rudiger N, et al. Upregulation of interleukin-12 and -17 in active inflammatory bowel disease. Scand J Gastroenterol 2003;38:180–5.

[30] Fujino S, Andoh A, Bamba S, et al. Increased expression of interleukin 17 in inflammatory bowel disease. Gut 2003;52:65–70.

[31] Iweala OI, Nagler CR. Immune privilege in the gut: the establishment and maintenance of non-responsiveness to dietary antigens and commensal flora. Immunol Rev 2006;213: 82–100.

[32] Marks DJ, Harbord MW, MacAllister R, et al. Defective acute inflammation in Crohn's disease: a clinical investigation. Lancet 2006;367:668–78.

[33] Monteleone G, Mann J, Monteleone I, et al. A failure of transforming growth factor-beta1 negative regulation maintains sustained NF-kappaB activation in gut inflammation. J Biol Chem 2004;279:3925–32.

[34] Monteleone G, Kumberova A, Croft NM, et al. Blocking Smad7 restores TGF-beta1 signaling in chronic inflammatory bowel disease. J Clin Invest 2001;108:601–9.

[35] Te Velde AA, Verstege MI, Hommes DW. Critical appraisal of the current practice in murine TNBS-induced colitis. Inflamm Bowel Dis 2006;12:995–9.

[36] Neurath MF, Fuss I, Pasparakis M, et al. Predominant pathogenic role of tumor necrosis factor in experimental colitis in mice. Eur J Immunol 1997;27:1743–50.

[37] Neurath MF, Fuss I, Kelsall BL, et al. Antibodies to interleukin 12 abrogate established experimental colitis in mice. J Exp Med 1995;182:1281–90.

[38] Mannon PJ, Fuss IJ, Mayer L, et al. Anti-interleukin-12 antibody for active Crohn's disease. N Engl J Med 2004;351:2069–79.

[39] Zhang Z, Zheng M, Bindas J, et al. Critical role of IL-17 receptor signaling in acute TNBS-induced colitis. Inflamm Bowel Dis 2006;12:382–8.

[40] Mangan PR, Harrington LE, O'Quinn DB, et al. Transforming growth factor-beta induces development of the T(H)17 lineage. Nature 2006;441:231–4.

[41] Bettelli E, Carrier Y, Gao W, et al. Reciprocal developmental pathways for the generation of pathogenic effector TH17 and regulatory T cells. Nature 2006;441:235–8.

[42] Becker C, Dornhoff H, Neufert C, et al. Cutting edge: IL-23 cross-regulates IL-12 production in T cell-dependent experimental colitis. J Immunol 2006;177:2760–4.

[43] Boirivant M, Fuss IJ, Chu A, et al. Oxazolone colitis: a murine model of T helper cell type 2 colitis treatable with antibodies to interleukin 4. J Exp Med 1998;188:1929–39.

[44] Berg DJ, Zhang J, Weinstock JV, et al. Rapid development of colitis in NSAID-treated IL-10-deficient mice. Gastroenterology 2002;123:1527–42.

[45] Fuss IJ, Boirivant M, Lacy B, et al. The interrelated roles of TGF-beta and IL-10 in the regulation of experimental colitis. J Immunol 2002;168:900–8.

[46] Boirivant M, Pallone F, Di GC, et al. Inhibition of Smad7 with a specific antisense oligonucleotide facilitates TGF-beta1-mediated suppression of colitis. Gastroenterology 2006;131: 1786–98.

[47] Kuhn R, Lohler J, Rennick D, et al. Interleukin-10-deficient mice develop chronic enterocolitis. Cell 1993;75:263–74.

[48] Shull MM, Ormsby I, Kier AB, et al. Targeted disruption of the mouse transforming growth factor-beta 1 gene results in multifocal inflammatory disease. Nature 1992;359: 693–9.

[49] Davidson NJ, Leach MW, Fort MM, et al. T helper cell 1-type CD4+ T cells, but not B cells, mediate colitis in interleukin 10-deficient mice. J Exp Med 1996;184:241–51.

[50] Li MO, Wan YY, Sanjabi S, et al. Transforming growth factor-beta regulation of immune responses. Annu Rev Immunol 2006;24:99–146.

[51] Gorelik L, Flavell RA. Immune-mediated eradication of tumors through the blockade of transforming growth factor-beta signaling in T cells. Nat Med 2001;7:1118–22.

[52] Li MO, Sanjabi S, Flavell RA. Transforming growth factor-beta controls development, homeostasis, and tolerance of T cells by regulatory T cell-dependent and -independent mechanisms. Immunity 2006;25:455–71.

[53] Powrie F, Carlino J, Leach MW, et al. A critical role for transforming growth factor-beta but not interleukin 4 in the suppression of T helper type 1-mediated colitis by CD45RB(low) CD4+ T cells. J Exp Med 1996;183:2669–74.

[54] Asseman C, Mauze S, Leach MW, et al. An essential role for interleukin 10 in the function of regulatory T cells that inhibit intestinal inflammation. J Exp Med 1999;190:995–1004.

[55] Rudensky AY, Campbell DJ. In vivo sites and cellular mechanisms of T reg cell-mediated suppression. J Exp Med 2006;203:489–92.

[56] Podolsky DK, Lobb R, King N, et al. Attenuation of colitis in the cotton-top tamarin by anti-alpha 4 integrin monoclonal antibody. J Clin Invest 1993;92:372–80.

[57] Sandborn WJ, Colombel JF, Enns R, et al. Natalizumab induction and maintenance therapy for Crohn's disease. N Engl J Med 2005;353:1912–25.

[58] Tysk C, Lindberg E, Jarnerot G, et al. Ulcerative colitis and Crohn's disease in an unselected population of monozygotic and dizygotic twins. A study of heritability and the influence of smoking. Gut 1988;29:990–6.

[59] Halfvarson J, Bodin L, Tysk C, et al. Inflammatory bowel disease in a Swedish twin cohort: a long-term follow-up of concordance and clinical characteristics. Gastroenterology 2003; 124:1767–73.

[60] Kufer TA, Banks DJ, Philpott DJ. Innate immune sensing of microbes by Nod proteins. Ann N Y Acad Sci 2006;1072:19–27.

[61] Gaya DR, Russell RK, Nimmo ER, et al. New genes in inflammatory bowel disease: lessons for complex diseases? Lancet 2006;367:1271–84.

[62] Lala S, Ogura Y, Osborne C, et al. Crohn's disease and the NOD2 gene: a role for Paneth cells. Gastroenterology 2003;125:47–57.

[63] Ogura Y, Lala S, Xin W, et al. Expression of NOD2 in Paneth cells: a possible link to Crohn's ileitis. Gut 2003;52:1591–7.

[64] Kobayashi KS, Chamaillard M, Ogura Y, et al. Nod2-dependent regulation of innate and adaptive immunity in the intestinal tract. Science 2005;307:731–4.

[65] Girardin SE, Boneca IG, Viala J, et al. Nod2 is a general sensor of peptidoglycan through muramyl dipeptide (MDP) detection. J Biol Chem 2003;278:8869–72.

[66] Maeda S, Hsu LC, Liu H, et al. Nod2 mutation in Crohn's disease potentiates NF-kappaB activity and IL-1beta processing. Science 2005;307:734–8.

[67] Radlmayr M, Torok HP, Martin K, et al. The c-insertion mutation of the NOD2 gene is associated with fistulizing and fibrostenotic phenotypes in Crohn's disease. Gastroenterology 2002;122:2091–2.

[68] Abreu MT, Taylor KD, Lin YC, et al. Mutations in NOD2 are associated with fibrostenosing disease in patients with Crohn's disease. Gastroenterology 2002;123:679–88.

[69] Ahmad T, Marshall SE, Jewell D. Genetics of inflammatory bowel disease: the role of the HLA complex. World J Gastroenterol 2006;12:3628–35.

[70] Rutgeerts P, Van AG, Vermeire S. Optimizing anti-TNF treatment in inflammatory bowel disease. Gastroenterology 2004;126:1593–610.

[71] Peltekova VD, Wintle RF, Rubin LA, et al. Functional variants of OCTN cation transporter genes are associated with Crohn disease. Nat Genet 2004;36:471–5.

[72] Panwala CM, Jones JC, Viney JL. A novel model of inflammatory bowel disease: mice deficient for the multiple drug resistance gene, mdr1a, spontaneously develop colitis. J Immunol 1998;161:5733–44.

[73] Annese V, Valvano MR, Palmieri O, et al. Multidrug resistance 1 gene in inflammatory bowel disease: a meta-analysis. World J Gastroenterol 2006;12:3636–44.

[74] Hue S, Ahern P, Buonocore S, et al. Interleukin-23 drives innate and T cell-mediated intestinal inflammation. J Exp Med 2006;203:2473–83.

[75] Kullberg MC, Jankovic D, Feng CG, et al. IL-23 plays a key role in Helicobacter hepaticus-induced T cell-dependent colitis. J Exp Med 2006;203:2485–94.

[76] Uhlig HH, McKenzie BS, Hue S, et al. Differential activity of IL-12 and IL-23 in mucosal and systemic innate immune pathology. Immunity 2006;25:309–18.

[77] Duerr RH, Taylor KD, Brant SR, et al. A genome-wide association study identifies IL23R as an inflammatory bowel disease gene. Science 2006;314:1461–3.

[78] Ishii K, Kurita-Taniguchi M, Aoki M, et al. Gene-inducing program of human dendritic cells in response to BCG cell-wall skeleton (CWS), which reflects adjuvancy required for tumor immunotherapy. Immunol Lett 2005;98:280–90.

[79] Akira S, Uematsu S, Takeuchi O. Pathogen recognition and innate immunity. Cell 2006; 124:783–801.

[80] Franchimont D, Vermeire S, El HH, et al. Deficient host-bacteria interactions in inflammatory bowel disease? The toll-like receptor (TLR)-4 Asp299gly polymorphism is associated with Crohn's disease and ulcerative colitis. Gut 2004;53:987–92.

[81] Torok HP, Glas J, Tonenchi L, et al. Polymorphisms of the lipopolysaccharide-signaling complex in inflammatory bowel disease: association of a mutation in the Toll-like receptor 4 gene with ulcerative colitis. Clin Immunol 2004;112:85–91.

[82] Torok HP, Glas J, Tonenchi L, et al. Crohn's disease is associated with a toll-like receptor-9 polymorphism. Gastroenterology 2004;127:365–6.

[83] Fukata M, Michelsen KS, Eri R, et al. Toll-like receptor-4 is required for intestinal response to epithelial injury and limiting bacterial translocation in a murine model of acute colitis. Am J Physiol Gastrointest Liver Physiol 2005;288:G1055–65.

[84] Fukata M, Chen A, Klepper A, et al. Cox-2 is regulated by Toll-like receptor-4 (TLR4) signaling: role in proliferation and apoptosis in the intestine. Gastroenterology 2006;131: 862–77.

[85] Ince MN, Elliott DE, Setiawan T, et al. Heligmosomoides polygyrus induces TLR4 on murine mucosal T cells that produce TGFbeta after lipopolysaccharide stimulation. J Immunol 2006;176:726–9.

[86] Bohm SK, Kruis W. Probiotics: do they help to control intestinal inflammation? Ann N Y Acad Sci 2006;1072:339–50.

[87] Lee J, Mo JH, Shen C, et al. Toll-like receptor signaling in intestinal epithelial cells contributes to colonic homoeostasis. Curr Opin Gastroenterol 2007;23:27–31.

[88] Rachmilewitz D, Katakura K, Karmeli F, et al. Toll-like receptor 9 signaling mediates the anti-inflammatory effects of probiotics in murine experimental colitis. Gastroenterology 2004;126:520–8.

[89] Pierik M, Joossens S, Van SK, et al. Toll-like receptor-1, -2, and -6 polymorphisms influence disease extension in inflammatory bowel diseases. Inflamm Bowel Dis 2006;12:1–8.

[90] Sutmuller RP, den Brok MH, Kramer M, et al. Toll-like receptor 2 controls expansion and function of regulatory T cells. J Clin Invest 2006;116:485–94.

[91] Lodes MJ, Cong Y, Elson CO, et al. Bacterial flagellin is a dominant antigen in Crohn disease. J Clin Invest 2004;113:1296–306.

[92] Gewirtz AT, Vijay-Kumar M, Brant SR, et al. Dominant-negative TLR5 polymorphism reduces adaptive immune response to flagellin and negatively associates with Crohn's disease. Am J Physiol Gastrointest Liver Physiol 2006;290:G1157–63.

[93] Lengeling RW, Mitros FA, Brennan JA, et al. Ulcerative ileitis encountered at ileo-colonoscopy: likely role of nonsteroidal agents. Clin Gastroenterol Hepatol 2003;1:160–9.

[94] Maizels RM, Yazdanbakhsh M. Immune regulation by helminth parasites: cellular and molecular mechanisms. Nat Rev Immunol 2003;3:733–44.

[95] Elliott DE, Summers RW, Weinstock JV. Helminths and the modulation of mucosal inflammation. Curr Opin Gastroenterol 2005;21:51–8.

[96] Summers RW, Elliott DE, Urban JF Jr, et al. Trichuris suis therapy for active ulcerative colitis: a randomized controlled trial. Gastroenterology 2005;128:825–32.

[97] Summers RW, Elliott DE, Urban JF Jr, et al. Trichuris suis therapy in Crohn's disease. Gut 2005;54:87–90.

[98] Elliott DE, Setiawan T, Metwali A, et al. Heligmosomoides polygyrus inhibits established colitis in IL-10-deficient mice. Eur J Immunol 2004;34:2690–8.

SURGICAL
CLINICS OF
NORTH AMERICA

Surg Clin N Am 87 (2007) 697–725

Current Medical Therapy for Chronic Inflammatory Bowel Diseases

Cyrus P. Tamboli, MD, FRCPC

Department of Internal Medicine, Division of Gastroenterology, 4614 JCP, 200 Hawkins Drive, University Hospitals & Clinics, University of Iowa Roy J. & Lucille A. Carver College of Medicine, Iowa City, IA 52242-1081, USA

Chronic idiopathic inflammatory bowel disease (IBD) is a term for Crohn's disease (CD), ulcerative colitis (UC), and colonic IBD type unclassified (IBDU) [1]; the latter was referred to previously as indeterminate colitis (IC). The full spectrum of IBD may include disorders such as lymphocytic colitis, collagenous colitis, diverticular disease–associated colitis, and others. This article focuses upon current medical therapies for adult CD and UC. Detailed management issues, treatment of extraintestinal manifestations of IBD, and therapies not yet shown effective through large clinical trials are not reviewed here. Because the pathophysiology is characterized by an overactive immune response at the gut level, almost all currently accepted therapies are anti-inflammatory or immunosuppressive by design. Newer "biologic" agents achieve potent, targeted blockade of specific aspects of intestinal and systemic immune dysregulation, such as tumor necrosis factor α (anti–TNF-α agents). Although this has improved the lives of patients suffering from severe IBD dramatically, knowledge of the impact of such immunosuppression (even from corticosteroids) continues to evolve. Therefore, the clinician who uses these therapies should be well versed in their pharmacology, clinical indications, contraindications, and complications and be committed to routine surveillance for all of these issues.

Optimal medical management of IBD is multifaceted and individualized. Except for mild cases (primarily UC), most patients require combination therapy to achieve sustained response or remission. Fine-tuning of treatment is based upon clinical, biochemical, endoscopic, and histologic responses that depend upon considerations of drug doses, routes, and timings and drug–drug synergies. Despite advances in our ability to predict clinical course in specific patients, the individual response to IBD therapy

E-mail address: cyrus-tamboli@uiowa.edu

0039-6109/07/$ - see front matter © 2007 Elsevier Inc. All rights reserved.
doi:10.1016/j.suc.2007.03.014   *surgical.theclinics.com*

often is idiosyncratic. There also are many well-known factors influencing response, including adherence with difficult medication regimens [2], pharmacogenetics [3], clinical phenotype of IBD, drug–drug interactions, drug tolerances, tachyphylaxis, toxicities, and adverse reactions. In addition, the clinician should be aware of commonly occurring infectious complications (eg *Clostridium difficile* or cytomegalovirus colitis intra-abdominal abscesses) and malignancies that may mimic an IBD "flare-up."

Specific goals of medical therapy for IBD include the reduction of: abdominal pain, diarrhea, fatigue, anemia, nutrient deficiencies, mucosal inflammation, extraintestinal manifestations, hospitalizations, operations, and complications, such as abscesses, fistulae, infections, and malignancy. Improved quality-of-life also has been an important outcome measured in clinical trials. Several clinical indices have been used to measure these outcomes in research trials, but they are difficult to use in day-to-day practice. The correlation between symptoms of IBD and endoscopic appearances is controversial [1].

This article has categorized medical therapy for IBD into agents for inducing remission and those for maintaining remission. Ideally, an overlap occurs between the two, transitioning from sometimes highly aggressive combination therapy induction phases to less complex maintenance regimens, hopefully while avoiding relapse. Best medical management for IBD over the long-term requires a solid physician–patient relationship and explicit agreement upon its shared responsibilities. Adverse effects of the medical therapies described in this article are listed in Appendix 1.

Crohn's disease

Induction of remission

The initial presentation of active CD or a subsequent "flare-up" implies adverse change from baseline. Because CD may affect any portion of the gut from mouth to anus, symptoms vary widely and may present diagnostic challenges. Most commonly, CD affects the colon, terminal ileum, or both, which may lead to abdominal pain, cramping, diarrhea with or without blood, nausea, vomiting, fever, malaise and fatigue, anorexia, or weight loss. Upper gastrointestinal (GI) tract involvement (esophagus, stomach, and duodenum) may produce heartburn, dysphagia, dyspepsia, early satiety, nausea and vomiting, or epigastric abdominal pain. Extraintestinal manifestations may be present. If clinically indicated, abscess should be ruled out with abdominopelvic CT or MRI, especially before initiating corticosteroids or immunomodulators/anti–TNF-α agents. Therapy should be instituted as early as possible, and, ideally, after colonoscopy or sigmoidoscopy with biopsies, and possibly upper esophagogastroduodenoscopy. This is especially important at initial disease presentation, such that therapy may be tailored to disease location and severity, and to avoid diagnostic confusion after partially treated IBD. If infectious colitis is suspected (eg, in those already taking immunosuppressors), early colonoscopic biopsy review is helpful before therapy. The Crohn's Disease Activity Index (CDAI) score, derived from a 1-week diary [4], has been used as a guide to distinguishing mild, moderate, and severe disease in clinical trials (Box 1). CDAI scores between 150 and 220 are "mild" and scores between 221 and 400 are "moderate"; more than 400 points is considered "severe" disease, and remission is defined as CDAI score less than 150.

Mild disease

The most commonly used agents include sulfasalazine, oral or topical mesalamine (topical for colonic disease), oral antibiotics, and the topically active oral corticosteroid budesonide (for terminal ileal and right-sided colonic disease). Sulfasalazine was the earliest 5′-aminosalicylate (5′-ASA) drug to be used in IBD; it is made up of a mesalamine moiety linked to sulfapyridine by an azo-bond (Table 1), which is cleaved by the action of colonic bacteria to release the clinically active mesalamine component. Early studies showed 40% to 50% remission rates with sulfasalazine at dosages of 3 to 5 g/d in CD at 16 weeks in patients with some colonic involvement [5–7]. Because the active moiety in sulfasalazine is mesalamine [8], and therapeutic doses

---

Box 1. Crohn's Disease Activity Index

Number of liquid/very soft stools (weighting 2)
Abdominal pain (0 = none, 1 = mild, 2 = moderate, 3 = severe) (weighting 5)
General well-being (0 = well, 1 = slightly below par, 2 = poor, 3 = very poor, 4 = terrible) (weighting 7)
Extraintestinal features (1 per finding): perianal disease (fissure/fistula/abscess), external fistula, mucocutaneous or cutaneous lesions, iritis/uveitis, arthritis/arthralgia, fever (weighting 20)
Use of antidiarrheal drugs, yes = 1, no = 0 (weighting 30)
Abdominal mass: none = 0, equivocal = 2, definite = 5 (weighting 10)
47 − current hematocrit (men); 42 − current hematocrit (females) (weighting 6)
100 × (1 − body weight/standard weight) (weighting 1)

Total score between 0 and 750, sum score based on a 7-day aggregate of each item scored daily and current hematocrit measurement. Total CDAI = sum (individual scores × weighting factor). (*From* Best WR, Becktel JM, Singleton JW. Rederived values of the eight coefficients of the Crohn's Disease Activity Index (CDAI). *Gastroenterology.* 1979;77(4 Pt 2):843–6; with permission.)

Table 1
Oral sulfasalazine, mesalamine and its second generation derivatives

Drug (brand)	Compound	Release mechanism	Site of action	Available in United States
Sulfasalazine (Azulfidine)	5′-ASA + sulfapyridine, diazo bond	Diazo-bond cleavage by colonic bacterial azoreductase enzyme	Colon	Yes
Mesalamine (Asacol)	mesalamine (5′-ASA), Eudragit-S coated	Coating dissolution at pH>7	(Ileum[a]), colon	Yes
Mesalamine (Pentasa)	mesalamine (5′-ASA), ethylcellulose coated	Time- and pH-dependent slow release	(Jejunum[a]), ileum, colon	Yes
Mesalamine (Mesasal)	mesalamine (5′-ASA), Eudragit-L coated	Coating dissolution at pH>6	Ileum, colon	No
Olsalazine (Dipentum)	2 mesalamines (5′-ASA + 5′-ASA), diazo bond	Diazo-bond cleavage by colonic bacterial azoreductase enzyme	Colon	Yes
Balsalazide (Colazal)	Mesalamine (5′-ASA) + 4-aminobenzoyl-β-alanine	Diazo-bond cleavage by colonic bacterial azoreductase enzyme	Colon	Yes

[a] Questionable site of significant therapeutic action.

of sulfasalazine often are tolerated poorly, a variety of mesalamine derivatives without sulfapyridine have been developed. These drugs differ in their site of active drug release (see Table 1). The effectiveness of sulfasalazine only in the subgroups of patients who have colonic CD supports this "targeted" design for various azo-bonded formulations. The influence of diarrhea or malabsorption on luminal pH and transit time likely affects drug release for the other types of 5′-ASA formulations; however, these formulations often provide higher doses of 5′-ASA than sulfasalazine because of their better tolerance. One large randomized, placebo-controlled study showed an advantage of Pentasa, 4 g/d for 8 weeks, over placebo for inducing remission (CDAI <150) in ileal and ileocolonic CD [9]. A meta-analysis of Pentasa studies in active CD [10] also concluded that there was a modest improvement with Pentasa, 4 g/d, versus placebo; however, the clinical significance was less impressive. A similar CDAI remission rate of 45% was shown with Asacol, 3.2 g/d for 16 weeks, in ileocolonic CD [11]. Collectively, these studies suggest modest benefits (≤50% remission) from sulfasalazine at dosages greater than 3 g/d in colonic CD and for ileocolonic CD at dosages of more than 4 g/d (Pentasa) or 3.2 g/d (Asacol) versus placebo when used for minimum 8 weeks. Because sulfasalazine inhibits absorption of folic acid, the latter usually is coadministered at dosages of 1 to 2 mg/d.

Bacteria play a central role in the pathophysiology of animal models of IBD [12] and are considered important in CD. Thus, antibiotics have often been used; however, few randomized controlled therapeutic trials have been performed, limiting the available evidence. In one 6-week study, oral ciprofloxacin, 1 g/d, induced remission rates (55%) similar to mesalamine, 4 g/d, in mild-moderate CD [13]. Metronidazole seems to be ineffective in uncomplicated CD. At 400 mg orally twice daily for 16 weeks, remission was induced in 25% of patients who had CD (mean CDAI = 261) [7,14], which is not different from placebo remission rates in other studies. Although the result was similar to sulfasalazine, 3 g/d, no placebo group was used in this study, and no benefit was seen in the subgroup with small bowel disease. Another study also suggested the ineffectiveness of metronidazole for small bowel CD at dosages up to 20 mg/kg/d [15]; however, several open-label studies suggested metronidazole's effectiveness in perianal CD, and its use for this indication remains popular (see "Special situations" below). Also of interest in IBD is rifaximin: a new, broad-spectrum antibiotic that is not (<0.4%) absorbed from the GI tract, making it an attractive candidate for targeting intestinal flora or bacterial pathogens that may be associated with CD. Rifaximin has established itself for the treatment of GI disorders, such as traveler's diarrhea, irritable bowel syndrome, small-bowel bacterial overgrowth, and hepatic encephalopathy [16]. One double-blind, placebo-controlled study in 83 patients who had mild-moderate CD found that rifaximin, 800 mg twice daily for 12 weeks, induced remission in 52% of patients versus 33% for placebo (P = not significant). In the subgroup with an elevated C-reactive protein, however, remission rates were significantly better with rifaximin (63%) than with placebo (21%) [17]. Most 5'-ASA or antibiotic studies referenced above did not stratify responses of mild versus moderate CD, but overall, therapeutic gains are modest. Thus, it is recommended that if sulfasalazine or mesalamine is used for induction of remission in CD at all, they should be limited to mild cases. Patients started on these agents require close observation for nonresponse or clinical deterioration, either of which warrants a switch to more aggressive therapy (usually within 2–3 weeks). Treatment of rectal or left-sided colonic CD with topical mesalamine or corticosteroid agents is discussed in the section on UC.

Moderate disease

Sulfasalazine or mesalamine derivatives should not be used as monotherapy if colonoscopy reveals deep or long ulcerations, edema, fissures, or fistulae or if there is significant transmural inflammation. Clinical findings may include persisting abdominal pain, diarrhea, tenderness, fever, weight loss, right lower quadrant mass, leukocytosis, or anemia, but most patients with moderate disease remain ambulatory and do not exhibit signs of hypovolemia or systemic toxicity. In some, mesalamine may have been tried but with disease progression. The mainstays of induction treatment in this subset are corticosteroids, either as topically acting oral budesonide or systemically in the form of oral prednisone or equivalent. Corticosteroids exhibit multiple effects, including inhibition of proinflammatory cytokines, such as interleukin (IL)-1, -2, -6, and -8, interferon-gamma, and TNF-α. The challenge is to achieve remission without early relapse following a steroid taper, while minimizing adverse effects that are duration- and dose-dependent (see Appendix 1). Recent studies have shown that complications following corticosteroid treatment in CD are at least as great as those associated with more "potent" immunomodulator therapies [18]. One exception may be budesonide, an oral, topically acting steroid similar in structure to 16a-hydroxyprednisolone. It is formulated as a delayed "controlled ileal release" capsule (Entocort-EC in North America), with acid-resistant microcapsules. The external Eudragit-L coating is designed to release at pH greater than 5, along with a second time-release ethylcellulose coating making it aimed at the distal small bowel. Presumably because of budesonide's high (90%) first-pass hepatic metabolism, traditional corticosteroid-related adverse effects are less common; however, hypothalamic-pituitary-adrenal-axis suppression still does occur with budesonide. Several studies have demonstrated its efficacy in ileal/ascending colonic CD, as well as confirming its fewer steroid-related side effects. A placebo-controlled trial [19] in mild-moderate CD showed remission rates of approximately 50% at 8 weeks of treatment with 9 mg/d. Another study found a difference in remission versus placebo at 2 weeks, but not at 8 weeks [20]. A third study [21] showed that over 16 weeks, budesonide, 9 mg/d, had a higher remission rate (62%) than mesalamine, 4 g/d (36%). Budesonide is not superior to traditional corticosteroids for induction of remission, so it is best reserved for mild-moderate ileal/ascending colonic CD. Similarly, combining mesalamine with any type of corticosteroid for the induction therapy of moderate-severe CD is not superior to steroid treatment alone. The treatment of moderate Crohn's colitis is similar to that for moderately active UC, and the reader is referred to that section for further details.

Severe disease

   In addition to severe signs and symptoms, this subgroup of patients can, for the purpose of therapeutic decision-making, include those who are steroid dependent (immediate or frequent relapse upon tapering) and steroid refractory (little or no response to oral corticosteroids). Perianal fistulizing CD is considered separately. For this article, only remission rates for the various agents are reported. The reader is reminded that when reading the literature, partial improvement (as measured by higher "response" rates) may be an equally important clinical outcome in this subset of patients for whom first-line therapies fail. Nonetheless, remission rates in moderate-severe CD with inductive systemic corticosteroids approach 80%. Two large studies [5,6] have confirmed this using prednisone, 0.5 to 0.75 mg/kg/d, or 6-methylprednisolone, 48 mg/d (dosage equivalent 60 mg/d prednisone) for at least 4 months. No head-to-head studies comparing various doses have been performed, but higher doses of prednisolone, up to 1 mg/kg/d, have slightly higher remission rates at the expense of additional adverse effects. A typical induction regimen used in North America is oral prednisone, 40 to 60 mg/d, with tapering to discontinuation over 8 to 16 weeks. Other investigators recommend 12 weeks as the maximal extent of steroid induction therapy. This period is best viewed as a "bridge" to longer-term immunomodulator maintenance therapies (Fig. 1) that require 12 weeks or more to effectively modulate inflammatory T-cell subsets [22]. Although it may minimize toxicity, premature tapering is associated with early relapse and possibly the later development of steroid refractoriness. For similar reasons, initial dosages of prednisone less than 40 mg/d generally are not recommended if a decision has been made to use this drug. Patients who respond usually begin to do so within 3 weeks. If no meaningful response or clinical deterioration is seen by this time ("steroid refractory") at full doses, the traditional therapeutic "step-up" model (Fig. 2) would suggest addition of immunomodulators, infliximab, or both. One example of a prednisone tapering schedule reduces the dosage by 10 mg/d every week at dosages greater than 40 mg/d, then reduces by 5 mg/d each week between dosages of 20 and 40 mg/d, then reduces by 2.5 mg/d each week between dosages of 10 and 20 mg/d, and then reduces by 1 mg/d each week once at less than 10 mg/d. Faster tapers have been used. Some clinicians advise a routine corticotrophin-stimulation test for adrenal insufficiency before steroid discontinuation, but this seldom is necessary unless considerable difficulty in weaning is encountered or if steroid withdrawal symptoms may mimic disease relapse.

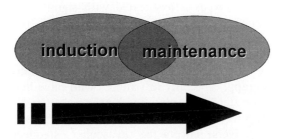

Fig. 1. Overlapping induction and maintenance therapy in IBD. Goal of IBD Therapy: Remission.

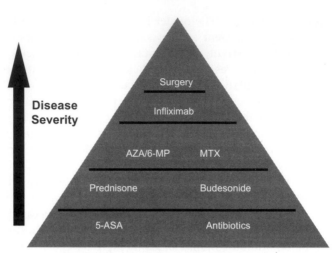

Fig. 2. Crohn's disease: traditional "step-up" therapeutic pyramid.

If the presentation is more fulminant with hypovolemia or other indications for hospitalization, intravenous (IV) steroids usually are administered (eg, methylprednisolone, 48–60 mg/d, or hydrocortisone, 300–400 mg), although the incremental benefit of the IV route over oral steroids for severe CD is unclear. One study showed equal therapeutic effectiveness (82% and 93% response, respectively) for corticotrophin, 120 units/d IV, and hydrocortisone, 300 mg/d [23].

Enteral nutritional therapy has been proposed as a safer and equally effective alternative to induce remission in moderate-severe CD. It has been more popular in Europe than in North America. A meta-analysis of randomized trials showed remission rates using this approach to be approximately 60% [24], which mainly included studies using elemental diets (amino acids); however, polymeric diets also have been used. The rationale for such therapies has been that patients who have CD often exhibit significant nutritional deficiencies, regular diets may present antigenic stimuli responsible for continued inflammatory responses, and traditional induction therapy with corticosteroids is associated with significant adverse effects. Most of the evidence for the elemental diet approach is from the pediatric population, but there is evidence of its effectiveness in adults [25–28]. Incremental benefit is obtained from using specifically defined, low-fat elemental diets [29,30]. Low-fat elemental diets are a valuable alternative to corticosteroid induction therapy, especially in patients who have highly active small bowel CD in whom steroid therapy has higher risks (eg, the elderly; those with concomitant infection, possible intra-abdominal abscess, or a history of steroid-related adverse effects [eg, avascular osteonecrosis]). Because most patients find elemental diets unpalatable, this usually requires temporary insertion of a feeding tube.

The thiopurine antimetabolites, azathioprine and 6-mercaptopurine (6-mp), have long been used in severe CD as induction and maintenance agents and have a large body of evidence supporting their use. These drugs also have well-known metabolic pathways (Fig. 3). Both agents are effective at inducing "response" ($\sim$ 55% with azathioprine, 2–3 mg/kg/d or 6-mp, 1.0–1.5 mg/kg/d) in CD, although the onset of action is slower than for corticosteroids: With continued therapy, response rates increase after 17 weeks [31]. Remission rate definitions differ among various studies, but there is consensus that using azathioprine or 6-mp as an induction agent enables better adherence to a fixed schedule of steroid tapering and the ability to maintain remission at daily steroid dosages less than 10 mg/d (the "steroid-sparing" effect). See Appendix 1 for the adverse effects of thiopurine metabolites. Thiopurine S-methyltransferase (TPMT) is an enzyme involved in metabolizing 6-mp to clinically inactive metabolites 6-thiouric acid, 6-methylmercaptopurine (6-mmp), and 6-mmp ribonucleotides (see Fig. 3). Approximately 89% of the population shows high levels of enzyme activity, approximately 11% have intermediate levels of activity, and 0.1% have low levels of activity. This latter group is at risk for severe leukopenia that is due to toxic accumulations of 6-thioguanine nucleotides whose concentrations correlate with clinical efficacy and leukopenia. Thus, it is recommended by leading IBD experts that a TPMT enzymatic assay be checked routinely before thiopurine

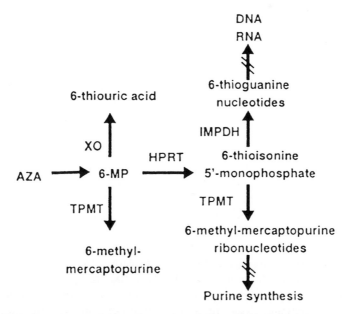

Fig. 3. Metabolic pathways of thiopurine antimetabolites. (*From* Colombel JF, Tamboli CP, Hugot, JP. Clinical genetics of inflammatory bowel diseases: genetic epidemiology, genotype-phenotype correlations and pharmacogenetics. In: Sartor RB, Sandborn WJ, editors. Kirsner's inflammatory bowel diseases, 6th edition. Elsevier Publishing Inc.; 2004. p. 273.)

metabolite therapy, with low metabolic activity being a contraindication to therapy [32]. TPMT enzyme testing does not obviate the need for routine complete blood cell counts and hepatic enzymes for as long as a patient uses these medications. Frequent checks are required initially. Nonadherence is a contraindication to using these drugs. For a review of thiopurine antimetabolite pharmacotherapy in IBD see Ref. [33]. Another antimetabolite, methotrexate, has been used extensively in rheumatoid arthritis and psoriasis, and, more recently, in CD. It is a dihydrofolate reductase inhibitor, blocking DNA synthesis, but likely possessing additional unknown anti-inflammatory mechanisms in IBD. When given as 25 mg intramuscularly (IM) every week for 16 weeks, it is effective at inducing remission (39% versus 19% with placebo) in steroid-refractory CD [34]. Usually, methotrexate is used as a "third-line" agent following steroid failure and thiopurine metabolite failure or intolerance, but there have been no large head-to-head trials comparing the induction efficacy of methotrexate with thiopurine metabolites. Oral methotrexate is ineffective for inducing remission in active CD, so parenteral administration is required. Some European centers have used subcutaneous (SC) methotrexate as an alternative. Methotrexate is coadministered with folic acid, 1 to 2 mg/d, to reduce nausea and stomatitis.

Infliximab, a chimeric immunoglobulin given intravenously that neutralizes TNF-α, has revolutionized the therapy of severe CD. Besides binding and neutralization of TNF-α, infliximab also fixes complement and induces inflammatory T-cell apoptosis, both of which may contribute to its therapeutic efficacy in IBD [35]. In those who are unresponsive to steroid induction or with the need for rapid induction, improvement of symptoms may be seen within several days of the first infusion. A single IV dose of infliximab, 5 mg/kg, had remission rates of 33% at week 4 in patients who had CD with CDAI greater than 220, most of whom were steroid and thiopurine metabolite resistant [36]. Subsequent to this study, considerable additional research and clinical experience showed that single-dose infusions, which are repeated after a long interval "on-demand" for relapses, are associated more with infusion reactions, loss of therapeutic response, and development of antibodies to infliximab (ATI) [37]. Additionally, ATI are more common when infliximab is given without the patient being on long-term immunomodulators or having preinfliximab treatment with corticosteroids [38]. Therefore, current guidelines discourage infliximab as monotherapy. A standard induction protocol for most forms of severe CD is infliximab, 5 mg/kg IV over several hours, which is repeated at weeks 2 and 6. If response is seen following the second dose, maintenance infusions are given every 8 weeks following the 6-week induction period. Mean time to loss of response is approximately 1 year [39]. Dosage escalation to 10 mg/kg for each infusion has been used to overcome drug "resistance" that develops in many individuals over time, but at the possible expense of increased complications. Intra-abdominal abscesses are a contraindication to commencing infliximab, until definitively managed by drainage or resection. Similarly, screening for latent pulmonary tuberculosis (TB) is mandatory before initiation of therapy; severe reactivations of TB were described in the early infliximab experience [40]. Surveillance for complications, including infection and malignancy, also demands periodic clinical and laboratory follow-ups. Details regarding clinical prediction of responses to infliximab are beyond the scope of this article, but the fibrostenosing CD phenotype (usually of terminal ileum) does not respond to infliximab; those patients are managed best with surgical resection or strictureplasty of affected segments if obstruction is occurring.

Adalimumab (Humira) is now the second TNF-α inhibitor to be approved by the US Food and Drug Administration (FDA) as induction and maintenance therapy for moderate-severe CD in those having inadequate response to conventional therapy. It is a recombinant human IgG1 monoclonal antibody that shares similar mechanisms of action with its predecessor, infliximab. Unlike infliximab, however, adalimumab does not contain mouse (chimeric) protein fractions, rather it is made up solely of human-derived heavy and light chain variable regions. Theoretically, this should reduce patient antibody formation toward the drug and associated drug reactions, with better sustained efficacy over time; however, further study and experience with adalimumab is required to corroborate this concept. In a large randomized controlled trial, adalimumab was effective at inducing remission (36% remission at week 2) when given as 160 mg SC initially, followed by 80 mg SC at week two [41]. Lower doses were less effective. Patients had moderate-severe active CD and already were on steroids or immunosuppressors (eg, azathioprine), but were "TNF-α blocker naive." This 36% remission rate result is similar to that for infliximab found in other studies; however, it is unclear whether adalimumab should supersede infliximab as the first "step-up" agent to induce remission in severe CD after failing corticosteroids.

There has been debate over choosing a "top-down" versus "step-up" approach for treatment of CD [42]. The "top-down" approach advocates aggressive therapy with TNF-α blockers before corticosteroids, because many patients eventually progress to the need for surgery, have frequent hospitalizations, and a poor quality of life. It is proposed that similar to rheumatoid arthritis therapy, a "disease-modifying" approach adopted early on in the course of disease may prevent future complications; however, no large trials have been published examining initial therapy with infliximab. Because concerns principally remain about long-term toxicities, the top-down approach has not become the standard of care. This will continue to be a topic of great interest in CD pharmacotherapeutics over the next several years.

Maintenance of remission

Following successful induction of remission, the natural history of CD is of further relapses and remissions for most patients. At 10 years, relapse rates as high as 76% have been documented for colorectal CD, with median time to relapse following induction being 2 years. It is difficult to interpret the literature regarding the role of mesalamine in maintaining remission in CD; however, the benefit seems to be greater in the postoperative setting (see "Special situations" below). When remission follows corticosteroid induction (probably implying a more severe CD subset), mesalamine in the form of Pentasa, 4 g/d, is not effective for maintaining remission at 1 year [43]. A meta-analysis of mesalamine as maintenance therapy concurs with the slight benefit in maintaining ileal CD in remission, or for postoperative (but not medically induced) remissions [44]. Oral budesonide, 6 mg/d, prolongs remission in CD up to 6 months, but not at 1 year [45]. It has been used off-label as an alternative to traditional immunosuppressors if necessary. Methotrexate, 15 mg IM once weekly, maintains remission significantly better than placebo (65% versus 39%) when remission is induced by methotrexate, 25 mg IM weekly [46]. Hepatic or significant renal disease is a contraindication to methotrexate. Several studies have shown the benefit of CD remission maintenance using oral azathioprine, 2 mg/kg/d, or 6-mp, 1.5 mg/kg/d, even when remission is induced by corticosteroids [47]. Although the results are less clear when remission follows azathioprine induction, there still seems to be a benefit over placebo [48]. Azathioprine and 6-mp are the most popular options for maintaining remission in moderate CD; however, long-smoldering concerns regarding a potential lymphoma risk associated with thiopurine metabolites have resurfaced recently [49].

In those in whom remission is induced with primary infusions at weeks 0, 2, and 6, infliximab maintains remission in CD for a mean of 40 weeks (versus 14 weeks with placebo) when given as 5 mg/kg infused IV every 8 weeks [50]. Generally, it is advisable to comaintain immunomodulator use, typically with azathioprine, 6-mp, or methotrexate, because this reduces infliximab immunogenicity and may prolong therapeutic responses [37]. In the Chrohn's Trial of the Fully Human Antibody Adalimumab for Remission Maintenance (CHARM) trial, adalimumab was shown to be effective in moderate-severe CD, with up to 41% maintaining remission at week 56 (versus only 12% with placebo) when given as 40 mg SC weekly [51]. Dosing adalimumab at 40 mg SC every other week was just as efficacious (36%). A second smaller trial Clinical Assessment of Adalimumab Safety and Efficacy Studied as Induction Therapy in Crohn's Disease (CLASSIC II) also confirmed high remission rates with adalimumab, 40 mg SC (79% remission when given every other week or 83% when given weekly), when treatment immediately follows remission induction with adalimumab [52]. The higher remission rates in CLASSIC II compared with CHARM may be due to differences in study design, sample size, and baseline patient characteristics. TNF-α blocker–naive patients may have higher response rates, and the CHARM trial enrolled many more patients than did CLASSIC II. It is unclear whether coadministration of immunomodulators with adalimumab is necessary or safe over the longer term, but efficacy and safety profiles (including serious infections) within CHARM were similar over 1 year with and without immunomodulators [51].

In summary, effective maintenance of remission has been shown for several of the currently used standard therapies in CD, with the exact drug choice being dictated by previous responses, drug toxicity/intolerance, and disease severity. The greatest clinical challenges for maintenance therapy are those patients with severe disease who become refractory to infliximab, typically after 1 or 2 years of continuous injections, and who already are optimized with traditional immunomodulator therapy. These patients become candidates for adalimumab, for newer experimental therapies in clinical trials, or for using less commonly prescribed agents that were shown to be useful in small studies.

Crohn's disease: special situations

Perianal fistulizing Crohn's disease

Sulfasalazine, mesalamine, and corticosteroids are ineffective at primarily controlling fistulizing CD [53]. Antibiotics have been used frequently for this indication (most commonly ciprofloxacin or metronidazole), but short-term clinical improvement is likely related to control of local sepsis, rather than to an inherent property for healing fistulous tracts. Azathioprine and 6-mp have been suggested to speed healing of fistulae (54% response rate overall), as shown by examining a pooled subgroup of CD patients within a meta-analysis of all thiopurine antimetabolite trials [54]; however, these results have been challenged by a retrospective study showing much poorer outcomes [55]. Infliximab has been examined specifically for its efficacy in fistulizing CD, both for induction [56] and maintenance settings [50]. These studies show approximately 50% of patients initially had "response," defined as more than 50% closure of draining fistulae with infliximab, 5 mg/kg at weeks 0, 2, and 6, followed by maintenance infusions, 5 mg/kg every 8 weeks for up to 54 weeks. Similar results are obtained with other immunomodulators, such as tacrolimus [57]; however, long-term data are unavailable, and it is well recognized radiologically that fistulous tracts often persist following infliximab, despite reduced drainage [58]. Clinical experience has suggested that adjunctive surgical therapy for complex fistulizing disease (eg, Seton placement, endorectal advancement flap, diversion procedures) achieves better outcomes and avoids infective complications than medical management alone. Therefore, a multimodality, medical-surgical team approach to dealing with most CD fistulae represents the current standard of care.

Medical management of postoperative recurrence

Historically, more than 70% of patients who have CD require surgery at some point [59]. Whether TNF-α antagonists or other biologic agents will reduce this figure requires further long-term study. Following resection, endoscopic evidence of inflammation is the strictest definition of postoperative recurrence, with the highest anticipated rates from studies using this definition. Conversely, having reoperation is the most liberal definition of postoperative recurrence and is expected to be much lower. Therefore, postoperative recurrence rates vary greatly among prophylactic studies. Because postoperative recurrence using any definition is high without prophylaxis (up to 100% 3 years postoperatively), it is generally desirable to continue medications in the postoperative setting. Mesalamine has a slightly more established role in CD here. A meta-analysis of several trials has concluded that a subset of patients who have ileal CD may have reduced postoperative recurrence rates when mesalamine is used at 4 g/d [60]. Metronidazole, although effective at up to 1 year in preventing endoscopic postoperative recurrence, is not used generally because of adverse effects during sustained therapy. Azathioprine, 2 mg/kg/d for 24 months, was effective at reducing clinical and surgical postoperative recurrence in those who had a previous *bowel resection* [61], but it had postoperative recurrence rates similar to mesalamine in other postoperative subgroups. Higher postoperative recurrence rates may occur in smokers (especially women), those with perforating or fistulizing disease, and possibly those with younger age at diagnosis or short disease duration before surgery [62]. Thus, it is particularly recommended that these patients undertake medical prophylaxis for postoperative recurrence.

Ulcerative colitis

In addition to severity, disease location influences therapeutic strategies for UC. Extent of disease follows more predictable patterns in UC than for CD, with well-recognized boundaries of extent being the sigmoid colon (proctitis) and splenic flexure (left-sided or "distal" colitis). For this reason, management strategies are presented here by disease location and severity; however, clinical end points have varied far more across UC clinical trials than for CD. A review of UC clinical trial end points describes 11 instruments that have been used for measuring clinical disease activity, 9 instruments based on endoscopic disease activity, and at least two composite scoring indices, with at least 10 different definitions of remission cited across the studies [63]. This must be considered when interpreting the "remission rates" referenced below. A general guide to assessing disease severity for this article may be given by the Truelove and Witts Severity Index (Box 2) [64], but therapeutic decision making must remain individualized.

Induction of remission

Mild-moderate distal disease
Usually, but not always, mild disease is restricted to the rectum or left colon. This makes topical therapy with mesalamine suppositories or enemas valuable in UC management. In fact, topical mesalamine is superior to topical corticosteroids for inducing remission in mild-moderate UC extending up to the splenic flexure [65,66]. Typically, mesalamine, 4 g in a 60 mL

Box 2. The Truelove and Witts Severity Index

Severe
Six or more bowel movements per day
Mean evening body temperature greater than 37.5°C
Mean pulse rate greater than 90 beats per minute
Hemoglobin less than 10.5 g/dL
Erythrocyte sedimentation rate (ESR) greater than 30 mm/h

Mild
Less than four bowel movements per day; scant amounts blood
No fever or tachycardia
Mild or absent anemia
ESR less than 30 mm/h

Moderate
Somewhere in between mild and severe

Adapted from Truelove SC, Witts LJ. Cortisone in ulcerative colitis; final report on a therapeutic trial. Br Med J 1955;2(4947):1042.

---

enema suspension, is administered once nightly. Lying on the left side is useful to allow drug migration proximally. Patients usually require encouragement with this treatment, because rectal retention is poor in the early phases when inflammation is greater. A 10% hydrocortisone foam or 100 mg hydrocortisone enema also induces remission and may be tolerated better; however, compared with topical mesalamine these are no more effective for induction, are less effective for maintenance, and carry higher risks for side effects [67–69]. A promising area for drug development is for alternative mesalamine formulations, such as gels and foams with better retention properties. For isolated proctitis, 1000 mg/d mesalamine suppositories are effective at inducing remission in 69% of patients after 4 weeks [70]. This is now available as a 1000-mg single suppository dose in North America. Topical budesonide enemas and foams are as effective as other topical therapies for mild-moderate UC induction, with remission rates up to 66% [71]; however, they are not readily available in North America.

In addition to topical therapy, all oral mesalamine formulations and sulfasalazine are effective in mild-moderate UC [72–75]. More than 40 years ago, sulfasalazine, 4.0 to 6.0 g/d, was shown to be effective [76,77]; however, at these dosages it often is poorly tolerated. Response with sulfasalazine or mesalamine is usually seen within 8 weeks. For mesalamine, typical dosages have ranged between 2.0 and 4.8 g/d. A combination of oral (2.4 g/d) and topical mesalamine (4 g/d rectal enema) is more effective then either drug alone for distal disease [78]. This is a useful strategy for more resistant cases.

Mild-moderate extensive disease

Traditionally, mesalamine was always prescribed at 2.4 g/d for inducing remission [75] in mild-moderate UC, but recent studies have considered improved release formulations and more aggressive dosing schedules [79]. Dosages of mesalamine of less than 2.0 g/d are ineffective for inducing remission. It also is probable that pH-dependent–release mesalamine formulations are less reliably effective than other formulations (see Fig. 2). Balsalazide, a newer diazo-bonded mesalamine preparation (mesalamine bonded to an inert carrier), may be more effective at dosages of 6.75 g/d than pH-dependent–release mesalamine at 2.4 g/d [80] for mild UC. There is also a dose-response gradient with pH-dependent mesalamine, however, with induction occurring more effectively at 4.8 g/d than the FDA-approved dosage of 2.4 g/d, or 1.6 g/d, which is no more effective than placebo [81]. A more recent study also suggested that 4.8 g/d of pH-dependent mesalamine is more effective to induce remission in moderately active UC (72% remission) than is 2.4 g/d (59% remission) after 6 weeks of therapy [82]. As with distal colitis, a combination of oral (4.0 g/d) and topical mesalamine is superior to oral mesalamine monotherapy (64% versus 43% remission at 8 weeks, $P = .03$), even when using a reduced-dosage 1.0 g/d rectal mesalamine enema [83]. This again suggests that higher overall doses of mesalamine delivered directly to inflamed colonic mucosa may be more effective at inducing remission. From these studies, it also is clear that remission rates continue to increase for up to 8 weeks of induction therapy; therefore, therapy should not be discontinued prematurely. A new, once-daily high-concentration multi matrix system (MMX) mesalamine formulation may improve patient adherence. When given once daily at 2.4 g/d or 4.8 g/d, MMX mesalamine induced clinical remission in 41% of patients versus 22% with placebo [84]. The FDA has given approval for this formulation as therapy for mild-moderate active UC.

If the initial induction regimen with oral or topical mesalamine is ineffective or clinical deterioration ensues early on, oral corticosteroids may be used. Several studies showed that prednisone, 40 to 60 mg/d, is effective induction therapy [64,85,86]. Remission rates are 55% to 65% at 30 to 35 days [86,87]. The exact timing and method of steroid tapering remains more an art than a science; see the section on induction of remission in moderate-severe CD for typical schedules, which also are used in UC. Although oral budesonide was shown to be effective in active UC, most of these studies did not use the controlled ileal release formulation.

Severe (usually extensive) and fulminant disease

As regards refractory distal colitis, it should be remembered that disease severity and disease extent (location) in UC do not always coincide. In other words, severe or refractory chronic ulcerative proctitis may be disabling, and on rare occasion it is an indication for total restorative proctocolectomy. The therapeutic approaches listed above should be tried aggressively first, however. Commonly, these have not been accelerated enough or maximized before being deemed ineffective, and this is important when making surgical decisions, following discussions of risks/benefits/costs with the patient. A "top-down" therapeutic strategy using TNF-α blockers has not been studied for severe UC naive to other therapies. Notwithstanding these comments, up to 15% of patients who have UC will have severe colitis and are less likely to respond to first-line conventional therapies; it is these patients with whom surgeons will be most acquainted. If the patient presents with a more fulminant course, hospitalization is required and IV corticosteroids should be instituted. IV prednisolone, 60 mg/d, induces remission in 64% of patients after 5 days [88,89]. On average, 50% response rates are seen across all studies [48]. A 10-day trial is considered sufficient to determine response, with little incremental benefit (and possibly toxic complications) beyond this. Bolus infusions fare as well as continuous infusions [90]. If oral and topical mesalamine and oral or IV corticosteroids have failed, traditionally the next step is total proctocolectomy. In selected patients, IV cyclosporine (as rescue therapy in patients failing IV corticosteroids; see later discussion) or infliximab can be considered, but the elderly and those with comorbid conditions, such as chronic cardiovascular or renal disease, are at higher risk from complications. Antibiotics have been studied in small trials, some showing benefit [91] and others showing no benefit [92–94]. One editor's letter reported no significant remission induction benefit over placebo in severe UC with oral rifaximin, 400 mg twice a day for 10 days [95], but there was some clinical improvement. This study only included 28 patients. No larger studies are available at this time. Despite some negative results (and similar to its use in CD in the absence of robust evidence), clinical intuition suggests that IV antibiotics might help to prevent sepsis in the setting of a severely inflamed colon. Therefore, they are added commonly to the induction regimen for hospitalized patients; however, worsening symptoms also may indicate superinfection with bacteria, such as *Clostridium difficile*, for which broad-spectrum antibiotics, including quinolones, are clearly a risk factor [96]. Repeat stool cultures and toxin assays for *C difficile* should be obtained.

Regarding antimetabolite immunomodulators, methotrexate cannot be recommended for UC induction therapy, based only on the results of one negative double-blind placebo-controlled study using 12.5 mg orally per week for 9 months [97]. Azathioprine and 6-mp have been studied more extensively in this role, but there is no consensus of results. These two agents do not improve outcome in the short-run for patients hospitalized with severe UC, but if a response is seen with other medical management, they may be considered for early introduction as maintenance agents [48]. IV cyclosporine was shown to "salvage" up to 82% of severe UC nonresponders to IV corticosteroids [98], averting colectomy and permitting discharge from hospital. Smaller doses may be as effective as larger ones [99]; however, its use does not remain widespread because of the significant potential for toxicities (see Appendix 1) [100] and the fact that colectomy is not averted over the longer term in many patients [101]. Effective transitioning to maintenance therapy probably requires intensive combination regimens involving simultaneous oral antibiotics (prophylactic for *Pneumocystis carinii*), corticosteroids, azathioprine, and oral cyclosporine.

Infliximab promises to revolutionize therapy for treatment-refractory, but ambulatory patients who have UC. When given as 5 mg/kg infusions at weeks 0, 2, and 6 to patients failing conventional medical management (including corticosteroids), infliximab induced "response" in 64% to 69% of patients at week 8 (versus 29%–37% for placebo, $P<.001$) [102]. Remission occurred in 39% of patients given infliximab at week 8 versus 15% with placebo in "ACT 1" of the study. Infliximab is approved by the FDA for induction therapy in UC. This new evidence is likely to reduce referrals for total proctocolectomy over the short range. Infliximab also has been used as a substitute for IV cyclosporine in hospitalized patients who had severe UC that was refractory to IV corticosteroids. A small series reported 77% clinical response to a single infliximab infusion of 5 mg/kg, with 80% of responders remaining in clinical remission after 2 years [103]. A slightly larger randomized, double-blind, placebo-controlled trial showed that in 45 hospitalized patients who had severe steroid-refractory UC, 67% of the placebo group required proctocolectomy within 1 month versus 29% of those receiving a single infusion of infliximab, 5 mg/kg ($P = .017$) [104]. Follow-up was to 90 days. Although the pretreatment severity details are not directly available for comparison, this result is similar to the IV cyclosporine trials. Thus, it is doubtful that IV cyclosporine, with its considerable potential for toxicities, can remain justifiable as a "last-resort" medical alternative to proctocolectomy in hospitalized patients who have severe UC. How long infliximab might be able to avert proctocolectomy in the long-term is unclear. As a comparison, the mean duration of infliximab efficacy in CD is only about 1 year [39] (see "Maintenance of UC remission" below). As well, the outcome and postoperative complications associated with urgent proctocolectomy following failed infliximab therapy should receive research attention in the combined medical-surgical arena. A small series suggests no increase in postoperative complications with failed IV cyclosporine followed by proctocolectomy [105], and postoperative complications do not seem to be higher using infliximab in CD [106]; however, the total volume of data available in this regard is small.

Maintenance of ulcerative colitis remission

5'-aminosalicylates and sulfasalazine are first-line therapies as maintenance agents for UC. There is strong evidence for this effect from multiple studies. An updated pooled analysis from a Cochrane Collaboration review of the literature showed an odds ratio (OR) for relapse of 0.47 (95% confidence interval [CI]: 0.36–0.62) for mesalamine versus placebo, but also a superior effect of sulfasalazine versus mesalamine, even at sulfasalazine dosages of 2 g/d [107]. A dosage-dependent effect was not observed for maintenance mesalamine, but this is not as well established because of lower statistical power from existing trials. In distal colitis, topical mesalamine also maintains remission, even when followed for 2 years (for summary of UC maintenance topical mesalamine trials see Ref. [108]). In one study, remission at 2 years was maintained in 74% of patients using 4-g mesalamine enemas every third night versus 32% remission with oral mesalamine, 1.5 g/d [109]. Other studies have confirmed the efficacy of twice or thrice weekly topical mesalamine. Thus, reduced-frequency rectal mesalamine schedules that decrease total medication inconveniences, risks, and costs may be an attractive alternative to maintaining remission in mild-moderate distal UC for those patients who are willing to continue it. As with CD, corticosteroids should not be used for maintenance therapy. In addition to side effects, relapse rates at 10 months are unacceptably high (50%) [110]. The data are not convincing regarding methotrexate as maintenance therapy in UC; therefore, this drug also is not currently recommended. As cited above, a 9-month randomized trial in UC used methotrexate, 12.5 mg/wk orally [97], which is a different route and lower dosage than shown to be effective for maintaining remission in CD [46]. Further studies are required here. There is evidence for a benefit of maintenance therapy with azathioprine, although the evidence is weaker than for its role in CD. A pooled analysis reported a significant OR for likelihood of relapse (OR, 0.41; 95% CI: 0.24–0.70) [111] when compared with placebo, but significant concerns persist because of the weakness of evidence relative to the potential risks of long-term immunosuppression. A recent randomized trial compared azathioprine, 2 mg/kg/d, with mesalamine, 3.2 g/d for 6 months, in patients who had UC and failed corticosteroid tapers [112]. This study strengthens the case for azathioprine. Adverse effects required withdrawal of treatment in only two individuals. Fifty-three percent of the group that received azathioprine treatment achieved clinical and endoscopic remission versus 19% for mesalamine ($P<.01$). TNF-α blockers are also being used for UC maintenance therapy. Infliximab also has found a new role here [102], with remission being maintained at week 54 in 45% of those receiving infusions of 5 mg/kg versus 20% remission rates with placebo. The long-term extent of response to infliximab remains unclear.

Ulcerative colitis: special situations

Pouchitis

Pouchitis is an idiopathic, nonspecific inflammation of the ileal pouch reservoir created during an ileal-pouch anal anastomosis (IPAA), usually for medically refractory UC. Endoscopy may reveal erythema, granularity, and friability of the mucosa, erosions, or ulcerations. Histology may reveal acute inflammation with neutrophils, crypt abscesses, and mucosal disruption superimposed on features of chronic inflammation. There has been great diversity regarding diagnostic criteria for pouchitis, making direct comparisons of therapeutic studies difficult. The etiology of pouchitis remains unknown. Some cases eventually may become diagnosed as CD, but this is uncommon. Following IPAA, about 50% of patients have at least one episode of pouchitis after 8 to 10 years of follow-up [113]. Of these, 10% who experience a single episode will not have further recurrence. Conversely, two thirds of this group experiences more than one episode of acute pouchitis, especially if the first episode occurs within 2 years of IPAA creation. These patients usually respond well to antibiotic treatment [114,115]. Up to one fifth of patients who have pouchitis have a form of "chronic" pouchitis, some of whom are refractory to standard antibiotics; however, a combination of ciprofloxacin plus rifaximin or metronidazole antibiotic therapy may lead to improvement, even in this setting [116,117]. As well, probiotics have a proven role for chronic pouchitis. Of many studies for probiotic therapy in IBD to date, the best evidence is for prevention of chronic pouchitis relapse. A double-blind, randomized, placebo-controlled clinical trial using VSL#3 (VSL#3 in USA Sigma-Tau Consumer Products, Gaithersburg, MD 20877; VSL#3 in Europe: Sigma-Tau Industrie Farmaceutiche Riunite S.p.A., Roma, Italy) was conducted in patients initially in remission after 1 month of antibiotic treatment. VSL#3, 3.0 g twice daily, was given for 9 months. Relapse occurred in 15% of patients who were treated with VSL#3 versus 100% of patients in the placebo group ($P < .001$) [118]. Adverse effects are negligible. An algorithm for the treatment of pouchitis has been proposed [119]: if one establishes the diagnosis of acute pouchitis, metronidazole, 250 mg three times daily, or ciprofloxacin, 500 mg two times daily, should be given for at least 2 weeks. The subset of patients who relapse may be treated with prolonged courses of the same antibiotics or with combination antibiotics. Remission should be maintained with probiotics; however, positive randomized clinical trial evidence is only available using the VSL#3 formulation. Similarly, chronic refractory pouchitis may be treated with aggressive antibiotic combinations, then with probiotics once in remission. If no response is seen, topical corticosteroids may be tried. Those remaining refractory to all medical therapy may require pouch revision or excision. A small first study of infliximab plus azathioprine for chronic refractory pouchitis suggests good clinical response [120], but larger positive studies are required before this approach can be recommended.

Appendix 1

Adverse effects of medical therapies for inflammatory bowel disease

Sulfasalazine
   Dyspepsia
   Nausea, vomiting

Fever, malaise
Allergy (rash, hives, arthralgia, hemolysis, anaphylaxis)
Toxic epidermal necrolysis (Stevens-Johnson syndrome)
Drug-induced lupus syndrome
Headache
Oligospermia, male infertility (reversible upon discontinuation)
Hepatotoxicity
Nephrotoxicity
Pulmonary toxicity
Myelosuppression
Megaloblastic anemia (folic acid malabsorption)

Mesalamine
Diarrhea (especially olsalazine)
Abdominal pain
Dyspepsia
Nausea and vomiting
Rash
Headache
Hair loss, alopecia
Nephritic syndrome, interstitial nephritis (rare)
Pericarditis, myocarditis (rare)
Pancreatitis
Hepatitis

Ciprofloxacin
Nausea and vomiting
Headache
Paresthesiae, seizures
Rash, photosensitivity, exfoliative dermatitis
Allergy, hypersensitivity
Elevated liver enzymes
Interstitial nephritis
Anxiety/psychosis
Diarrhea, pseudomembranous colitis
Tendon rupture

Metronidazole
Nausea, vomiting
Dysgeusia (altered taste, metallic taste)
Stomatitis, dry mouth, glossitis
Illness (nausea, vomiting, abdominal pain, fever: 'Disulfiram-like reaction')
   with ethanol coingestion
Paresthesiae (sometimes irreversible)
Diarrhea, pseudomembranous colitis

718 TAMBOLI

Neutropenia, leukopenia
Electrocardiogram changes
Cystitis, dysuria

Rifaximin
Diarrhea
Abdominal pain, cramps
Nausea, vomiting
Fatigue

Corticosteroids (prednisone > budesonide)
Mood changes, insomnia
Increased appetite, weight gain
Cushingoid appearance ("moon face," "buffalo hump")
Edema
Hyperglycemia, diabetes mellitus
Acne, striae
Hirsutism
Alopecia
Infection, impaired wound healing
Osteoporosis
Avascular bone necrosis
Cataracts
Narrow-angle glaucoma
Adrenal axis suppression (including budesonide)
Hypertension
Hypercholesterolemia
Hypokalemia
Myopathy
Growth retardation in children

Thiopurine antimetabolites (azathioprine and 6-mercaptopurine)
Allergy (rash, hives, anaphylaxis)
Pancreatitis (<5%)
Leukopenia, bone marrow suppression
Infection
Elevated liver enzymes, hepatotoxicity
"Flu"-like symptoms, malaise, myalgia
Nausea, vomiting
Malignancy (lymphoma)
Skin rash
Arthralgia

Methotrexate
Anorexia, malaise, diarrhea
Fever, chills

Nausea, vomiting
Stomatitis, gingivitis, pharyngitis
Rash, photosensitivity
Toxic epidermal necrolysis (Stevens-Johnson syndrome)
Leukopenia
Infection
Megaloblastic anemia (folate metabolism antagonism)
Alopecia
Hepatotoxicity, hepatic fibrosis
Neuropathy
Nephrotoxicity
Interstitial pneumonitis
Pericarditis
Pleural effusion
Malignancy (?)

Cyclosporine
Opportunistic infection (*eg. Pneumocystis carinii*)
Hypomagnesemia
Headache
Tremor, paresthesiae, seizures
Hypercholesterolemia
Hypertension
Nephrotoxicity - common (sometimes irreversible)
Hepatotoxicity
Gingival hyperplasia
Hirsutism

Infliximab, adalimumab
Headache
Fatigue, myalgia
Acute infusion reactions (local site irritation, rash, fever, arthralgia, back
   pain)
Allergy (rash, hypersensitivity, anaphylaxis)
Delayed infusion reactions (rash, arthralgia, renal dysfunction, lupus-like
   syndrome)
Infections (including reactivation tuberculosis), fungal infections
Reactivated chronic hepatitis B infection
Respiratory: naso-sinopulmonary infections, dyspnea, bronchitis
Neurotoxicity (multiple sclerosis, peripheral demyelination, optic neuritis)
Malignancy (?), lymphoma
Pancytopenia
Worsening congestive heart failure

References

[1] Silverberg MS, Satsangi J, Ahmad T, et al. Toward an integrated clinical, molecular and serological classification of inflammatory bowel disease: report of a working party of the 2005 Montreal World Congress of Gastroenterology. Can J Gastroenterol 2005; 19(Suppl A):5–36.

[2] Kane SV. Systematic review: adherence issues in the treatment of ulcerative colitis. Aliment Pharmacol Ther 2006;23(5):577–85.

[3] Dubinsky MC. Azathioprine, 6-mercaptopurine in inflammatory bowel disease: pharmacology, efficacy, and safety. Clin Gastroenterol Hepatol 2004;2(9):731–43.

[4] Best WR, Becktel JM, Singleton JW. Rederived values of the eight coefficients of the Crohn's Disease Activity Index (CDAI). Gastroenterology 1979;77(4 Pt 2):843–6.

[5] Malchow H, Ewe K, Brandes JW, et al. European Cooperative Crohn's Disease Study (ECCDS): results of drug treatment. Gastroenterology 1984;86(2):249–66.

[6] Summers RW, Switz DM, Sessions JT Jr, et al. National Cooperative Crohn's Disease Study: results of drug treatment. Gastroenterology 1979;77(4 Pt 2):847–69.

[7] Ursing B, Alm T, Barany F, et al. A comparative study of metronidazole and sulfasalazine for active Crohn's disease: the cooperative Crohn's Disease Study in Sweden. II. Result. Gastroenterology 1982;83(3):550–62.

[8] Azad Khan AK, Piris J, Truelove SC. An experiment to determine the active therapeutic moiety of sulphasalazine. Lancet 1977;2(8044):892–5.

[9] Singleton JW, Hanauer SB, Gitnick GL, et al. Mesalamine capsules for the treatment of active Crohn's disease: results of a 16-week trial. Pentasa Crohn's Disease Study Group. Gastroenterology 1993;104(5):1293–301.

[10] Hanauer SB, Stromberg U. Oral Pentasa in the treatment of active Crohn's disease: a meta-analysis of double-blind, placebo-controlled trials. Clin Gastroenterol Hepatol 2004;2(5): 379–88.

[11] Tremaine WJ, Schroeder KW, Harrison JM, et al. A randomized, double-blind, placebo-controlled trial of the oral mesalamine (5-ASA) preparation, Asacol, in the treatment of symptomatic Crohn's colitis and ileocolitis. J Clin Gastroenterol 1994;19(4):278–82.

[12] Sartor RB. Mechanisms of disease: pathogenesis of Crohn's disease and ulcerative colitis. Nat Clin Pract Gastroenterol Hepatol 2006;3(7):390–407.

[13] Colombel JF, Lemann M, Cassagnou M, et al. A controlled trial comparing ciprofloxacin with mesalazine for the treatment of active Crohn's disease. Groupe d'Etudes Therapeutiques des Affections Inflammatoires Digestives (GETAID). Am J Gastroenterol 1999; 94(3):674–8.

[14] Rosen A, Ursing B, Alm T, et al. A comparative study of metronidazole and sulfasalazine for active Crohn's disease: the cooperative Crohn's Disease Study in Sweden. I. Design and methodologic considerations. Gastroenterology 1982;83(3):541–9.

[15] Sutherland L, Singleton J, Sessions J, et al. Double blind, placebo controlled trial of metronidazole in Crohn's disease. Gut 1991;32(9):1071–5.

[16] Gerard L, Garey KW, DuPont HL. Rifaximin: a nonabsorbable rifamycin antibiotic for use in nonsystemic gastrointestinal infections. Expert Rev Anti Infect Ther 2005;3(2): 201–11.

[17] Prantera C, Lochs H, Campieri M, et al. Antibiotic treatment of Crohn's disease: results of a multicentre, double blind, randomized, placebo-controlled trial with rifaximin. Aliment Pharmacol Ther 2006;23(8):1117–25.

[18] Lichtenstein GR, Feagan BG, Cohen RD, et al. Serious infections and mortality in association with therapies for Crohn's disease: TREAT registry. Clin Gastroenterol Hepatol 2006;4(5):621–30.

[19] Greenberg GR, Feagan BG, Martin F, et al. Oral budesonide for active Crohn's disease. Canadian Inflammatory Bowel Disease Study Group. N Engl J Med 1994;331(13):836–41.

[20] Tremaine WJ, Hanauer SB, Katz S, et al. Budesonide CIR capsules (once or twice daily divided-dose) in active Crohn's disease: a randomized placebo-controlled study in the United States. Am J Gastroenterol 2002;97(7):1748–54.

[21] Thomsen OO, Cortot A, Jewell D, et al. A comparison of budesonide and mesalamine for active Crohn's disease. International Budesonide-Mesalamine Study Group. N Engl J Med 1998;339(6):370–4.

[22] Present DH, Meltzer SJ, Krumholz MP, et al. 6-Mercaptopurine in the management of inflammatory bowel disease: short- and long-term toxicity. Ann Intern Med 1989;111(8): 641–9.

[23] Chun A, Chadi RM, Korelitz BI, et al. Intravenous corticotrophin vs. hydrocortisone in the treatment of hospitalized patients with Crohn's disease: a randomized double-blind study and follow-up. Inflamm Bowel Dis 1998;4(3):177–81.

[24] Fernandez-Banares F, Cabre E, Esteve-Comas M, et al. How effective is enteral nutrition in inducing clinical remission in active Crohn's disease? A meta-analysis of the randomized clinical trials. JPEN J Parenter Enteral Nutr 1995;19(5):356–64.

[25] O'Morain C, Segal AW, Levi AJ. Elemental diet as primary treatment of acute Crohn's disease: a controlled trial. Br Med J (Clin Res Ed) 1984;288(6434):1859–62.

[26] Giaffer MH, North G, Holdsworth CD. Controlled trial of polymeric versus elemental diet in treatment of active Crohn's disease. Lancet 1990;335(8693):816–9.

[27] Mansfield JC, Giaffer MH, Holdsworth CD. Controlled trial of oligopeptide versus amino acid diet in treatment of active Crohn's disease. Gut 1995;36(1):60–6.

[28] Verma S, Brown S, Kirkwood B, et al. Polymeric versus elemental diet as primary treatment in active Crohn's disease: a randomized, double-blind trial. Am J Gastroenterol 2000;95(3): 735–9.

[29] Suzuki H, Hanyou N, Sonaka I, et al. An elemental diet controls inflammation in indomethacin-induced small bowel disease in rats: the role of low dietary fat and the elimination of dietary proteins. Dig Dis Sci 2005;50(10):1951–8.

[30] Middleton SJ, Rucker JT, Kirby GA, et al. Long-chain triglycerides reduce the efficacy of enteral feeds in patients with active Crohn's disease. Clin Nutr 1995;14(4): 229–36.

[31] Sandborn W, Sutherland L, Pearson D, et al. Azathioprine or 6-mercaptopurine for inducing remission of Crohn's disease. Cochrane Database Syst Rev 2000;(2):CD000545.

[32] Dubinsky MC, Reyes E, Ofman J, et al. A cost-effectiveness analysis of alternative disease management strategies in patients with Crohn's disease treated with azathioprine or 6-mercaptopurine. Am J Gastroenterol 2005;100(10):2239–47.

[33] Siegel CA, Sands BE. Review article: practical management of inflammatory bowel disease patients taking immunomodulators. Aliment Pharmacol Ther 2005;22(1):1–16.

[34] Feagan BG, Rochon J, Fedorak RN, et al. Methotrexate for the treatment of Crohn's disease. The North American Crohn's Study Group Investigators. N Engl J Med 1995;332(5): 292–7.

[35] Sands BE. New therapies for the treatment of inflammatory bowel disease. Surg Clin North Am 2006;86(4):1045–64.

[36] Targan SR, Hanauer SB, van Deventer SJ, et al. A short-term study of chimeric monoclonal antibody cA2 to tumor necrosis factor alpha for Crohn's disease. Crohn's Disease cA2 Study Group. N Engl J Med 1997;337(15):1029–35.

[37] Baert F, Noman M, Vermeire S, et al. Influence of immunogenicity on the long-term efficacy of infliximab in Crohn's disease. N Engl J Med 2003;348(7):601–8.

[38] Farrell RJ, Alsahli M, Jeen YT, et al. Intravenous hydrocortisone premedication reduces antibodies to infliximab in Crohn's disease: a randomized controlled trial. Gastroenterology 2003;124(4):917–24.

[39] Hanauer SB, Feagan BG, Lichtenstein GR, et al. Maintenance infliximab for Crohn's disease: the ACCENT I randomised trial. Lancet 2002;359(9317):1541–9.

[40] Keane J, Gershon S, Wise RP, et al. Tuberculosis associated with infliximab, a tumor necrosis factor alpha-neutralizing agent. N Engl J Med 2001;345(15):1098–104.

[41] Hanauer SB, Sandborn WJ, Rutgeerts P, et al. Human anti-tumor necrosis factor monoclonal antibody (adalimumab) in Crohn's disease: the CLASSIC-I trial. Gastroenterology 2006;130(2):323–33.

[42] Hanauer SB. Crohn's disease: step up or top down therapy. Best Pract Res Clin Gastroenterol 2003;17(1):131–7.

[43] Modigliani R, Colombel JF, Dupas JL, et al. Mesalamine in Crohn's disease with steroid-induced remission: effect on steroid withdrawal and remission maintenance, Groupe d'Etudes Therapeutiques des Affections Inflammatoires Digestives. Gastroenterology 1996;110(3):688–93.

[44] Camma C, Giunta M, Rosselli M, et al. Mesalamine in the maintenance treatment of Crohn's disease: a meta-analysis adjusted for confounding variables. Gastroenterology 1997;113(5):1465–73.

[45] Greenberg GR, Feagan BG, Martin F, et al. Oral budesonide as maintenance treatment for Crohn's disease: a placebo-controlled, dose-ranging study. Canadian Inflammatory Bowel Disease Study Group. Gastroenterology 1996;110(1):45–51.

[46] Feagan BG, Fedorak RN, Irvine EJ, et al. A comparison of methotrexate with placebo for the maintenance of remission in Crohn's disease. North American Crohn's Study Group Investigators. N Engl J Med 2000;342(22):1627–32.

[47] Pearson DC, May GR, Fick G, et al. Azathioprine for maintaining remission of Crohn's disease. Cochrane Database Syst Rev 2000;(2):CD000067.

[48] Lichtenstein GR, Abreu MT, Cohen R, et al. American Gastroenterological Association Institute technical review on corticosteroids, immunomodulators, and infliximab in inflammatory bowel disease. Gastroenterology 2006;130(3):940–87.

[49] Kandiel A, Fraser AG, Korelitz BI, et al. Increased risk of lymphoma among inflammatory bowel disease patients treated with azathioprine and 6-mercaptopurine. Gut 2005;54(8): 1121–5.

[50] Sands BE, Anderson FH, Bernstein CN, et al. Infliximab maintenance therapy for fistulizing Crohn's disease. N Engl J Med 2004;350(9):876–85.

[51] Colombel JF, Sandborn WJ, Rutgeerts P, et al. Adalimumab for maintenance of clinical response and remission in patients with Crohn's disease: the CHARM trial. Gastroenterology 2007;132(1):52–65.

[52] Sandborn WJ, Hanauer SB, Rutgeerts PJ, et al. Adalimumab for maintenance treatment of Crohn's disease: results of the CLASSIC II Trial. Gut 2007; in press.

[53] Gelbmann CM, Rogler G, Gross V, et al. Prior bowel resections, perianal disease, and a high initial Crohn's disease activity index are associated with corticosteroid resistance in active Crohn's disease. Am J Gastroenterol 2002;97(6):1438–45.

[54] Pearson DC, May GR, Fick GH, et al. Azathioprine and 6-mercaptopurine in Crohn disease. A meta-analysis. Ann Intern Med 1995;123(2):132–42.

[55] Lecomte T, Contou JF, Beaugerie L, et al. Predictive factors of response of perianal Crohn's disease to azathioprine or 6-mercaptopurine. Dis Colon Rectum 2003;46(11): 1469–75.

[56] Present DH, Rutgeerts P, Targan S, et al. Infliximab for the treatment of fistulas in patients with Crohn's disease. N Engl J Med 1999;340(18):1398–405.

[57] Sandborn WJ, Present DH, Isaacs KL, et al. Tacrolimus for the treatment of fistulas in patients with Crohn's disease: a randomized, placebo-controlled trial. Gastroenterology 2003;125(2):380–8.

[58] Parsi MA, Lashner BA, Achkar JP, et al. Type of fistula determines response to infliximab in patients with fistulous Crohn's disease. Am J Gastroenterol 2004;99(3):445–9.

[59] Caprilli R, Gassull MA, Escher JC, et al. European evidence-based consensus on the diagnosis and management of Crohn's disease: special situations. Gut 2006;55(Suppl 1):i36–58.

[60] Cottone M, Camma C. Mesalamine and relapse prevention in Crohn's disease. Gastroenterology 2000;119(2):597.

[61] Ardizzone S, Maconi G, Sampietro GM, et al. Azathioprine and mesalamine for prevention of relapse after conservative surgery for Crohn's disease. Gastroenterology 2004;127(3): 730–40.

[62] Van Assche G, Rutgeerts P. Medical management of postoperative recurrence in Crohn's disease. Gastroenterol Clin North Am 2004;33(2):347–60.

[63] D'Haens G, Sandborn WJ, Feagan BG, et al. A review of activity indices and efficacy end points for clinical trials of medical therapy in adults with ulcerative colitis. Gastroenterology 2007;132(2):763–86.

[64] Truelove SC, Witts LJ. Cortisone in ulcerative colitis; final report on a therapeutic trial. Br Med J 1955;2(4947):1041–8.

[65] Danish 5-ASA Group. Topical 5-aminosalicylic acid versus prednisolone in ulcerative proctosigmoiditis. A randomized, double-blind multicenter trial. Dig Dis Sci 1987;32(6): 598–602.

[66] Marshall JK, Irvine EJ. Rectal corticosteroids versus alternative treatments in ulcerative colitis: a meta-analysis. Gut 1997;40(6):775–81.

[67] Sutherland LR. Topical treatment of ulcerative colitis. Med Clin North Am 1990;74(1): 119–31.

[68] Watkinson G. Treatment of ulcerative colitis with topical hydrocortisone hemisuccinate sodium; a controlled trial employing restricted sequential analysis. Br Med J 1958; 2(5103):1077–82.

[69] Truelove SC, Hambling MH. Treatment of ulcerative colitis with local hydrocortisone hemisuccinate sodium; a report on a controlled therapeutic trial. Br Med J 1958;2(5103): 1072–7.

[70] Campieri M, De Franchis R, Bianchi Porro G, et al. Mesalazine (5-aminosalicylic acid) suppositories in the treatment of ulcerative proctitis or distal proctosigmoiditis. A randomized controlled trial. Scand J Gastroenterol 1990;25(7):663–8.

[71] Gross V, Bar-Meir S, Lavy A, et al. Budesonide foam versus budesonide enema in active ulcerative proctitis and proctosigmoiditis. Aliment Pharmacol Ther 2006;23(2):303–12.

[72] Sutherland LR, May GR, Shaffer EA. Sulfasalazine revisited: a meta-analysis of 5-aminosalicylic acid in the treatment of ulcerative colitis. Ann Intern Med 1993;118(7):540–9.

[73] Meyers S, Sachar DB, Present DH, et al. Olsalazine sodium in the treatment of ulcerative colitis among patients intolerant of sulfasalazine. A prospective, randomized, placebo-controlled, double-blind, dose-ranging clinical trial. Gastroenterology 1987;93(6): 1255–62.

[74] Sninsky CA, Cort DH, Shanahan F, et al. Oral mesalamine (Asacol) for mildly to moderately active ulcerative colitis. A multicenter study. Ann Intern Med 1991;115(5):350–5.

[75] Sutherland L, Macdonald JK, Lennard-Jones JE, et al. Oral 5-aminosalicylic acid for induction of remission in ulcerative colitis. Cochrane Database Syst Rev 2006;(2):CD000543.

[76] Baron JH, Connell AM, Lennard-Jones JE, et al. Sulphasalazine and salicylazosulphadimidine in ulcerative colitis. Lancet 1962;1:1094–6.

[77] Dick AP, Grayson MJ, Carpenter RG, et al. Controlled trial of sulphasalazine in the treatment of ulcerative colitis. Gut 1964;5:437–42.

[78] Safdi M, DeMicco M, Sninsky C, et al. A double-blind comparison of oral versus rectal mesalamine versus combination therapy in the treatment of distal ulcerative colitis. Am J Gastroenterol 1997;92(10):1867–71.

[79] Hanauer SB. Review article: high-dose aminosalicylates to induce and maintain remissions in ulcerative colitis. Aliment Pharmacol Ther 2006;24(Suppl 3):37–40.

[80] Green JR, Lobo AJ, Holdsworth CD, et al. Balsalazide is more effective and better tolerated than mesalamine in the treatment of acute ulcerative colitis. The Abacus Investigator Group. Gastroenterology 1998;114(1):15–22.

[81] Schroeder KW, Tremaine WJ, Ilstrup DM. Coated oral 5-aminosalicylic acid therapy for mildly to moderately active ulcerative colitis. A randomized study. N Engl J Med 1987; 317(26):1625–9.

[82] Hanauer SB, Sandborn WJ, Kornbluth A, et al. Delayed-release oral mesalamine at 4.8 g/ day (800 mg tablet) for the treatment of moderately active ulcerative colitis: the ASCEND II trial. Am J Gastroenterol 2005;100(11):2478–85.

[83] Marteau P, Probert CS, Lindgren S, et al. Combined oral and enema treatment with Pentasa (mesalazine) is superior to oral therapy alone in patients with extensive mild/moderate active ulcerative colitis: a randomised, double blind, placebo controlled study. Gut 2005; 54(7):960–5.

[84] Kamm MA, Sandborn WJ, Gassull M, et al. Once-daily, high-concentration MMX mesalamine in active ulcerative colitis. Gastroenterology 2007;132(1):66–75 [quiz: 432–3].

[85] Lennard-Jones JE, Longmore AJ, Newell AC, et al. An assessment of prednisone, salazopyrin, and topical hydrocortisone hemisuccinate used as out-patient treatment for ulcerative colitis. Gut 1960;1:217–22.

[86] Baron JH, Connell AM, Kanaghinis TG, et al. Out-patient treatment of ulcerative colitis. Comparison between three doses of oral prednisone. Br Med J 1962;2(5302): 441–3.

[87] Faubion WA Jr, Loftus EV Jr, Harmsen WS, et al. The natural history of corticosteroid therapy for inflammatory bowel disease: a population-based study. Gastroenterology 2001;121(2):255–60.

[88] Truelove SC, Willoughby CP, Lee EG, et al. Further experience in the treatment of severe attacks of ulcerative colitis. Lancet 1978;2(8099):1086–8.

[89] Truelove SC, Jewell DP. Intensive intravenous regimen for severe attacks of ulcerative colitis. Lancet 1974;1(7866):1067–70.

[90] Bossa F, Fiorella S, Caruso N, et al. Continuous infusion versus bolus administration of steroids in severe attacks of ulcerative colitis: a randomized, double-blind trial. Am J Gastroenterol 2007;102(3):601–8.

[91] Burke DA, Axon AT, Clayden SA, et al. The efficacy of tobramycin in the treatment of ulcerative colitis. Aliment Pharmacol Ther 1990;4(2):123–9.

[92] Chapman RW, Selby WS, Jewell DP. Controlled trial of intravenous metronidazole as an adjunct to corticosteroids in severe ulcerative colitis. Gut 1986;27(10):1210–2.

[93] Dickinson RJ, O'Connor HJ, Pinder I, et al. Double blind controlled trial of oral vancomycin as adjunctive treatment in acute exacerbations of idiopathic colitis. Gut 1985;26(12): 1380–4.

[94] Mantzaris GJ, Petraki K, Archavlis E, et al. A prospective randomized controlled trial of intravenous ciprofloxacin as an adjunct to corticosteroids in acute, severe ulcerative colitis. Scand J Gastroenterol 2001;36(9):971–4.

[95] Gionchetti P, Rizzello F, Ferrieri A, et al. Rifaximin in patients with moderate or severe ulcerative colitis refractory to steroid-treatment: a double-blind, placebo-controlled trial. Dig Dis Sci 1999;44(6):1220–1.

[96] Loo VG, Poirier L, Miller MA, et al. A predominantly clonal multi-institutional outbreak of Clostridium difficile-associated diarrhea with high morbidity and mortality. N Engl J Med 2005;353(23):2442–9.

[97] Oren R, Arber N, Odes S, et al. Methotrexate in chronic active ulcerative colitis: a double-blind, randomized, Israeli multicenter trial. Gastroenterology 1996;110(5):1416–21.

[98] Lichtiger S, Present DH, Kornbluth A, et al. Cyclosporine in severe ulcerative colitis refractory to steroid therapy. N Engl J Med 1994;330(26):1841–5.

[99] Van Assche G, D'Haens G, Noman M, et al. Randomized, double-blind comparison of 4 mg/kg versus 2 mg/kg intravenous cyclosporine in severe ulcerative colitis. Gastroenterology 2003;125(4):1025–31.

[100] Kornbluth A, Present DH, Lichtiger S, et al. Cyclosporin for severe ulcerative colitis: a user's guide. Am J Gastroenterol 1997;92(9):1424–8.

[101] Carbonnel F, Boruchowicz A, Duclos B, et al. Intravenous cyclosporine in attacks of ulcerative colitis: short-term and long-term responses. Dig Dis Sci 1996;41(12):2471–6.

[102] Rutgeerts P, Sandborn WJ, Feagan BG, et al. Infliximab for induction and maintenance therapy for ulcerative colitis. N Engl J Med 2005;353(23):2462–76.

[103] Kohn A, Prantera C, Pera A, et al. Infliximab in the treatment of severe ulcerative colitis: a follow-up study. Eur Rev Med Pharmacol Sci 2004;8(5):235–7.

[104] Jarnerot G, Hertervig E, Friis-Liby I, et al. Infliximab as rescue therapy in severe to moderately severe ulcerative colitis: a randomized, placebo-controlled study. Gastroenterology 2005;128(7):1805–11.

[105] Hyde GM, Jewell DP, Kettlewell MG, et al. Cyclosporin for severe ulcerative colitis does not increase the rate of perioperative complications. Dis Colon Rectum 2001;44(10):1436–40.

[106] Colombel JF, Loftus EV Jr, Tremaine WJ, et al. Early postoperative complications are not increased in patients with Crohn's disease treated perioperatively with infliximab or immunosuppressive therapy. Am J Gastroenterol 2004;99(5):878–83.

[107] Sutherland L, Macdonald JK. Oral 5-aminosalicylic acid for maintenance of remission in ulcerative colitis. Cochrane Database Syst Rev 2006;(2):CD000544.

[108] Bergman R, Parkes M. Systematic review: the use of mesalazine in inflammatory bowel disease. Aliment Pharmacol Ther 2006;23(7):841–55.

[109] Mantzaris GJ, Hatzis A, Petraki K, et al. Intermittent therapy with high-dose 5-aminosalicylic acid enemas maintains remission in ulcerative proctitis and proctosigmoiditis. Dis Colon Rectum 1994;37(1):58–62.

[110] Powell-Tuck J, Buckell NA, Lennard-Jones JE. A controlled comparison of corticotropin and hydrocortisone in the treatment of severe proctocolitis. Scand J Gastroenterol 1977; 12(8):971–5.

[111] Timmer A, McDonald J, Macdonald J, et al. Azathioprine and 6-mercaptopurine for maintenance of remission in ulcerative colitis. Cochrane Database Syst Rev 2007;(1):CD000478.

[112] Ardizzone S, Maconi G, Russo A, et al. Randomised controlled trial of azathioprine and 5-aminosalicylic acid for treatment of steroid dependent ulcerative colitis. Gut 2006; 55(1):47–53.

[113] Tamboli CP, Caucheteux C, Cortot A, et al. Probiotics in inflammatory bowel disease: a critical review. Best Pract Res Clin Gastroenterol 2003;17(5):805–20.

[114] Hurst RD, Molinari M, Chung TP, et al. Prospective study of the incidence, timing and treatment of pouchitis in 104 consecutive patients after restorative proctocolectomy. Arch Surg 1996;131(5):497–500 [discussion: 501–2].

[115] Shen B, Achkar JP, Lashner BA, et al. A randomized clinical trial of ciprofloxacin and metronidazole to treat acute pouchitis. Inflamm Bowel Dis 2001;7(4):301–5.

[116] Gionchetti P, Rizzello F, Venturi A, et al. Antibiotic combination therapy in patients with chronic, treatment-resistant pouchitis. Aliment Pharmacol Ther 1999;13(6):713–8.

[117] Mimura T, Rizzello F, Helwig U, et al. Four-week open-label trial of metronidazole and ciprofloxacin for the treatment of recurrent or refractory pouchitis. Aliment Pharmacol Ther 2002;16(5):909–17.

[118] Gionchetti P, Rizzello F, Venturi A, et al. Oral bacteriotherapy as maintenance treatment in patients with chronic pouchitis: a double-blind, placebo-controlled trial. Gastroenterology 2000;119(2):305–9.

[119] Gionchetti P, Amadini C, Rizzello F, et al. Diagnosis and treatment of pouchitis. Best Pract Res Clin Gastroenterol 2003;17(1):75–87.

[120] Viscido A, Habib FI, Kohn A, et al. Infliximab in refractory pouchitis complicated by fistulae following ileo-anal pouch for ulcerative colitis. Aliment Pharmacol Ther 2003;17(10): 1263–71.

**ELSEVIER
SAUNDERS**

Surg Clin N Am 87 (2007) 727–741

SURGICAL
CLINICS OF
NORTH AMERICA

Novel and Future Medical Management of Inflammatory Bowel Disease

Robert W. Summers, MD

*Division of Gastroenterology and Hepatology, Department of Internal Medicine,
4545 JCP, University of Iowa, Carver College of Medicine,
200 Hawkins Drive, Iowa City, IA 52242, USA*

If possible, therapeutic strategies should be based on a sound and thorough mechanistic understanding of the disease etiology; however, the cause of inflammatory bowel disease (IBD) remains unknown. Both genetic and environmental factors are involved, but the understanding of their roles and relative importance in pathogenesis is far from clear. The high incidence in identical twins, particularly in Crohn's disease, is the strongest evidence of a genetic influence. The rapid increase in incidence that occurs when immigrants move from a low- to a high-incidence area is the strongest evidence of an environmental influence. Advances in understanding of genetic or environmental factors have yet to have an impact on therapy; however, over the past decade, significant advances in clarifying the immune processes involved in IBD pathogenesis and how they regulate inflammation are being translated into more effective therapy. Still, treatment remains largely empirical, relying upon anti-inflammatory 5-aminosalicylate compounds (5-ASA), corticosteroids, and immunomodulatory drugs. For many patients, these current time-tested therapies perform very well to keep active disease under good control. On the other hand, inadequacies in both efficacy and safety and potentially serious complications and side effects provide a strong impetus to seek new approaches to disease management. Mesalamine and other 5-ASA drugs may induce allergic reactions and renal injury, and they are frequently ineffective in inducing or maintaining a remission. Although corticosteroids are among the most effective agents to reduce active inflammation, they are not effective maintenance drugs, and they cause dozens of adverse side effects and complications that seriously limit their

This work was supported by grants from the Crohn's and Colitis Foundation of America and the Broad Medical Foundation.

E-mail address: robert-summers@uiowa.edu

doi:10.1016/j.suc.2007.03.004
surgical.theclinics.com

utility. Azathioprine and 6-mercaptopurine are only 60% to 70 % effective, and either may cause significant liver injury, bone marrow depression, or pancreatitis. Methotrexate may induce pulmonary or hepatic fibrosis, and it is less effective than other immunomodulatory agents. Beside the drug complications and side effects, the major failing of standard therapy is the fact that the medications just do not work in many patients. Although they have beneficial effects and frequently keep IBD in remission, the treatments fail to be successful in preventing exacerbations, inducing and maintaining disease remission, and modifying the long-term course of the disease.

In this article, new and potentially important treatments are discussed. These measures include the newer biologic agents, probiotics, helminth ova therapy, leukocytophoresis, and bone- marrow and mesenchymal stem-cell transplantation.

Biologic agents

Biologic agents include a wide variety of circulating substances (antibodies against proinflammatory cytokines, T-cell antibodies, anti-inflammatory cytokines, antagonists of adhesion molecules, growth factors, colony stimulating factors, fusion proteins, antisense oligonucleotides, hormones, immunostimulatory DNA (ISS-DNA, CpG oligodeoxynucleotides) that act through influencing key elements of the immune cascade. Most are blocking antibodies directed against proinflammatory cytokines, others reduce local inflammation by reducing migration of leukocytes across vascular endothelium by blocking key leukocyte adhesion factors, and still others appear to stimulate the innate immune system. As knowledge of how to regulate the immune system increases, additional approaches will be explored.

Infliximab

Infliximab is a chimerc IgG_1 monoclonal antibody to tumor necrosis factor (TNF) that is composed of 75% human and 25% mouse sequences. It was rapidly accepted as the prototype biologic agent in Crohn's disease therapy after a single dose produced a response in about 65% of those treated [1]. Its mechanism is still incompletely understood, but two important modes of action are prevention of TNF signaling and induction of apoptosis of lymphocytes and monocytes. At a dose of 5 or 10 mg/kg, remission occurred in 39% and 45%, respectively, at 30 weeks, compared with 21% on placebo [2]. Even though it may be ineffective or responsible for serious complications, its impact on the management of Crohn's disease has been profound. It can dramatically and rapidly improve symptom improvement, reduce local inflammation, close fistulae, and decrease the need for corticosteroids; however, its efficacy is frequently lost because of immunogenicity, and at 1 year, only 25% of patients were responding to infliximab and off corticosteroids. Its use in ulcerative colitis was recently approved. After 8 weeks of therapy with 5 mg/kg, approximately 38 % of patients were in clinical remission, and the remission was maintained at approximately 20% at 8, 30, and 54 weeks, with evidence of mucosal healing in about 50% of patients at 30 weeks [3]. The recommended dose for Crohn's disease or fistulizing Crohn's disease is 5 mg/kg with an intravenous induction regimen at 0, 2 and 6 weeks followed by maintenance of 5 mg/kg every 8 weeks thereafter.

Adverse side effects include infusion reactions, serum sickness-like reactions, deterioration of congestive heart failure, and central nervous system (CNS) demyelinating disease. It can be responsible for emergence of serious infections, including bacterial sepsis, disseminated tuberculosis, and invasive fungal and other opportunistic infections. Rare cases of hepatosplenic T-cell lymphomas have been reported in adolescent and young adult patients who have Crohn's disease. All cases have been reported in patients on concomitant therapy with immunosuppressive agents. Thus there is increasing interest in attempting to withdraw immunosuppressive agents at a year in order to reduce the risk of developing some of these serious complications of treatment.

Adalimumab

Adalimumab is a fully "human" IgG_1 antibody against $TNF\alpha$. It also binds to soluble and membrane-bound TNF, fixes complement, and induces apoptosis of mononuclear leukocytes. It is given subcutaneously to persons who have Crohn's disease, beginning with a dose of 160 mg at week 0, 80 mg at week 2, followed at biweekly intervals with 40 mg by 40 mg every other week beginning at week 4. Initial studies indicate that the agent is well-tolerated and has beneficial effects that are similar to infliximab. Clinical remission occurred in 36% and 24% given 160 mg followed by 80 mg every 2 weeks, or 80 mg followed by 40 mg every 2 weeks, respectively, when compared with 12% of patients given placebo [4,5]. It appears to be both safe and effective in patients who have failed infliximab, and its use is not associated with cross-reactivity in patients who have experienced this in response to infliximab infusions. Because it is a humanized antibody, it is less immunogenic, and the rate of antibody formation is low. The response rate is not increased in patients treated with immunosuppressives compared with those who are only on adalimumab. Although unproven, it may not require concomitant immunosuppressant therapy. Increased susceptibility to infection is likely to occur as with other anti-TNF agents. It has not been adequately tested in ulcerative colitis.

Certolizumab

Certolizumab pegol (CDP571) is a pegylated 95% humanized Fab fragment of an anti-$TNF\alpha$ monoclonal antibody. It too is given subcutaneously at a dosage of 400 mg every 2 weeks. It has a high affinity to TNF, but because it lacks an Fc fragment, it does not induce apoptosis. Nevertheless, studies in Crohn's disease have demonstrated that it can induce a response and maintain remission [6–9]. At 26 weeks, 48% of treated patients were in remission, compared with 29% treated with placebo. It also is effective in infliximab failures, and it does not induce more adverse effects than placebo-treated patients. It appears to be more effective in maintaining clinical remission when used early in the disease course, but it has not been tested in ulcerative colitis.

The adverse effects of the above agents are very much like those that occur with infliximab. It is of interest that several other anti-TNF antibodies failed to demonstrate adequate benefit in Crohn's disease, including CDP571, onercept, and etanercept. The reasons for failure are not well-understood, but might be dose-related, or more likely, caused subtle differences in the mechanism of action.

Natalizumab

Natalizumab is a humanized IgG_4 monoclonal antibody against $\alpha 4$ integrin, and it inhibits interactions between $\alpha 4$ integrin and adhesion molecules expressed on leukocytes and gut vascular endothelial cells. Thus the agent reduces adhesion, recruitment, and diapedesis of leukocytes into sites of chronic inflammation. Immunogenicity of this agent appears to be low. The first controlled trial in Crohn's disease demonstrated that 300 mg monthly infusions were effective in inducing a clinical remission of about 33% at 8 weeks of treatment, and maintaining it at about 40% at 8, 36, and 60 weeks compared with placebo [10]. Although intermittent use may promote immunogenicity, like many other biologic agents, it is hoped that intermittent treatment interruption may be possible with this agent. Natilzumab therapy of multiple sclerosis was well-accepted until three cases in about 3000 treated patients developed fatal progressive multifocal leukoencephalopathy (PML). This disorder is caused by an opportunistic infection caused by the Jacob-Creutzfeld virus, and it uniformly occurred in patients on both natalizumab and an immunosuppressant. The agent was removed from the market, but then reinstated to be used without a concomitant immunosuppressant, and with a stringent registry designed to detect subtle neurological symptoms that might suggest early PML. Whether or not the agent will be approved for Crohn's disease is unknown, but it will depend on the outcome of several ongoing clinical trials and the results of the strict surveillance that is proceeding in multiple sclerosis.

Visilizumab

Visilizumab is a humanized monoclonal antibody that binds to the CD3 antigen on activated T cells; it is a component of the T-cell receptor complex that does not fix complement. The proposed mechanisms of action from in vitro studies include apoptosis of activated T-cells and downmodulation of cytokine release from resting T cells. It is given as an injection for 2 days, and has been reported to be efficacious in both moderate to severe ulcerative colitis and Crohn's disease [11,12]. At higher doses of greater than 15 mcg/kg, it can cause an acute "cytokine release syndrome" that is short-lived and can be partially ameliorated by giving aspirin. Acceptance will depend on confirmatory evidence from controlled clinical trials.

Probiotics

Trillions of bacteria divided into hundreds of different species inhabit the gastrointestinal tract. Many of these organisms are not even identified or categorized. They are in intimate relationship with the enteral immunologic system and play a key role in priming and forming the developing immune system and in maintaining its homeostasis. The vast majority of bacteria are commensal and do not induce an immune inflammatory reaction; however, they still have the capacity to modulate the immune response and induce intestinal epithelial cells to suppress chemotaxis, downregulate proinflammatory cytokine expression, and increase IL-10 production [13]. The host–bacterial interaction is almost certain to play a role in the pathogenesis of IBD, a role that is called dysbiosis. Antibiotics may affect this relationship in a beneficial way, but a more precise method to influence the ratio of "good" versus "bad" bacteria is to administer large doses of specific microorganisms via the digestive tract.

The beneficial role of probiotics is best exemplified in the case of pouchitis. After colectomy and ileal pouch-anal anastomosis, symptomatic inflammation occurs in the pouch in about 50% of cases. Although antibiotics are usually effective, about 10% of cases are either refractory or frequently recurrent. A preparation containing four species of lactobacilli has been shown to be effective in achieving symptomatic and endoscopic remission in about 85% of cases treated with VSL#3 [14,15]. More investigation is ongoing with other agents and doses, and improvement in results may to occur.

Helminth ova therapy

As noted above, the development of abnormally amplified intestinal inflammation appears to be caused in part by hyperreactive and misdirected immune responses to enteric bacteria. The idea for a new approach to IBD therapy arose from theoretical, epidemiological, and experimental roots. IBD occurs in families of patients with a higher than expected frequency and there is a higher relative risk in identical twins, especially for Crohn's disease [16]. A mutation in the caspase activation and recruitment domain 15 (CARD15)/ nuclear oligomerization domain 2 (NOD2) intracellular protein product increases the susceptibility of developing Crohn's disease [17]; however, no single gene is responsible for either ulcerative colitis or Crohn's disease, although other genes are being explored. CARD15 accounts for only a few persons who have the disease; most patients who have Crohn's disease do not have the defect, and most persons who have a mutated form do not develop Crohn's disease. As yet, no treatment discoveries have emerged from finding genetic mutations.

Genetic traits affect the risk of developing IBD, but only environmental factors can explain the increasing worldwide incidence of these diseases. Both geography and living conditions have been shown to influence the development of IBD. For many years, an increased North-South incidence gradient, and an increased higher-to-lower socioeconomic status gradient have been recognized as IBD risk factors, but the reason for this observation remains unexplained. IBD is common in industrialized and highly hygienic areas of the world, but uncommon in areas where living quarters are crowded and unsanitary. Helminths have been largely eliminated in most of the Western industrialized world, but continue to colonize people in many parts of the world, including much of Central and South America, Asia, and Africa. It is possible that eradication of helminthic colonization of the gut has increased the risk of developing autoimmune disorders such as IBD by eliminating a protective parasitic influence, and that reintroducing helminths in persons who have active disease would inhibit dysregulated immune-mediated mucosal injury [18].

Helminths have the capacity to prevent excessive inflammatory responses [19]. Parasitic worms inhibit immune responsiveness in naturally colonized humans and various types of experimental colitis in laboratory animals [20]. One proposed mechanism was that helminths altered the Th1-Th2 balance. They have been demonstrated to induce lymphocyte subtypes that produce increased cytokines. Thymus derived lymphocytes that express CD4 surface molecules are known as helper T cells. The Th1 and Th2 subsets are prolific cytokine producers. Helminths induce Th2 type anti-inflammatory cytokines such as interleukin (IL)-4, IL-5, IL-9, and IL-13. These Th2 cytokines are often manifest clinically by increased immunoglobulin E (IgE), increased numbers of mast cells and eosinophils and increased IL-10. Helminths also inhibit production of Th1 cytokines, IL-2, Il-12, TNFa, and interferon g (IFNg). Although these changes occur, this explanation of the inhibitory helminthic mechanisms is incomplete, and does not explain how helminths would improve diseases that are not characterized by Th1 hyperreactivity, such as ulcerative colitis, or allergic disorders, such as asthma. Recent observations demonstrate that helminths also induce regulatory substances and cytokines such as prostaglandin E_2 (PGE_2), IL-10, and tumor growth factor (TGF)-β that exert immune suppression. It appears that regulatory T cells exert a major role in maintaining balance between pro- and anti-inflammatory factors, and achieve immune tolerance largely through the suppression of effector cells and downmodulating their effector function. Thus helminths possess an important capacity to limit immune reactivity and induce peripheral tolerance by increasing production of regulatory T cells. A transcription factor, FoxP3, in these naturally occurring regulatory T cell plays a role in their development, and also induces secondary suppressor T cells that secrete high levels of IL-10 or TGF-β. These immunomodulatory mechanisms of helminths in rodents have been explored in a series of studies, and are summarized in a recent article [21]. In addition to mechanistic studies, a number of laboratories have demonstrated reduction or prevention of gastrointestinal inflammation when experimental animal models of colitis or gastritis were treated with intestinal helminths [22–26].

A helminth chosen for clinical trials should have the following characteristics

Colonization should be self-limited, and spontaneous elimination should occur in only a few weeks.

There should be no systemic phase, and the helminth should not multiply in the host.

The helminth should not be directly transmissible, and eggs should not be infective until they incubate outside the body for several months.

The helminth should be readily obtainable from animals grown in a controlled, pathogen- free environment.

The organism *Trichuris suis*, known as the porcine whipworm, possesses all of the above criteria that support its safety profile. In a small pilot study, a single dose of 2500 *T suis* eggs was given to a small group of seven patients who had either ulcerative colitis or Crohn's disease. All seven subjects experienced a temporary improvement followed by a relapse; however, longer courses of therapy produced clinical improvement for several months without any detectable adverse effects. These results prompted larger clinical trials [27].

A larger open trial was performed in 29 patients who had active Crohn's disease (Crohn's disease activity index [CDAI] ranged between 220 and 450) by giving them 2500 *T suis* ova by mouth every 3 weeks for a total of 24 weeks [28]. Most patients had long-standing disease and were refractory to standard therapy. Patients ingested 2500 *T suis* ova every 3 weeks, and dosing of all other medications was held constant. Four patients withdrew at or before week 12 because of disease activity, and 1 withdrew between weeks 12 and 24 because of pregnancy. At week 12, 22 patients (76%) responded (as defined by a decrease in CDAI by greater than 100 points or a decrease in CDAI of more than 150), and 18 of /29 (62%) were in remission (as defined by a CDAI of less than 150). At week 24, 23 patients (79%) experienced a response, and 21 of 29 (72%) were in remission. The mean initial CDAI of the responders was 286 ± 51. It decreased to 96 ± 51 at week 12 and 99 ± 37 at week 24. Thus the mean improvement in CDAI for these patients was 190 and 188 at weeks 12 and 24, respectively. There were no side effects or complications attributable to therapy, and of multiple laboratory values monitored, only the eosinophil count increased from 152 $\pm$ 23 to 212 $\pm$ 54 ($P < .05$). Disease location, disease duration, use of other IBD therapies, and tobacco use did not affect outcome. No adverse clinical effects occurred as a result of therapy, and no patients had to be treated with an anthelmintic for worsening disease activity or suspicion of adverse side effects attributable to the parasite.

A double-blind controlled clinical trial was performed in 54 subjects who had active ulcerative colitis [29]. Subjects were treated with an orally administered a dose of 2500 eggs in a sport drink with charcoal, or the placebo vehicle every 2 weeks for 12 weeks. *T suis* ova induced major improvement in these patients in comparison with those treated with placebo. Using intention-to-treat, a favorable response (defined as a fall in the ulcerative colitis disease activity index ≥ 4) occurred in 13/30 (43%) of the subjects treated with ova and 4/24 (17%) of the placebo-treated subjects, $P = .04$. The initial ulcerative colitis disease activity index (UCDAI) of the 13 patients who responded to ova decreased from 8.8 $\pm$ 0.4 to 2.8 $\pm$ 0.4 at 12 weeks. The differences in remission rates between the two groups did not achieve statistical significance. Of the 13 ova-treated patients who responded, 6 attained a UCDAI of 2 or less, compared with two of the four placebo-responders. Subset analysis was limited because of the small sample size; however, there was a trend that patients who had total colonic involvement and shorter durations of disease activity were more likely to respond to ova therapy. The data from another clinical index (Simple Index) that could be measured at every clinic visit indicated that the therapeutic response to the agent occurred in about 6 weeks. The study was continued for an additional 12 weeks (Phase II) by treating each group of patients with the alternate therapy while maintaining the double blind. In this crossover phase, fewer patients (49) entered, because 5 chose not to continue, and only patients who had active disease at the beginning of Phase II were analyzed. At the end of Phase II, 56% given *T suis* ova responded, whereas only 13% improved with placebo ($P = .02$). Combining data from both 12 week periods (Phases I and II) showed a 47% response with ova and 15% with placebo. It was of interest that of the 13 subjects who responded to the active treatment in Phase I, 6 remained in remission for the 12 week of placebo therapy, 6 suffered relapse, and 1 dropped out. There were no side effects, complications, or changes in laboratory values attributable to the therapeutic agent in either the first or second 12-week periods.

Conclusions from clinical trials with *Trichurus suis ova*

The studies described above included over 100 patients who had initially active disease, and demonstrated that *T suis* ova therapy is safe and effective in both ulcerative colitis and Crohn's disease. Many had disease that was long-standing and refractory to conventional medications, and benefit occurred whether the treatment was given alone or in conjunction with other

IBD drugs. Many patients were treated effectively well beyond the study periods, some for more than 3 years. Thus the agent appears to be effective not only in treating active disease, but also in maintaining remission. Withdrawal of the treatment resulted in relapse over variable time periods, and thus the therapy appears to have a suppressive effect on the immune system. Finally, no adverse clinical effects occurred that could be ascribed to therapy, and thus safety and tolerability appear to be high. Another helminth, hookworm or *Necator americanus*, is also being investigated in a controlled trial of active Crohn's disease in Nottingham, England [30]. Because the use of helminths is an entirely new approach to therapy, many issues remain for use of helminths in IBD. Some of these are listed in Box 1.

Alternative and complementary medications

Although physicians do not prescribe the majority of alternative and complementary therapies in IBD, it is becoming increasingly recognized that their use by patients over the past 20 years has increased significantly, in up to 68% of patients in the United States and Canada. Unfortunately, the usefulness of these treatments is almost impossible to ascertain because of the paucity of adequate controlled clinical trials. Thus, both physicians and their patients are forced to rely on anecdotal reports of benefit or harm. Most patients do not regard the lack of scientific evidence as a problem, and many would likely continue using these approaches even if clinical trials showed that they were ineffective. Unfortunately, some of the treatments not only are of no benefit, but they may cause significant problems, including aggravation of symptoms and interference with the effects of other medications, and their lack of approval by regulatory agencies allows the inclusion of harmful impurities. The supplements listed in Box 2 are the most likely to be of benefit and the least likely to be harmful. Herbal therapies may be the most hazardous, and the naturopathic therapies may be the

---

Box 1. Considerations on use of helminths in inflammatory bowel disease

Confirmation of results in larger trials
Active versus maintenance therapy
Dose response and timing of doses
Use in high-risk subjects as prophylaxis
Efficacy of other helminths
Effects of secretory extracts/fractions
Short- and long-term safety
Use in other immune-mediated diseases
Adjunctive/complementary therapy
Investigation of mechanisms of action

Box 2. Alternative approaches to treatment of inflammatory bowel disease

Supplements
Protein
Zinc
Selenium
Vitamins A, E, B complex
Vitamin B12 and folic acid
Lycopene
Glutamine
N-acetyl glucosamine
Omega 3 fatty acids
Flavinoids

Herbs
Cat's claw
Gingko
Goldenseal
Marijuana
Slippery elm
Tumeric (curcumin)
Wild indigo
Green tea
Aloe-derived mucopolysaccharide
St. John's wort
Boswellia serrata
Echinacea
Tylophora

Naturopathies
Hypnotherapy
Chiropractic
Aroma therapy
Acupuncture, acupressure
Reflexology
Homeopathy
Bioelectromagnetism
Relaxation therapy
Massage relaxation therapy
Hydrotherapy
Clinical nutrition
Physiotherapy
Touch therapy

most like placebo. It is imperative that health care workers ask their patients if they are using unproven or unapproved treatments and be aware of the potential problems that they may cause. Unfortunately, there is little scientific information to judge the effect of these approaches to treatment; however, physicians should keep an open mind about their potential. Without data, it is not possible to evaluate their effect or recommend their use.

Leukocyte filtration

The discussion to this point has focused on administering various therapies by mouth, injection, or infusion. Investigation has also explored modifying the immune environment by other means, including leukocytophoresis, extracorporeal photoapheresis, and bone-marrow and stem-cell transplantation. Most of the work has been done on selective leukocyte apheresis [31–33]. The two most common techniques employed passing peripheral blood through an external column or filters and returning it through another line. The Adacolumn (JIMRO, Gunma, Japan) is made of cellulose diacetate beads and removes 65% of granulocytes, 55% of monocytes, and 2% of lymphocytes. Cellsorba (Ashahi Kasai Medical, Tokyo, Japan) is composed of two nonwoven polyester fiber filters, and it traps 100% of granulocytes, 60% of lymphocytes, and 35% of platelets. Centrifugal cell separators have also been used, but the number of cases and the methods used make interpretation of the data difficult. Granulocytes, monocytes, and lymphocytes play an important role in initiating and maintaining the inflammatory reaction. Removing these cells favorably modifies the cellular immune response. The process does more than decreasing the number of cells. The programmed leukocytes removed are replaced by naïve immunocytes from the marrow or peripheral blood. The process also decreases expression of adhesion molecules and reactive oxygen species, reduces cytokine production, and alters the function of white blood cells and dendritic cells.

Unfortunately, few controlled clinical trials have been done, patient groups have been heterogeneous, and many of the published studies are methodologically flawed, so that it is difficult to evaluate the results of therapy. Therapy is usually given weekly or biweekly. Results with the Adacolumn in ulcerative colitis range from responses of 60% to 80%, and remission rates of 20% to 90 % after 3 to 20 weeks of therapy are reported. With the Cellsorba system, the improvement or response rates range from 60% to 80%, and remission from a single study was reported as 65%. Studies are very limited in Crohn's disease, but suffer from similar methodological deficiencies. With the Adacolumn, responses or improvement occurred in 50% to 100%, and remission occurred in 15% to 60%. With Cellsorba, about 75% improved and 50% entered remission. The duration of response in either ulcerative colitis or Crohn's disease is essentially impossible to determine because of the uncontrolled nature of the studies—it ranges from 2 months to nearly 2 years. One constant feature of all of the reports is the almost total absence of adverse effects. Such a study is in progress in the United States and the most recent review of these methods is useful [31].

Bone-marrow and stem-cell transplantation

There is a limited body of information regarding bone-marrow and stem-cell transplantation. A report of six patients who had Crohn's disease and leukemia and who were treated with allogeneic marrow transplantation was published in 1998. Four of five patients followed for 6 to 15 years remained free of Crohn's disease (one patient died of sepsis and one had a relapse of Crohn's disease after 1.5 years). Two patients who had long-standing ulcerative colitis, psoriasis, and leukemia underwent allogeneic stem cell transplantation, and all three of these disorders were in remission for 4 years after transplantation. Not all patients reported have experienced remission of their IBD, and some have experienced deterioration of their condition or death; thus the outcome of long-term benefit is not established, and a number of issues remain before this becomes an acceptable form of therapy.

Summary

The clinical appearance of biologic agents represents a milestone in the understanding of the inflammatory process. They permit modification of the basic elements of the immune process. There is a vigorous debate over when in the clinical course of the disease the biologic agents should be administered. Both the traditional "step-up" versus the more recent "top-down" approach have proponents and opponents. The top-down approach has taken its lead from the discipline of rheumatology, where it is argued how important it is to prevent irreversible anatomic joint changes in the joints by giving biologic agents early in the course of the disease. Arguments for the step-up approach include the frequent loss of prolonged beneficial effect, the development of systemic and local immune reactions to administration, the risk of developing serious infections, and the extremely high cost of administration. These provide strong arguments that the agents should be given when other more standard agents are no longer effective. The occurrence of lymphomas may be increased in patients on concomitant immunosuppressive therapy, and if it can be avoided, that complication may occur less frequently. The controversy about timing is not settled, and it is likely that multiple strategies will be tested to find the most cost-effective approach.

Probiotics are attractive because they represent a "natural," safe, and relatively inexpensive approach; however, it is difficult to be enthusiastic about their potential when the majority of controlled studies have failed to demonstrate any therapeutic benefit in IBD. It remains possible that the results may have been influenced by the bacterial species used. Some species or combination of species might have a greater immunomodulatory effect, and the quantity of the bacteria administered might have a profound effect on the clinical outcome. The stage and location of the disease may also affect the response to treatment. Because the use of probiotics in the treatment of active Crohn's disease or ulcerative colitis has not been successful, further investigation is necessary before this mode of therapy is employed in any disorder except pouchitis.

Helminth ova therapy is also an attractive therapy because of its apparent safety, "natural" mechanism, and ease of administration. Preliminary experience has been encouraging, but larger studies are required to confirm not only efficacy, but also safety. It is not approved by the Food and Drug Administration, and must be considered an experimental therapy. Many details of its use remain to be elucidated, but further investigations are being planned. Helminth therapy could be complementary to drug therapies, and may be used in combination with other more traditional therapeutic agents commonly used to manage IBD. It is possible that *T suis* ova therapy might be especially beneficial as maintenance therapy, because it is likely that it may be easier to maintain a noninflamed bowel than to reign in a highly active one.

Alternative and complementary therapies are increasingly being used by patients, and usually without their physicians' knowledge or recommendations. Because of the lack of factual information about the efficacy and safety of these approaches, it is very important for clinical trials to be done so that physicians and their patients can make informed decisions about their use.

The removal of the immunocytes from the circulation is relatively new, and much remains to be investigated before leukophoresis becomes a standard of treatment. Although the results of many reports are encouraging, the potential of this therapy cannot be evaluated until adequate multicenter, placebo-controlled clinical trials are done according to current standards acceptable to judge clinical outcomes in comparison with standard drug trials.

Bone-marrow and stem-cell transplantation is an extreme procedure with many inherent hazards. Issues such as separating the effect of intense immunosuppression from the effect of the transplantation, the type of transplantation (bone marrow or peripheral stem cell), the choice of conditioning regimens, the type of patients selected, the degree of informed consent, and patient protection all must be considered before this approach is considered for more widespread use; however, it is possible that this approach may be applicable under certain conditions.

It is anticipated that safer and more effective treatments will emerge as our understanding of the interactions between genetics, the environment, and regulation and dysregulation of the immune process increases. There are reasons to be optimistic, because new agents will be chosen according to strict criteria to satisfy the regulatory agencies; from these explorations, continued therapeutic advances will be made that will result in improved quality of life, reduced permanent anatomic damage, and fewer surgical procedures. With advances, however, problems may also arise, because the newer agents are more effective in modifying basic immunological processes. By reducing inflammation, we may interfere with immune surveillance of malignant processes, render the patient even more vulnerable to serious infections, and unveil unanticipated problems that the immune system is meant to keep in check.

References

[1] Targan SR, Hanauer SB, van Deventer SJ, et al. A short-term study of chimeric monoclonal antibody cA2 to tumor necrosis factor alpha for Crohn's disease. Crohn's Disease cA2 Study Group. N Engl J Med 1997;337:1029–35.

[2] Rutgeerts P, D'Haens G, Targan S, et al. Efficacy and safety of retreatment with anti-tumor necrosis factor antibody (infliximab) to maintain remission in Crohn's disease. Gastroenterology 1999;117:761–9.

[3] Rutgeerts P, Sandborn WJ, Feagan BG, et al. Infliximab for induction and maintenance therapy for ulcerative colitis. N Engl J Med 2005;353:2462–76.

[4] Hanauer SB, Sandborn WJ, Rutgeerts P, et al. Human anti-tumor necrosis factor monoclonal antibody (adalimumab) in Crohn's disease: the CLASSIC-I trial. Gastroenterology 2006; 130:323–33.

[5] Sandborn WJ, Hanauer SB, Rutgeerts PJ, et al. Adalimumab for maintenance treatment of Crohn's disease: results of the CLASSIC II trial. Gut 2007; in press.

[6] Schreiber S, Khaliq-Kareemi M, Lawrance I, et al. Certolizumab pegol, a humanized anti-TNF pegylated FAb' fragment, is safe and effective in the maintenance of response and remission following induction in active Crohn's disease; a Phase III study (Precise). Gut 2005; 54(Suppl VII):A82.

[7] Loftus EV Jr. Biologic therapy in Crohn's disease: review of the evidence. Rev Gastroenterol Disord 2007;(Suppl 1):S3–12.

[8] Schreiber S, Rutgeerts P, Fedorak RN, et al. A randomized, placebo-controlled trial of certolizumab pegol (CDP870) for the treatment of Crohn's disease. Gastroenterology 2005;129:807–18.

[9] Sandborn WJ, Feagan BG, Stonov S, et al. Certolizumab pegol administered subcutaneously is effective and well-tolerated in patients with active Crohn's disease: results from a 26-week, placebo-controlled Phase III study (Precise I) [abstract # 7445]. Gastroenterology 2006;130 A-107.

[10] Sanborn WJ, Colombel JF, Enns R, et al. Natalizumab induction and maintenance therapy for Crohn's disease. N Engl J Med 2005;353:1912–25.

[11] Plevy SE, Salzberg BA, Regueiro M, et al. A humanized anti-CD3 monoclonal antibody, visilizumab, for treatment of severe steroid-refractory ulcerative colitis: preliminary results of Phase I study. Gastroenterology 2003;134(4):A62.

[12] Plevy SE, Salzbert B, vanAssche G, et al. A humanized anti-CD3 monoclonal antibody, visilizumab, for treatment of severe steroid-refractory ulcerative colitis: results of a Phase I study. Gastroenterology 2004;126(4):A75.

[13] Haller D, Serrant P, Peruisseau G, et al. Il-10 producing CD14 low monocytes by commensal bacteria. Microbiol Immunol 2002;46:195–205.

[14] Gionchetti P, Rizzello F, Venturi A, et al. Oral bacteriotherapy as maintenance treatment in patients with chronic pouchitis: a double-blind, placebo-controlled trial. Gastroenterology 2000;119:305–9.

[15] Mimura T, Rizzello G, Helwig U, et al. Once daily high dose probiotic therapy (VSL#3) for maintaining remission in recurrent or refractory pouchitis. Gut 2004;53:108–14.

[16] Probert CS, Jayanthi V, Hughes AO, et al. Prevalence and family risk of ulcerative colitis and Crohn's disease: an epidemiological study among Europeans and South Asians in Leicestershire. Gut 1993;34:1547–51.

[17] Ogua Y, Bonen DK, Inohara N, et al. A frameshift in NOD2 associated with susceptibility to Crohn's disease. Nature 2001;411:603–6.

[18] Elliott DE, Urban JF, Argo CK, et al. Does the failure to acquire helminthic parasites predispose to Crohn's disease. FASEB J 2000;14:1848–55.

[19] Maizels RM, Yazdanbakhsh M. Immune regulation by helminth parasites: cellular and molecular mechanisms. Nat Rev Immunol 2003;3:733–44.

[20] Weinstock JV, Summers R, Elliott DE. Helminths and harmony: mounting evidence suggests that helminths help regulate mucosal inflammation. Gut 2004;53:7–9.

[21] Weinstock JV, Summers RW, Elliott DE. Role of helminths in regulating mucosal inflammation. Springer Semin Immunopathol 2005;27:249–71.

[22] Fox JG, Beck P, Dangler CA, et al. Concurrent enteric helminth infection modulates inflammation and gastric immune responses and reduces helicobacter-induced gastric atrophy. Nat Med 2000;6:536–42.

[23] Khan WI, Blennerhasset PA, Varghese AK, et al. Intestinal nematode infection ameliorates experimental colitis in mice. Infect Immun 2002;70:5931–7.

[24] Elliott DE, Li J, Blum A, et al. Exposure to schistosome eggs protects mice from TNBS colitis. Am J Physiol 2003;284:G385–91.

[25] Elliott DE, Li J, Setiawan T, et al. Heligomonsomoides polygyrus inhibits established colitis in IL-10-deficient mice. Eur J Immunol 2004;34:2690–8.

[26] Moreels TG, Nieuwendijk RJ, De Man JG, et al. Concurrent infection with *Schistosoma mansoni* attenuates inflammation-induced changes in colonic morphology, cytokine levels, and smooth muscle contractility of trinitrobenzene sulphonic acid induced colitis in rats. Gut 2004;53:99–107.

[27] Summers RW, Elliott DE, Qadir JF, et al. *Trichuris suis* seems to be safe and possibly effective in the treatment of inflammatory bowel disease. Am J Gastroenterol 2003;98:2034–41.

[28] Summers RW, Elliott DE, Urban JF, et al. *Trichuris suis* therapy in Crohn's disease. Gut 2005;54:87–90.

[29] Summers RW, Elliott DE, Urban JF, et al. *Trichuris suis* therapy for active ulcerative colitis: a randomized controlled trial. Gastroenterology 2005;128:825–32.

[30] Croese J, O'Neil J, Masson J, et al. A proof of concept study establishing *Necator americanus* in Crohn's patients and reservoir donors. Gut 2006;55:136–7.

[31] Sands BE, Sandborn WJ, Wolf DC, et al. Pilot feasibility studies of leukacytopheresis with the Adacolumn Apheresis system in patients with active ulcerative colitis or Crohn's disease. J Clin Gastroenterol 2006;40(6):482–9.

[32] Pineda AA. Developments in the apheresis procedure for the treatment of inflammatory bowel disease. Inflam Bowel Dis 2006;(Suppl 1):510–4.

[33] Sandborn WJ. Preliminary data on the use of apheresis in inflammatory bowel disease. Inflam Bowel Dis 2006;(Suppl 1):15–21.

SURGICAL
CLINICS OF
NORTH AMERICA

Surg Clin N Am 87 (2007) 743–762

Endoscopy/Surveillance in Inflammatory Bowel Disease

Anis A. Ahmadi, MD, Steven Polyak, MD*

*Inflammatory Bowel Diseases Program, Division of Gastroenterology,
Department of Medicine, University of Florida, 1600 SW Archer Road,
Box 100214, Gainesville, FL 32610, USA*

Patients who have chronic colitis from inflammatory bowel disease (IBD) have an increased risk of colorectal cancer (CRC). In the past, to ameliorate this risk, prophylactic total colectomy was offered to patients who had chronic ulcerative colitis (UC); however, research has identified less-invasive management options through a better understanding of the pathogenesis of cancer in chronic inflammation, a more uniform histologic diagnosis by pathologists, and proper surveillance colonoscopy techniques. To best understand the management of dysplasia in IBD, the authors first review the pathogenesis of neoplasia in IBD. In addition, we review the risk factors for CRC in IBD, surveillance guidelines and their limitations, surveillance techniques, ileal pouch dysplasia, and chemoprevention. Although the data for CRC risk in Crohn's disease (CD) are not as vast, it has been suggested that the risks are comparable to UC.

Epidemiology

The association between CRC and IBD was first recognized in 1925 by Crohn and Rosenberg [1] in a patient who had UC. Work over the next 30 years further confirmed the strong link between UC and CRC [2,3]. In 1967, the discovery that dysplasia found on random biopsy was associated with CRC at other sites in UC patients gave birth to the initial surveillance program [4].

The overall prevalence of CRC in UC has been estimated at 3.7%, with an overall annual incidence of 0.3% [5]. In a large comprehensive meta-analysis

---

* Corresponding author.
E-mail address: polyasf@medicine.ufl.edu (S. Polyak).

0039-6109/07/$ - see front matter © 2007 Elsevier Inc. All rights reserved.
doi:10.1016/j.suc.2007.03.013 *surgical.theclinics.com*

of 116 studies involving 54,478 patients who had UC, the cumulative risk of CRC in UC patients was 8.3% at 20 years and 18.4% at 30 years [5]; however, more recent population-based studies have found a lower annual incidence (0.06–0.2%) of CRC in the setting of UC [6–9]. This decrease in risk is believed to be the result of better patient compliance with maintenance therapy and surveillance colonoscopy, aggressive surgical management, and unforeseen chemoprevention.

Crohn's disease has also been found to carry an increased risk of CRC when studies separately analyzed isolated colonic involvement [10–12]. In a large population-based study from Sweden, Ekbom and colleagues [10] reviewed 1655 patients, and reported a relative risk of 5.6 for CRC in patients who had Crohn's colitis alone. Overall, this increased risk of CRC preferentially affects men and women before the age of 50, prompting practitioners to identify those who need to be screened.

Risk factors for colorectal cancer in inflammatory bowel disease

Identification of risk factors associated with the development of dysplasia and CRC can help stratify patients who have IBD, and allow for more effective surveillance. Patients with greater than 8 years of colitis involving more than one third of the colon have long been known to be at increased risk. It is important to note that duration of disease should reflect the onset of IBD symptoms, and not necessarily the time of endoscopic or radiologic diagnosis (Box 1).

The greatest risk for CRC is in patients who have disease extending proximal to the hepatic flexure, with the lowest risk seen in patients who have isolated rectal involvement only [13]. Extent of colitis is defined either macroscopically or microscopically, whichever reveals the furthest extent of inflammation. Generally, patients who have left-sided colitis develop CRC approximately a decade later than patients who have pancolitis [18]. The field effect described by many in chronic colitis implicates that the entire

---

Box 1. Risk factors that are essential in stratifying patients appropriately for surveillance

Longer duration of disease [13]
Greater extent of colitis [13]
Primary sclerosing cholangitis [14]
Family history of CRC [15]
Younger age at diagnosis [13]
Severity of inflammation [16]
Backwash ileitis [17]

colon is at risk for developing dysplasia and CRC. In fact, Mathy and colleagues [19] demonstrated that neoplastic lesions can arise in areas of microscopic colitis that are otherwise grossly normal.

Initially shown in 1992, the concomitant presence of primary sclerosing cholangitis (PSC) is known to impart a high risk of CRC in patients who have UC [20]. In a Swedish population-based cohort of 104 patients who had PSC, Kornfeld and colleagues [21] found that the cumulative risk of CRC was 33% at 20 years, and 40% at 30 years after the diagnosis of UC. A family history of sporadic CRC carries a twofold higher risk of CRC when compared with IBD patients who have no family history of CRC [22,23]. Conflicting data exist regarding the risk of CRC and age at onset of IBD [5,8]. One would hypothesize that this increased risk is associated with a longer duration of disease; however, even after controlling for duration of disease, a Swedish population-based cohort of 3117 patients diagnosed with UC between 1922 and 1983 found a fourfold increase in CRC risk in patients diagnosed with UC before age 15 compared with patients diagnosed with UC between ages 15 and 29 [13].

Introduced by the group at St. Mark's Hospital, inflammation severity has been found to be associated with an increased risk for dysplasia and cancer [16]. Recently, other case-control and cohort studies have confirmed that both histologic inflammation and endoscopic evidence of inflammation (ie, presence of pseudopolyps, strictures, backwash ileitis, and so on) are independently associated with an increased risk of CRC [15,24,25]. Taken together, these risk factors have contributed to our understanding of the natural history of dysplasia in chronic colitis.

Pathogenesis of colorectal cancer in chronic colitis

Most sporadic colorectal cancers arise from the development of chromosomal instability (85%) caused by loss of adenomatous polyposis coli (APC), p53, and *K-ras* tumor suppressor function. The remainder develops from impaired DNA repair mechanisms resulting in DNA mutations and microsatellite instability (15%). A third overlapping pathway involves the hypermethylation of the promoter regions of regulatory genes, inhibiting their expression [26,27]. These same events also occur in chronic colitis-associated carcinogenesis, but in different order and frequency [28,29], illustrated in Fig. 1. The chronic inflammation that results in recurrent epithelial regeneration and oxidative stress may contribute to these alterations in colon carcinogenesis [30,31].

Macroscopic classification of dysplasia

Dysplasia is histologically defined as the unequivocal neoplastic alteration of the epithelium without invasion into the lamina propria [32]. The

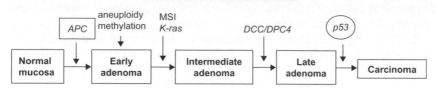

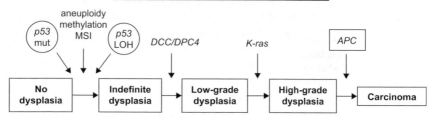

Fig. 1. Outline of events involved in the pathogenesis of sporadic (*top*) and chronic colitis-associated (*bottom*) carcinoma. The main differences in the order of events are highlighted here. Specifically, in sporadic CRC, loss of APC function occurs early, whereas in chronic ulcerative colitis-associated carcinogenesis it occurs infrequently and late. Additionally, p53 mutations occur late in sporadic CRC, in contrast to colitis-associated carcinogenesis, where it occurs early and more frequently. Other variations seen in chronic inflammation are less frequent *K-ras* mutations and earlier development of microsatellite instability. (*From* Itzkowitz SH, Harpaz N. Diagnosis and management of dysplasia in patients with inflammatory bowel diseases. Gastroenterol 2004;126:1641; with permission from the American Gastroenterological Association.)

macroscopic appearance of dysplastic lesions in IBD is heterogeneous and can be elevated, polypoid, plaquelike, flat, localized, or multifocal [33,34]. Originally described by Blackstone and colleagues [33], grossly visible lesions noted endoscopically within areas of colitis have been labeled dysplasia-associated lesions or masses (DALMs). In contrast, flat dysplasia refers to lesions that are undetectable endoscopically, and are found on nontargeted biopsies microscopically [35]. DALMs are further categorized into adenomalike and non-adenomalike lesions (Fig. 2), which can at times be difficult to differentiate and which have different management implications [36]. Non-adenomalike DALMs carry a risk for synchronous occurrence of CRC as high as 43% to 58%, and thus are referred for total colectomy [33,37]. Further management of these lesions is described below.

Microscopic classification of dysplasia

There are two classification systems used to describe dysplasia in IBD: the IBD Dysplasia Morphology Study Group system, and the Vienna classification system [32,38]. In the United States, the IBD Dysplasia

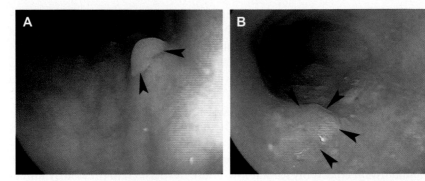

Fig. 2. Examples of DALMs in the setting of colitis. (*A*) A 5-mm adenomalike DALM seen in a patient with mildly active chronic ulcerative colitis. The features are consistent with a distinct, well-circumscribed, smooth, sessile or pedunculated polyp that is usually completely resectable and is not surrounded by dysplastic tissue. These adenoma-like DALMs are similar in appearance to sporadic polyps, but when sessile and sitting in a field of active inflammation, the visual differentiation can be difficult. (*B*) An 8-mm non-adenomalike DALM seen in a patient with mild to moderately active chronic ulcerative colitis. The features are consistent with a less well-defined nodule or raised plaque, representative of non-adenomalike DALMs. The blurred margins can make complete endoscopic resection uncertain without histologic evaluation. (*Courtesy of* the Inflammatory Bowel Diseases Center at the University of Florida & Shands Hospital, Gainesville, FL.)

Morphology Study Group classification system is predominantly used. According to this system, dysplasia is divided into three categories: (1) negative for dysplasia,(2) indefinite for dysplasia, and (3) positive for dysplasia. The positive-for-dysplasia group is further broken down into low-grade dysplasia and high-grade dysplasia [32]. The histologic features used to determine dysplasia type are similar to the classification of neoplastic tissue in general, and entail nuclear, cytoplasmic, and architectural abnormalities [32,39].

Unfortunately, subtle changes in histology can make the distinction between low- and high-grade dysplasia difficult, leaving some degree of subjectivity in pathologic interpretation [32]. In addition, determining the presence of dysplasia in a diffuse background of regenerating epithelium or active inflammation can be challenging. This is the reason for the category of indefinite for dysplasia [40]. Prospective studies evaluating interobserver agreement among pathologists have revealed a significant degree of variability in diagnosing dysplasia [41,42]. Most disagreement has been noted in distinguishing low-grade dysplasia from high-grade dysplasia, and low-grade dysplasia from indefinite for dysplasia [41,42]. For these reasons, it is recommended that biopsies that are indefinite or positive for dysplasia be confirmed by an additional gastrointestinal pathologist [43].

Natural history of dysplasia

The key to endoscopic surveillance in colitis is dysplasia. Unfortunately, carcinogenesis in IBD does not always follow a progressive pattern from no dysplasia to low-grade dysplasia, to high-grade dysplasia, and finally to cancer [27]. Ullman and colleagues [44] showed that cancer can arise in patients who have no prior dysplasia, or without progressing from low-grade dysplasia to high-grade dysplasia first. In the mid 1990s, Connell and colleagues [45] noted an increased risk of developing advanced pathology in the 5-year period following the diagnosis of low-grade dysplasia. Additionally, a review of 10 prospective surveillance studies involving a total of 1225 patients before 1994 demonstrated a 19% and 42% frequency of synchronous CRC in patients diagnosed with low- and high-grade dysplasia, respectively [37]. More recently, the group at Mount Sinai found that 23% of patients who underwent colectomy for flat low-grade dysplasia had previously unrecognized advanced pathology [44]. Thus, findings of flat low-grade dysplasia could prompt the need for colectomy; however, a consensus has not been reached on the proper management of flat low-grade dysplasia, because two large cohort studies from Europe found only a 2% to 10% frequency of advanced pathology over a 10-year period in patients who had flat low-grade dysplasia [46,47].

Current surveillance guidelines

The known association of dysplasia and CRC in chronic colitis has served as the basis to formulating screening and surveillance strategies aimed at early detection and mortality reduction from CRC in IBD. Recommendations for CRC prevention are mainly based on retrospective and case-control studies, along with expert opinion and consensus, rather than on prospective trials. Table 1 [48–56] summarizes key studies that have provided the data on the association of dysplasia and CRC in chronic colitis, supporting the need for secondary prevention. The last two studies in Table 1 provide evidence that surveillance colonoscopy can reduce mortality from CRC in UC; however, the 2004 Cochrane Database systematic pooled data of the last three studies in Table 1 did not show "clear evidence that surveillance colonoscopy prolongs survival" (RR = 0.81, 95% CI 0.17–3.83). This analysis did reveal indirect evidence that surveillance may be effective at reducing the risk of mortality from CRC associated with IBD (level of evidence B) [57].

In 2005, an international group of IBD experts, supported by the Crohn's and Colitis Foundation of America (CCFA), reviewed past surveillance guidelines and new studies on chronic colitis-associated colorectal cancer, and through consensus, developed the latest strategies regarding surveillance for CRC in IBD [43]. In summary, the group concluded that screening colonoscopies in both UC pancolitis/left-sided colitis and Crohn's colitis (involving at least one third of the colon) should begin 8 to 10 years after the onset of IBD symptoms; however, because of the increased CRC risk, all patients who have primary sclerosing cholangitis and IBD should begin

Table 1
Evidence for the need of surveillance for colorectal cancer in ulcerative colitis

Study	Type	N	Surveillance findings	Support surveillance	Statistics
Rosenstock et al 1985 [50]	R	248	39 LGD, 16 HGD/CRC	(+) Trend	N/A
Jones et al 1988 [51]	R	313	5 asymptomatic HGD/CRC, 84 lost to f/u developed CRC	(+) Trend	N/A
Leidenius et al 1991 [52]	R	66	8 LGD, 1 HGD	(+) Trend	N/A
Lynch et al 1993 [53]	P	160	40 LGD, 1 HGD, 1 CRC	No	N/A
Connell et al 1994 [45]	P	332	12 dysplasia, 11 asymptomatic CRC, missed 6 CRCs in 43 months f/u	(+) Trend	PV of LGD to HGD or CRC = 54%
Rozen et al 1995 [54]	P	154	16 IND, 10 LGD, 7 HGD, 4 CRC	(+) Trend	N/A
Lindberg et al 1996 [55]	P	143	4 IND, 32 LGD, 19 HGD (7 with synchronous CRC)	(+) Trend	PV of LGD to HGD or CRC = 41%
Lashner et al 1990 [56]	R	186	Deaths from CRC: surveillance 4/91, no surveillance 2/95	(-) Trend	RR = 2.09 95% CI 0.39–11.12
			CRC detected at earlier Duke's stage in surveillance group.		P = .039
Choi et al 1993 [49]	ROA	41	5-year survival rate: surveillance 77.2%, no surveillance 36.3%	Yes	P = .026
Karlen et al 1998 [48]	PBCC	142	Deaths from CRC: surveillance 2/40, no surveillance 18/102	(+) Trend	RR = 0.29 95% CI 0.06–1.31

Abbreviations: CI, confidence interval; f/u, follow-up; HGD, high-grade dysplasia; IND, indefinite for dysplasia; LGD, low-grade dysplasia; N/A, not applicable as these studies reported only observed frequencies; OA, outcome analysis; P, prospective; PBCC, population-based case-control; PV, predictive value; R, retrospective; ROA, retrospective outcome analysis; RR, relative risk; (+) Trend, statistics indicate a positive trend toward significance; (−) Trend, statistics indicate a negative trend toward significance.

yearly surveillance colonoscopies at the time primary sclerosing cholangitis is diagnosed. In addition, the group also agreed that although the majority of studies regarding dysplasia and screening are in the UC population, current practice endorses the same screening and surveillance recommendations for Crohn's colitis, because the CRC risk is similar in both entities [58,59]. Fig. 3 illustrates the current CCFA consensus guidelines for screening and surveillance. The timing of follow-up surveillance colonoscopy depends on initial biopsy findings. If biopsies are negative on the initial screening colonoscopy, repeat surveillance colonoscopy should be performed every 1 to 2 years. After two negative surveillance colonoscopies, further colonoscopies may be performed every 1 to 3 years until IBD has been present for 20 years, at which point surveillance colonoscopies should be repeated every 1 to 2 years. Patients found to have dysplasia on screening or surveillance

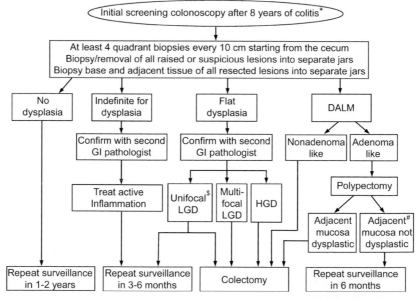

Fig. 3. Consensus screening and surveillance colonoscopy guidelines for CRC in IBD. *Other studies and previous guidelines advocate beginning surveillance after 15 years of left-sided disease; however, the CCFA consensus states that all IBD-associated colitis patients, excluding those who have proctosigmoiditis, begin at 8–10 years. Additionally, patients who have PSC start surveillance at the time primary sclerosing cholangitis is diagnosed. $\$$There is ongoing debate regarding the management of unifocal, flat, low-grade dysplasia; however, the consensus guidelines state that a prophylactic colectomy should be offered to these patients, and that consultation with a surgeon is advised. If the patient refuses colectomy and accepts the known risk for CRC in this situation, then a more aggressive surveillance regimen should be instituted. If recurrent flat, low-grade dysplasia is found on future surveillance, a colectomy is recommended. #Adenoma-like DALMs can be managed conservatively when dysplasia is not found elsewhere in the colon and the mucosa from the base of the resected polyp and adjacent biopsies are negative. HGD, high-grade dysplasia; LGD, low-grade dysplasia. (*Adapted from* Farrell RJ, Peppercorn MA. Ulcerative colitis. Lancet 2002;359:336; with permission.)

colonoscopy will require colectomy or more aggressive surveillance as described below. Patients who have solely proctosigmoiditis (with no colitis proximal to 35 cm) have CRC risks similar to those of the general population, and therefore should follow the standard CRC screening guidelines for the general population.

Biopsy techniques

Most surveillance guidelines recommend four-quadrant biopsies every 10 cm for a minimum of 30 to 40 biopsy specimens [27,60,61]. It is important to note that this accounts for less than 1% of the total colonic surface area, resulting in the potential for false-negative results [27]. In a retrospective analysis [60], it was demonstrated that 33 biopsies were required to detect dysplasia with 90% confidence, and 56 biopsies were necessary to detect dysplasia with 95% confidence [60]. In fact, some authors recommend sampling every 5 cm within the lower sigmoid colon and rectum, given the higher frequency of CRC in these areas. Ideally, 6 to 8 biopsies should be placed in separate containers and labeled by location; however, this is difficult to perform in clinical practice and quite costly, especially without adequate evidence of benefit from studies. Ideally, all irregular or suspicious lesions should be sampled separately. Raised lesions that resemble sporadic adenomas or DALMs should be completely resected, with biopsies of the base and surrounding tissue sampled as well.

Management of dysplasia

All dysplastic (low- and high-grade) and indefinite-for-dysplasia biopsy results should be reviewed by at least a second experienced gastrointestinal pathologist. As mentioned in the natural history section, there is no clear-cut management recommendation regarding unifocal, flat, low-grade dysplasia, primarily because of conflicting data regarding the progression of flat, low-grade dysplasia to cancer. Studies have revealed a low-grade to high-grade dysplasia or cancer progression rate ranging anywhere from 2% to 50% [37,44–47]. Therefore, it is important to discuss the risks and benefits of both aggressive surveillance (repeat surveillance colonoscopies every 3–6 months) and the option of a proctocolectomy with patients at the time low-grade dysplasia is identified. If multifocal flat, low-grade dysplasia, repetitive flat, low-grade dysplasia, or more advanced pathology is found during the aggressive surveillance program, however, the CCFA consensus strongly recommends a prophylactic total proctocolectomy [43]. Likewise, patients who have multifocal flat low-grade and high-grade dysplasia should all be referred for prophylactic total proctocolectomy.

Management recommendations for endoscopically visible lesions that contain dysplasia on histologic examination (DALMs) depend on their endoscopic appearance and degree of removal. Raised lesions that resemble sporadic adenomas (adenomalike DALM) should be resected during colonoscopy, with biopsies obtained from the base of the polyp and surrounding tissue, and placed in a separate container. If the base of the polyp or surrounding mucosa contains dysplasia, then these lesions should be treated as non-adenomalike DALMs and the patient should be referred for surgery. Otherwise, if there is no dysplasia in the adjacent or distant tissue, a repeat colonoscopy should be performed within 6 months [43]. Then, if no further dysplasia is identified, surveillance can be resumed every 1 to 2 years. On the other hand, if the lesion does not have the typical appearance of an adenoma, patients should be referred for a complete proctocolectomy [36,62].

As mentioned previously, the detection of dysplasia in the setting of active inflammation can be difficult both histologically and endoscopically. To help reduce this challenge, the CCFA consensus on surveillance in IBD recommends performing surveillance procedures at times of minimal disease activity. In the case of "indefinite for dysplasia," it is advised to aggressively treat the active colitis and follow up with a repeat colonoscopy in 3 to 6 months [63]. As noted above, a decision-making algorithm for management of dysplasia is presented in Fig. 3.

As discussed above, the risk of CRC in Crohn's colitis is similar to that of UC; therefore the consensus guidelines apply to both UC and Crohn's colitis; however, patients who have ileal Crohn's disease are not at an increased risk of CRC, and can therefore follow the general population CRC screening guidelines [5]. In the setting of localized colonic Crohn's disease, segmental resection of dysplastic or cancerous lesions has been reported, but currently there are no strong data supporting or refuting this type of management [64,65].

In addition to the above, three special considerations regarding surveillance colonoscopy need to be addressed further: (1) pseudopolyps, (2) UC-associated strictures, and (3) Crohn's-associated colonic strictures. In a case-control study, Velayos and colleagues [15] demonstrated that a prior diagnosis of pseudopolyps was associated with a 2.5-fold increase in odds (OR 2.5; 95% CI 1.4–4.6) for the development of CRC. In the setting of multiple or diffuse pseudopolyps, identification of suspicious lesions can be a daunting task. There are no formal recommendations regarding pseudopolyps besides the routine surveillance discussed previously. Other options include complete polypectomy of all lesions, chromoendoscopy-targeted biopsies, and colectomy versus segmental resection [43].

Strictures in UC should arouse a high suspicion of CRC, and should prompt a referral for colectomy versus repeat colonoscopy within 3 to 4 months, with more localized biopsies. In the setting of colonic Crohn's strictures, the risk of underlying malignancy is not as high as in UC, but is still present [66]. Therefore, efforts should be made to visualize the area proximal to the stricture either by CT colonography, barium enema, or endoscopy with more frequent localized biopsies. A review of 175 Crohn's colon strictures revealed a 6.8% frequency of colon cancer after 20 years of disease duration [66]. Therefore surgical resection should be considered if one is unable to fully evaluate the stricture or proximal colon [43,66].

Ileal pouch dysplasia

Patients who have a proctocolectomy and ileal pouch anal anastomosis (IPAA) are not entirely immune from the risk of cancer. Not only is there a risk of dysplasia in the rectal cuff, but also within the ileal pouch [67–70]. Several groups have demonstrated through retrospective reviews and case reports that the anal transition zone and rectal cuff of patients who have a stapled IPAA without mucosectomy are at increased risk for CRC [67,71,72]. It has been reported that the alternative procedure, a hand-sewn IPAA with mucosectomy, carries a risk, albeit lower, of CRC development, which is attributed to the fact that there is a 20% chance of leaving remnant rectal mucosa [68,73,74]. The hypothetical risk of malignancy at the cuff is 1% at 30 years and 2% if an additional 2 cm of rectal mucosa remains above the anal canal [75]. The risk is even higher for patients who had high-grade dysplasia or cancer in their original resection specimens [76].

Dysplasia within the ileal mucosa of the pouch is less common than dysplasia within the rectal cuff [69]. In a retrospective study of 60 UC patients who had an IPAA, Herline and colleagues [77] found only one case of dysplasia. All risk factors for CRC after IPAA, as suggested by nonprospective studies, are

IPAA with stapled anastomosis without mucosectomy [67]
History of dysplasia or CRC in resected colon [67]
Backwash ileitis before IPAA [17]
Chronic pouchitis [80]
Pouch mucosal atrophy [81]

No formal guidelines for surveillance of the ileal pouch currently exist; however, given the potential for the development of neoplastic changes, regular surveillance is advised [78,79]. Coull and colleagues [76] suggest surveillance of the rectal cuff should begin 10 years after an IPAA if no dysplasia or carcinoma was present in the original resection, whereas Borjesson and colleagues [69] suggest that routine surveillance of the pouch be performed every 5 years. It is unclear from the current literature when to begin surveillance in patients at highest risk. The authors suggest that those patients who have multiple risk factors (see list above) for the development of ileal pouch-associated dysplasia should start endoscopic surveillance even sooner than 5 years after IPAA. Nonetheless, it is important that the endoscopist biopsy both cuff mucosa and ileal mucosa at the time of surveillance.

As with flat low-grade dysplasia, management of ileal pouch dysplasia is also unclear. Coull and colleagues [76] suggest that patients who have low-grade dysplasia undergo closer surveillance with follow-up biopsies, whereas patients who have high-grade dysplasia should be referred for completion mucosectomy and perineal pouch advancement with a neo-ileal pouch-anal anastomosis. Certainly, patients who have carcinoma will require complete excision, if amenable.

Limitations of surveillance colonoscopy

Although colonoscopic screening and surveillance for CRC in IBD is widely accepted, it does have its limitations. First, a high sampling error exists, with less than 1% of the entire mucosal colonic surface area sampled if 32 biopsies are obtained [27]. Further contributing to sampling error is the fact that endoscopists have difficulty discerning flat dysplastic lesions, especially if there are extensive pseudopolyps. Second, there is a large degree of interobserver disagreement among pathologists when detecting dysplasia in a field of active inflammation and when distinguishing between low-grade and high-grade dysplasia [41,42]. For this reason, all biopsies revealing or concerning for dysplasia should be confirmed by a second gastrointestinal pathologist. A strong line of communication between endoscopist and pathologist is necessary, and all endoscopic abnormalities should be precisely conveyed to the pathologist [63]. Third, patients must understand the risk for CRC and the need to be compliant with surveillance programs to ensure maximum benefit and prevention. Last, the lack of agreement on recommendations regarding the management of flat low-grade dysplasia may prevent optimal follow-up or treatment.

Advances in imaging techniques and development of biomarkers for dysplasia detection

As previously mentioned, one of the technically challenging aspects in surveillance of CRC in IBD is the difficulty identifying flat dysplastic lesions endoscopically. Advances in endoscopic imaging techniques will potentially aid in dysplasia detection and improve surveillance outcomes. The most commonly used new technique is magnification chromoendoscopy, which involves the topical application of stains and dyes to enhance mucosal contrast and highlight changes that would otherwise be missed by traditional white light endoscopy [82].

The most commonly studied dyes in UC are indigo carmine and methylene blue in conjunction with narrow band imaging [83,84]. Four prospective studies, including one randomized controlled trial, published in 2003 to 2005, documented significantly better detection rates of dysplasia with magnification chromoendoscopy when compared with conventional colonoscopy with four quadrant biopsies at 10-cm intervals plus targeted biopsies of abnormal lesions [83–86]. The largest study, published by Hurlstone and colleagues [85] in 2005, compared magnification chromoendoscopy in surveillance of 350 UC patients to 350 disease-extent matched UC patients undergoing traditional surveillance. Sixty-nine dysplastic lesions were identified by chromoendoscopy, compared with only 24 dysplastic lesions in the traditional surveillance group ($P < .001$). Given these significant findings, the latest CCFA consensus guidelines endorse the use of chromoendoscopy for CRC screening and surveillance in IBD, but do not state specific recommendations. The future of advanced endoscopy holds great promise as an array of techniques, including fluorescence endoscopy, optical coherence tomography, and confocal laser endomicroscopy are further studied. Currently, there are limited data regarding the role of these techniques in the surveillance of chronic colitis [87].

The current challenges in detecting dysplasia, and the variability in histological interpretation, warrant the identification and evaluation of molecular techniques and biomarkers that might improve detection and diagnosis. The understanding of carcinogenesis in chronic inflammation has led to the investigation of genetic (chromosomal instability and microsatellite instability) and epigenetic factors (methylation) involved in this pathway. Fluorescence in-situ hybridization has been used to detect chromosomal instability in rectal biopsies from UC patients and potentially identify at-risk patients [88]. Despite conflicting results, telomerase activity from colon biopsies, another marker of chromosomal instability, has been reported to be highly sensitive in detecting CRC in UC patient [89]. Highly variable studies evaluating the detection of microsatellite instability in colon biopsies of UC patients have demonstrated differences from sporadic cancers, but have not correlated with advanced pathology prediction in UC [90]. Promoter hypermethylation was detected in the biopsies of UC patients in dysplastic epithelium and also in normal epithelium of colons that also had CRC or dysplasia, suggesting that this method might also predict at-risk patients [91]. Additionally, another marker, alpha-methylacyl-CoA racemase, which is highly expressed in different cancers, was found to have a sensitivity of 96% and a specificity of 100% for the detection of low-grade dysplasia in IBD colitis [92]. Translational efforts are now needed to determine the clinical utility of these promising markers in chronic colitis-associated colon cancer screening and surveillance.

Chemoprevention

The development of dysplasia in the setting of colitis occurs over time. With the identification of inflammation severity and duration of colitis as risk factors for CRC in IBD, chemopreventive measures throughout the course of disease may reduce this risk. Indeed, anti-inflammatory medications such as 5-aminosalicylates (5-ASA) have been the most widely studied agents for chemoprevention. The results have been conflicting, with all current data stemming from case-control, cross-sectional, and cohort studies

[93–97]. A recent meta-analysis of nine observational studies demonstrated that 5-ASA significantly reduced the risk for CRC (OR = 0.51, 95% CI 0.37–0.69) as well as combined CRC and dysplasia (OR = 0.51, 95% CI 0.38–0.69); however, no protective benefit of 5-ASA against the development of dysplasia alone was found (OR = 1.18, 95% CI 0.41–3.43) [94]. A 72% odds reduction (OR = 0.28, 95% CI 0.09–0.85) of neoplasia was found in patients taking an average dose of 1.2 g 5-ASA/day in a recent matched case-control study published by Rubin and colleagues [95] in November 2006. Interestingly, the authors also noted a significant dose–response relationship between cumulative dose of mesalamine and reduced CRC risk. Whether 5-ASA is truly chemopreventive remains to be seen, but overall, the data support a protective effect of 5-ASA against CRC in the setting of IBD.

Other medications studied for their potential chemopreventive effects include folate, ursodeoxycholic acid (UDCA), corticosteroids, nonsteroidal anti-inflammatory drugs (NSAIDs), calcium, statins, and immunomodulators [27]. Although not statistically significant, folate has shown trends in reduction of CRC in IBD [16,98–100]. In prior studies examining the treatment of primary sclerosing cholangitis with UDCA, there appeared to be a protective effect against CRC [101,102]; however, a recent historical cohort found no significant difference in the rate of neoplasia in patients who had UC/primary sclerosing cholangitis treated with and without UDCA [103]. Currently, it is advisable to use UDCA for chemoprotective measures in patients who have UC and concomitant primary sclerosing cholangitis, because of the high risk of CRC [93]. These data, however, cannot be extrapolated to UC without concomitant primary sclerosing cholangitis. At this time, there are insufficient data to justify the use of corticosteroids, NSAIDs, calcium, and statins in the chemoprevention of CRC in IBD. Although some studies have revealed a protective benefit with NSAIDs and corticosteroids, their poor side-effect profile limits the use of both for chemoprevention [15,96,104]. Studies evaluating immunomodulators, such as 6-mercaptopurine or azathioprine, have not revealed any protective effect against CRC [100,101,105].

Summary

The risk of CRC in both long-standing UC and Crohn's colitis is clear; however, an incomplete understanding of the risk factors for IBD-associated neoplasia, the natural history of dysplasia, the molecular pathogenesis of colitis-associated cancer, and the difficulty in the histologic diagnosis of dysplasia have limited the ability to interpret the implication of these precursor lesions. Influential observational studies have brought to light the benefit of colonoscopic screening and surveillance in chronic colitis as a means for secondary prevention. The lack of prospective studies and limited evidence have led to disagreements in the management of dysplasia, requiring expert opinion and consensus meetings to manifest our current endoscopic surveillance strategies using random biopsies. The ultimate goal is to reduce CRC-related morbidity and mortality through efficient and targeted modalities, and prevent unwarranted colectomies. Current research has also demonstrated that surveillance should not stop after colectomy with ileal pouch anal anastomosis. The future is already starting to take shape with a shift from conventional white light endoscopy to magnified chromoendoscopy to aid in finding dysplastic lesions. Additionally, the development of molecular methods may aid in the more accurate diagnosis of dysplasia, and the search for chemopreventive agents will reduce the risk of CRC. Most importantly, however, without compliant patient participation, all prevention and surveillance strategies will fail, making patient education and awareness a vital part of our practice.

References

[1] Crohn BB, Rosenberg H. The sigmoidoscopic picture of chronic ulcerative colitis. Am J Med Sci 1925;170:220–8.
[2] Svartz N, Ernberg T. Cancer coli in cases of colitis ulcerosa. Acta Med Scand 1949;135: 444–7.
[3] Rosenqvist H, Ohrling H, Lagercrantz R, et al. Ulcerative colitis and carcinoma coli. Lancet 1950;1:906–8.
[4] Morson BC, Pang LS. Rectal biopsy as an aid to cancer control in ulcerative colitis. Gut 1967;8:423–34.
[5] Eaden JA, Abrams KR, Mayberry JF. The risk of colorectal cancer in ulcerative colitis: a meta-analysis. Gut 2001;48:526–35.
[6] Jess T, Loftus EV, Velayos FS, et al. Risk of intestinal cancer in inflammatory bowel disease: a population-based study from Olmsted county, Minnesota. Gastroenterology 2006; 130:1039–46.
[7] Bernstein CN, Blanchard JF, Kliewer E, et al. Cancer risk in patients with inflammatory bowel disease: a population-based study. Cancer 2001;91:854–62.
[8] Winther KV, Jess T, Langholz E, et al. Long-term risk of cancer in ulcerative colitis: a population-based cohort study from Copenhagen county. Clin Gastroenterol Hepatol 2004;2: 1088–95.
[9] Lakatos L, Mester G, Erdelyi Z, et al. Risk factors for ulcerative colitis-associated colorectal cancer in a Hungarian cohort of patients with ulcerative colitis: results of a population-based study. Inflamm Bowel Dis 2006;12:205–11.
[10] Ekbom A, Helmick C, Zack M, et al. Increased risk of large-bowel cancer in Crohn's disease with colonic involvement. Lancet 1990;336:357–9.
[11] Jess T, Winther KV, Munkholm P, et al. Intestinal and extra-intestinal cancer in Crohn's disease: follow-up of a population-based cohort in Copenhagen county, Denmark. Aliment Pharmacol Ther 2004;19(3):287–93.
[12] Jess T, Gamborg M, Matzen P, et al. Increased risk of intestinal cancer in Crohn's disease: a meta-analysis of population-based cohort studies. Am J Gastroenterol 2005;100(12): 2724–9.
[13] Ekbom A, Helmick C, Zack M, et al. Ulcerative colitis and colorectal cancer. A population-based study. N Engl J Med 1990;323:1228–33.
[14] Loftus EV Jr, Harewood GC, Loftus CG, et al. PSC-IBD: a unique form of inflammatory bowel disease associated with primary sclerosing cholangitis. Gut 2005;54(1):91–6.

[15] Velayos FS, Loftus EV Jr, Jess T, et al. Predictive and protective factors associated with colorectal cancer in ulcerative colitis: a case-control study. Gastroenterology 2006; 130(7):1941–9.

[16] Rutter M, Saunders B, Wilkinson K, et al. Severity of inflammation is a risk factor for colorectal neoplasia in ulcerative colitis. Gastroenterology 2004;126:451–9.

[17] Heuschen UA, Hinz U, Allemeyer EH, et al. Backwash ileitis is strongly associated with colorectal carcinoma in ulcerative colitis. Gastroenterology 2001;120(4):841–7.

[18] Greenstein AJ, Sachar DB, Smith H, et al. Cancer in universal and left-sided ulcerative colitis: factors determining risk. Gastroenterology 1979;77:290–4.

[19] Mathy C, Schneider K, Chen YY, et al. Gross versus microscopic pancolitis and the occurrence of neoplasia in ulcerative colitis. Inflamm Bowel Dis 2003;9:351–5.

[20] Broome U, Lindberg G, Lofberg R. Primary sclerosing cholangitis in ulcerative colitis—a risk factor for the development of dysplasia and DNA aneuploidy? Gastroenterology 1992;102:1877–80.

[21] Kornfeld D, Ekbom A, Ihre T. Is there an excess risk for colorectal cancer in patients with ulcerative colitis and concomitant primary sclerosing cholangitis? A population based study. Gut 1997;41:522–5.

[22] Nuako KW, Ahlquist DA, Mahoney DW, et al. Familial predisposition for colorectal cancer in chronic ulcerative colitis: a case-control study. Gastroenterology 1998;115:1079–83.

[23] Askling J, Dickman PW, Karlen P, et al. Family history as a risk factor for colorectal cancer in inflammatory bowel disease. Gastroenterology 2001;120:1356–62.

[24] Rutter MD, Saunders BP, Wilkinson KH, et al. Cancer surveillance in longstanding ulcerative colitis: endoscopic appearances help predict cancer risk. Gut 2004;53:1813–6.

[25] Haskell H, Andrews CW Jr, Reddy SI, et al. Pathologic features and clinical significance of "backwash" ileitis in ulcerative colitis. Am J Surg Pathol 2005;29:1472–81.

[26] Itzkowitz SH, Yio X. Inflammation and cancer IV. Colorectal cancer in inflammatory bowel disease: the role of inflammation. Am J Physiol Gastrointest Liver Physiol 2004; 287(1):G7–17.

[27] Itzkowitz SH, Harpaz N. Diagnosis and management of dysplasia in patients with inflammatory bowel diseases. Gastroenterology 2004;126:1634–48.

[28] Redston MS, Papadopoulos N, Caldas C, et al. Common occurrence of APC and K-ras gene mutations in the spectrum of colitis-associated neoplasias. Gastroenterology 1995; 108:383–92.

[29] Burmer GC, Rabinovitch PS, Haggitt RC, et al. Neoplastic progression in ulcerative colitis: histology, DNA content, and loss of a p53 allele. Gastroenterology 1992;103: 1602–10.

[30] Sato F, Shibata D, Harpaz N, et al. Aberrant methylation of the HPP1 gene in ulcerative colitis-associated colorectal carcinoma. Cancer Res 2002;62:6820–2.

[31] Chang CL, Marra G, Chauhan DP, et al. Oxidative stress inactivates the human DNA mismatch repair system. Am J Physiol Cell Physiol 2002;283:C148–54.

[32] Riddell RH, Goldman H, Ransohoff DF, et al. Dysplasia in inflammatory bowel disease: standardized classification with provisional clinical applications. Hum Pathol 1983;14: 931–68.

[33] Blackstone MO, Riddell RH, Rogers BH, et al. Dysplasia-associated lesion or mass (DALM) detected by colonoscopy in long-standing ulcerative colitis: an indication for colectomy. Gastroenterology 1981;80:366–74.

[34] Butt JH, Konishi F, Morson BC, et al. Macroscopic lesions in dysplasia and carcinoma complicating ulcerative colitis. Dig Dis Sci 1983;28:18–26.

[35] Odze RD. Adenomas and adenoma-like DALMs in chronic ulcerative colitis: a clinical, pathological, and molecular review. Am J Gastroenterol 1999;94:1746–50.

[36] Rubin PH, Friedman S, Harpaz N, et al. Colonoscopic polypectomy in chronic colitis: conservative management after endoscopic resection of dysplastic polyps. Gastroenterology 1999;117:1295–300.

[37] Bernstein CN, Shanahan F, Weinstein WM, et al. Are we telling patients the truth about surveillance colonoscopy in ulcerative colitis? Lancet 1994;343:71–4.

[38] Schlemper RJ, Riddell RH, Kato Y, et al. The Vienna classification of gastrointestinal epithelial neoplasia. Gut 2000;47:251–5.

[39] Allen DC, Hamilton PW, Watt PC, et al. Architectural morphometry in ulcerative colitis with dysplasia. Histopathology 1988;12:611–21.

[40] Harpaz N, Talbot IC. Colorectal cancer in idiopathic inflammatory bowel disease. Semin Diagn Pathol 1996;13:339–57.

[41] Odze RD, Goldblum J, Noffsinger A, et al. Interobserver variability in the diagnosis of ulcerative colitis-associated dysplasia by telepathology. Mod Pathol 2002;15:379–86.

[42] Eaden J, Abrams K, McKay H, et al. Inter-observer variation between general and specialist gastrointestinal pathologists when grading dysplasia in ulcerative colitis. J Pathol 2001; 194:152–7.

[43] Itzkowitz SH, Present DH. Crohn's and Colitis Foundation of America Colon Cancer in IBD Study Group. Consensus conference. Colorectal cancer screening and surveillance in inflammatory bowel disease. Inflamm Bowel Dis 2005;11:314–21.

[44] Ullman T, Croog V, Harpaz N, et al. Progression of flat low-grade dysplasia to advanced neoplasia in patients with ulcerative colitis. Gastroenterology 2003;125:1311–9.

[45] Connell WR, Lennard-Jones JE, Williams CB, et al. Factors affecting the outcome of endoscopic surveillance for cancer in ulcerative colitis. Gastroenterology 1994;107(4):934–44.

[46] Befrits R, Ljung T, Jaramillo E, et al. Low-grade dysplasia in extensive, long-standing inflammatory bowel disease: a follow-up study. Dis Colon Rectum 2002;45(5):615–20.

[47] Lim CH, Dixon MF, Vail A, et al. Ten year follow up of ulcerative colitis patients with and without low grade dysplasia. Gut 2003;52(8):1127–32.

[48] Karlen P, Kornfeld D, Brostrom O, et al. Is colonoscopic surveillance reducing colorectal cancer mortality in ulcerative colitis? A population based case control study. Gut 1998;42: 711–4.

[49] Choi PM, Nugent FW, Schoetz DJ Jr, et al. Colonoscopic surveillance reduces mortality from colorectal cancer in ulcerative colitis. Gastroenterology 1993;105:418–24.

[50] Rosenstock E, Farmer RG, Petras R, et al. Surveillance for colonic carcinoma in ulcerative colitis. Gastroenterology 1985;89(6):1342–6.

[51] Jones HW, Grogono J, Hoare AM. Surveillance in ulcerative colitis: burdens and benefit. Gut 1988;29(3):325–31.

[52] Leidenius M, Kellokumpu I, Husa A, et al. Dysplasia and carcinoma in longstanding ulcerative colitis: an endoscopic and histological surveillance programme. Gut 1991;32(12): 1521–5.

[53] Lynch DA, Lobo AJ, Sobala GM, et al. Failure of colonoscopic surveillance in ulcerative colitis. Gut 1993;34(8):1075–80.

[54] Rozen P, Baratz M, Fefer F, et al. Low incidence of significant dysplasia in a successful endoscopic surveillance program of patients with ulcerative colitis. Gastroenterology 1995; 108(5):1361–70.

[55] Lindberg B, Persson B, Veress B, et al. Twenty years' colonoscopic surveillance of patients with ulcerative colitis. Detection of dysplastic and malignant transformation. Scand J Gastroenterol 1996;31(12):1195–204.

[56] Lashner BA, Kane SV, Hanauer SB. Colon cancer surveillance in chronic ulcerative colitis: historical cohort study. Am J Gastroenterol 1990;85(9):1083–7.

[57] Mpofu C, Watson AJ, Rhodes JM. Strategies for detecting colon cancer and/or dysplasia in patients with inflammatory bowel disease. Cochrane Database Syst Rev 2004;(2): CD000279.

[58] Gillen CD, Andrews HA, Prior P, et al. Crohn's disease and colorectal cancer. Gut 1994; 35(5):651–5.

[59] Greenstein AJ, Sachar DB, Smith H, et al. A comparison of cancer risk in Crohn's disease and ulcerative colitis. Cancer 1981;48(12):2742–5.

[60] Rubin CE, Haggitt RC, Burmer GC, et al. DNA aneuploidy in colonic biopsies predicts future development of dysplasia in ulcerative colitis. Gastroenterology 1992; 103(5):1611–20.

[61] Rubin DT, Kavitt RT. Surveillance for cancer and dysplasia in inflammatory bowel disease. Gastroenterol Clin North Am 2006;35(3):581–604.

[62] Odze RD, Farraye FA, Hecht JL, et al. Long-term follow-up after polypectomy treatment for adenoma-like dysplastic lesions in ulcerative colitis. Clin Gastroenterol Hepatol 2004;2: 534–41.

[63] Rubin DT, Turner JR. Surveillance of dysplasia in inflammatory bowel disease: the gastro-enterologist-pathologist partnership. Clin Gastroenterol Hepatol 2006;4:1309–13.

[64] Andersson P, Olaison G, Hallbook O, et al. Segmental resection or subtotal colectomy in Crohn's colitis? Dis Colon Rectum 2002;45(1):47–53.

[65] Tekkis PP, Purkayastha S, Lanitis S, et al. A comparison of segmental vs. subtotal/total colectomy for colonic Crohn's disease: a meta-analysis. Colorectal Dis 2006;8(2):82–90.

[66] Yamazaki Y, Ribeiro MB, Sachar DB, et al. Malignant colorectal strictures in Crohn's disease. Am J Gastroenterol 1991;86(7):882–5.

[67] Remzi FH, Fazio VW, Delaney CP, et al. Dysplasia of the anal transitional zone after ileal pouch-anal anastomosis: results of prospective evaluation after a minimum of ten years. Dis Colon Rectum 2003;46(1):6–13.

[68] Heppell J, Weiland LH, Perrault J, et al. Fate of the rectal mucosa after rectal mucosectomy and ileoanal anastomosis. Dis Colon Rectum 1983;26(12):768–71.

[69] Borjesson L, Willen R, Haboubi N, et al. The risk of dysplasia and cancer in the ileal pouch mucosa after restorative proctocolectomy for ulcerative proctocolitis is low: a long-term follow-up study. Colorectal Dis 2004;6(6):494–8.

[70] Gullberg K, Stahlberg D, Liljeqvist L, et al. Neoplastic transformation of the pelvic pouch mucosa in patients with ulcerative colitis. Gastroenterology 1997;112(5):1487–92.

[71] Gilchrist KW, Harms BA, Starling JR. Abnormal rectal mucosa of the anal transitional zone in ulcerative colitis. Arch Surg 1995;130(9):981–3.

[72] Laureti S, Ugolini F, D'Errico A, et al. Adenocarcinoma below ileoanal anastomosis for ulcerative colitis: report of a case and review of the literature. Dis Colon Rectum 2002; 45(3):418–21.

[73] Stern H, Walfisch S, Mullen B, et al. Cancer in an ileoanal reservoir: a new late complication? Gut 1990;31(4):473–5.

[74] Rotholtz NA, Pikarsky AJ, Singh JJ, et al. Adenocarcinoma arising from along the rectal stump after double-stapled ileorectal J-pouch in a patient with ulcerative colitis: the need to perform a distal anastomosis. Report of a case. Dis Colon Rectum 2001; 44(8):1214–7.

[75] Thompson-Fawcett MW, Mortensen NJ. Anal transitional zone and columnar cuff in restorative proctocolectomy. Br J Surg 1996;83(8):1047–55.

[76] Coull DB, Lee FD, Henderson AP, et al. Risk of dysplasia in the columnar cuff after stapled restorative proctocolectomy. Br J Surg 2003;90:72–5.

[77] Herline AJ, Meisinger LL, Rusin LC, et al. Is routine pouch surveillance for dysplasia indicated for ileoanal pouches? Dis Colon Rectum 2003;46(2):156–9.

[78] Bernstein CN. Ulcerative colitis with low-grade dysplasia. Gastroenterology 2004;127(3): 950–6.

[79] Negi SS, Chaudhary A, Gondal R, et al. Carcinoma of pelvic pouch following restorative proctocolectomy: report of a case and review of the literature. Dig Surg 2003; 20(1):63–5.

[80] Heuschen UA, Heuschen G, Autschbach F, et al. Adenocarcinoma in the ileal pouch: late risk of cancer after restorative proctocolectomy. Int J Colorectal Dis 2001;16(2):126–30.

[81] Veress B, Reinholt FP, Lindquist K, et al. Long-term histomorphological surveillance of the pelvic ileal pouch: dysplasia develops in a subgroup of patients. Gastroenterology 1995;109(4):1090–7.

[82] Jung M, Kiesslich R. Chromoendoscopy and intravital staining techniques. Baillieres Best Pract Res Clin Gastroenterol 1999;13(1):11–9.

[83] Kiesslich R, Fritsch J, Holtmann M, et al. Methylene blue-aided chromoendoscopy for the detection of intraepithelial neoplasia and colon cancer in ulcerative colitis. Gastroenterology 2003;124(4):880–8.

[84] Hurlstone DP, McAlindon ME, Sanders DS, et al. Further validation of high-magnification chromoscopic-colonoscopy for the detection of intraepithelial neoplasia and colon cancer in ulcerative colitis. Gastroenterology 2004;126(1):376–8.

[85] Hurlstone DP, Sanders DS, Lobo AJ, et al. Indigo carmine-assisted high-magnification chromoscopic colonoscopy for the detection and characterization of intraepithelial neoplasia in ulcerative colitis: a prospective evaluation. Endoscopy 2005;37(12):1186–92.

[86] Rutter MD, Saunders BP, Schofield G, et al. Pancolonic indigo carmine dye spraying for the detection of dysplasia in ulcerative colitis. Gut 2004;53(2):256–60.

[87] Kiesslich R, Neurath MF. Chromoendoscopy and other novel imaging techniques. Gastroenterol Clin North Am 2006;35(3):605–19.

[88] Rabinovitch PS, Dziadon S, Brentnall TA, et al. Pancolonic chromosomal instability precedes dysplasia and cancer in ulcerative colitis. Cancer Res 1999;59(20):5148–53.

[89] Myung SJ, Yang SK, Chang HS, et al. Clinical usefulness of telomerase for the detection of colon cancer in ulcerative colitis patients. J Gastroenterol Hepatol 2005;20(10):1578–83.

[90] Risques RA, Rabinovitch PS, Brentnall TA. Cancer surveillance in inflammatory bowel disease: new molecular approaches. Curr Opin Gastroenterol 2006;22(4):382–90.

[91] Issa JP, Ahuja N, Toyota M, et al. Accelerated age-related CpG island methylation in ulcerative colitis. Cancer Res 2001;61(9):3573–7.

[92] Dorer R, Odze RD. AMACR immunostaining is useful in detecting dysplastic epithelium in Barrett's esophagus, ulcerative colitis, and Crohn's disease. Am J Surg Pathol 2006; 30(7):871–7.

[93] Chan EP, Lichtenstein GR. Chemoprevention: risk reduction with medical therapy of inflammatory bowel disease. Gastroenterol Clin North Am 2006;35(3):675–712.

[94] Velayos FS, Terdiman JP, Walsh JM. Effect of 5-aminosalicylate use on colorectal cancer and dysplasia risk: a systematic review and metaanalysis of observational studies. Am J Gastroenterol 2005;100(6):1345–53.

[95] Rubin DT, LoSavio A, Yadron N, et al. Aminosalicylate therapy in the prevention of dysplasia and colorectal cancer in ulcerative colitis. Clin Gastroenterol Hepatol 2006;4(11): 1346–50.

[96] Eaden J, Abrams K, Ekbom A, et al. Colorectal cancer prevention in ulcerative colitis: a case-control study. Aliment Pharmacol Ther 2000;14(2):145–53.

[97] van Staa TP, Card T, Logan RF, et al. 5-Aminosalicylate use and colorectal cancer risk in inflammatory bowel disease: a large epidemiological study. Gut 2005;54(11): 1573–8.

[98] Lashner BA, Heidenreich PA, Su GL, et al. Effect of folate supplementation on the incidence of dysplasia and cancer in chronic ulcerative colitis. A case-control study. Gastroenterology 1989;97(2):255–9.

[99] Lashner BA. Red blood cell folate is associated with the development of dysplasia and cancer in ulcerative colitis. J Cancer Res Clin Oncol 1993;119(9):549–54.

[100] Lashner BA, Provencher KS, Seidner DL, et al. The effect of folic acid supplementation on the risk for cancer or dysplasia in ulcerative colitis. Gastroenterology 1997; 112(1):29–32.

[101] Tung BY, Emond MJ, Haggitt RC, et al. Ursodiol use is associated with lower prevalence of colonic neoplasia in patients with ulcerative colitis and primary sclerosing cholangitis. Ann Intern Med 2001;134(2):89–95.

[102] Sjoqvist U, Tribukait B, Ost A, et al. Ursodeoxycholic acid treatment in IBD-patients with colorectal dysplasia and/or DNA-aneuploidy: a prospective, double-blind, randomized controlled pilot study. Anticancer Res 2004;24(5B):3121–7.

[103] Wolf JM, Rybicki LA, Lashner BA. The impact of ursodeoxycholic acid on cancer, dysplasia and mortality in ulcerative colitis patients with primary sclerosing cholangitis. Aliment Pharmacol Ther 2005;22(9):783–8.

[104] Bansal P, Sonnenberg A. Risk factors of colorectal cancer in inflammatory bowel disease. Am J Gastroenterol 1996;91(1):44–8.

[105] Matula S, Croog V, Itzkowitz S, et al. Chemoprevention of colorectal neoplasia in ulcerative colitis: the effect of 6-mercaptopurine. Clin Gastroenterol Hepatol 2005; 3(10):1015–21.

SURGICAL
CLINICS OF
NORTH AMERICA

Surg Clin N Am 87 (2007) 763–785

Pathologist Surgeon Interface in Idiopathic Inflammatory Bowel Disease

Andrew D. Vanderheyden, MD, Frank A. Mitros, MD*

Department of Pathology, Roy J. and Lucille A. Carver College of Medicine, 200 Hawkins Drive, 5244B RCP, Iowa City, IA 52242, USA

The importance of close cooperation among gastroenterologists, surgeons, and pathologists in the care and management of patients who have idiopathic inflammatory bowel disease cannot be stressed too strongly. This cooperation is essential to establishing the correct diagnosis, as well as determining if surgery is indicated, and the timing and type of surgical procedure in those requiring such intervention. Each of these individual important decisions is often less than clear-cut. Historical, endoscopic, and laboratory results all affect the accuracy of interpretation by the pathologist, and a free exchange of information among these specialties is invaluable.

Before surgery

Endoscopic biopsies play a major role in the establishment of a diagnosis of idiopathic inflammatory bowel disease. This is true despite the fact that it is clearly not possible to consistently be certain of the presence of inflammatory bowel disease (as opposed to infection, toxin, and the like) on a single limited sample at a single point in time. A frequent error that leads to many difficult problems is the over-zealous diagnosis of ulcerative colitis, based on a single rectal biopsy that contains some crypt abscesses. Although crypt abscesses are characteristically seen in ulcerative colitis, they are also frequent in Crohn's disease and bacterial infection, and can even be seen in cases of lymphocytic colitis or *Clostridium difficile*-related toxic damage. There are several important ways to minimize error at the major decision-making points.

---

* Corresponding author.
  E-mail address: frank-mitros@uiowa.edu (F.A. Mitros).

0039-6109/07/$ - see front matter © 2007 Elsevier Inc. All rights reserved.
doi:10.1016/j.suc.2007.03.012   *surgical.theclinics.com*

Distinguishing inflammatory bowel disease from other cases of colitis

Perhaps the most important factor in making the distinction is establishing the presence of chronicity. This is best done by historical information. The presence of diarrhea of a few days duration, even if blood is present, may be seen in a wide variety of diseases. A history of "bloody diarrhea" with no further information may mislead an unwary pathologist. The conservative approach is to insist on 6 months of symptoms before establishing the diagnosis of inflammatory bowel disease. There is certainly a great difference between symptoms of several days duration and the same symptoms of several months duration—and that information should be conveyed to the pathologist. At times the presence of chronicity is established by previous colorectal biopsy, and the pathologist should seek a record of prior material in the files.

Chronicity can also be established histologically (Figs. 1–6) [1]. The presence of crypt branching is the strongest evidence in this regard. There should be irregular angles between the branches of the crypt, and these abnormal branches often nearly parallel the muscularis mucosae. Symmetric parallel branches may merely represent a normal variant, with adjacent crypts

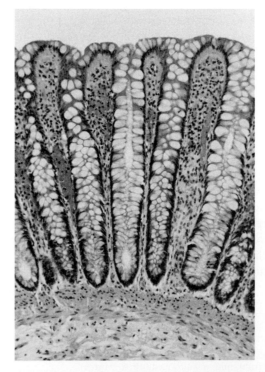

Fig. 1. Normal colonic mucosa. Note the cellularity of the lamina propria, composed of lymphocytes and plasma cells. The crypts are producing abundant mucin.

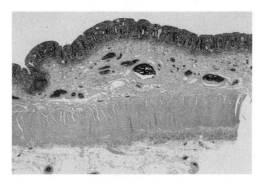

Fig. 2. This full-thickness histologic section in a patient with ulcerative colitis shows the mucosal predominance of the inflammatory process. The submucosa and below are entirely free of involvement.

sometimes appearing to be "bifid." Paneth cell metaplasia is another important finding. Paneth cells may extend into the proximal colon in adults and some distance further in pediatric patients. Their presence in rectosigmoid biopsies is excellent proof of chronic damage. Providing multiple biopsies simply designated as "random colon" precludes using the presence of Paneth metaplasia in a meaningful way. The lymphoplasmacytic infiltrate of the lamina propria is increased throughout its entire thickness in ulcerative colitis. In other processes, such as bacterial colitis, it is not uniformly increased [2,3]. In lymphocytic colitis and collagenous colitis the lymphoplasmacytic increase is "top-heavy," usually being limited to the top half of the lamina propria. The muscularis mucosae is often increased in thickness in inflammatory bowel disease. The intercryptal surface epithelium is an area that is relatively spared in inflammatory bowel disease, but is preferentially and characteristically damaged in some disease processes in the differential. These include ischemic damage, C. difficile toxin, and lymphocytic and

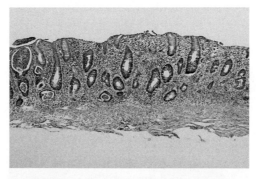

Fig. 3. A biopsy of active ulcerative colitis. The lamina propria cellularity is diffusely increased, the muscularis mucosae is thickened, and there are multiple crypt abscesses, most of which are located deep in the mucosa.

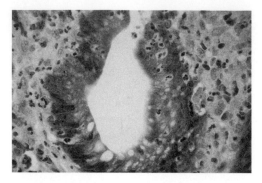

Fig. 4. This crypt shows penetration by neutrophils between the crypt epithelial cells, the characteristic appearance of cryptitis.

collagenous colitis. In the latter two there is also an increase in intra-epithelial lymphocytes in this area; in collagenous colitis there is also a thick, irregular collagen band under this surface epithelium. These latter two diseases are important in that they can produce chronicity similar to inflammatory bowel disease, though the diarrhea is watery rather than bloody, and the endoscopic appearance is normal or near normal [4]. Crypt abscesses can be present in both acute and chronic colitis. In inflammatory bowel disease they may be anywhere throughout the thickness of the mucosae. In bacterial colitis they are often quite superficial, and may produce a "string of pearls" appearance. In *C difficile* colitis there are often rounded tufts of vacuolated damaged surface cells, referred to by some as "summit lesions." In acute ischemic damage there may be hemorrhage and a peculiar hyalinization of the superficial lamina propria.

The distinction of ulcerative colitis from Crohn's disease

The distribution and character of the inflammation is the key distinguishing morphologic feature. With the exception of some mild mucosal

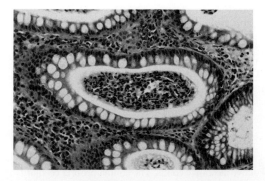

Fig. 5. Neutrophils fill the lumen of the crypt; this is a crypt abscess, commonly seen in ulcerative colitis, but not specific for that process.

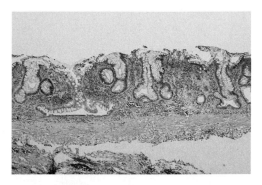

Fig. 6. Biopsies are often obtained in chronic ulcerative colitis. The characteristic crypt branching is clearly evident, as is a thickened muscularis mucosae.

inflammatory change in the terminal ileum ("backwash ileitis"), involvement of the ileum or proximal gastrointestinal tract clearly distinguishes ulcerative colitis from Crohn's disease. Absence of ileal involvement does not exclude Crohn's. If there is radiologic evidence of proximal gastrointestinal involvement, that information needs to be conveyed to the pathologist. Within segments of the gastrointestinal tract that are actively inflamed, the characteristic pattern of damage of ulcerative colitis and Crohn's disease differ in two important aspects (Figs. 7–13). The inflammation in ulcerative colitis is diffuse and mucosal-based, rarely extending beyond the most superficial aspects of the submucosa. The inflammation in Crohn's disease is almost always segmental (patchy), and importantly, is transmural and aggregated. The aggregate may be lymphoid follicles, or in a minority of cases, recognizably granulomatous. Unfortunately, mucosal biopsies do not go deep enough to readily allow this distinction to be made. In a small number of cases there may be "disproportionate inflammation," in which the inflammatory process is clearly more prominent in the submucosa than in the mucosa. When present, this provides excellent evidence for Crohn's disease.

The other important difference with regards to the pattern of damage is the distribution. Ulcerative colitis usually involves the entire colon, with more severe damage distally. A smaller number of cases involve only the distal or left side of the colon (left-sided predominant ulcerative colitis or ulcerative proctitis). To use this important distinguishing feature, the sites of the colonoscopic biopsies need to be carefully mapped and correlated with the endoscopic appearance. The biopsy of endoscopically normal-appearing areas in suspected Crohn's disease ("skip areas") can provide valuable information. Simply labeling biopsies as "random colon" or right colon and left colon with no endoscopic description dramatically reduces the ability of even an experienced pathologist to make the distinction between ulcerative colitis and Crohn's disease. It would be foolhardy to attempt to distinguish the two with a limited sample at a single point in time with little or no endoscopic and clinical information.

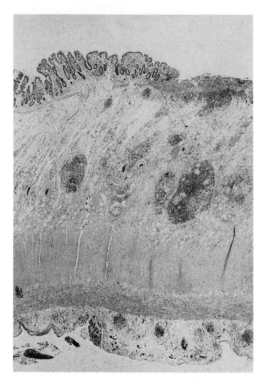

Fig. 7. This full-thickness histologic section from a patient with Crohn's disease of the colon shows an area of ulceration to the right, with normal mucosa present to the left. There is an aggregated transmural pattern of the inflammation, with prominent expansion of the submucosa and of the subserosal connective tissues.

Some specific histologic features may prove quite helpful. Granulomas are the best example of focal aggregated inflammation, and when present, provide excellent evidence for Crohn's disease. Granulomatous foci related directly to crypt abscesses, especially such an abscess with a break in the

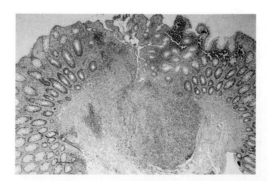

Fig. 8. This mucosal biopsy was taken from an aphthous ulcer in a patient with Crohn's disease; there is a small fissure overlying a physiologic submucosal lymphoid aggregate.

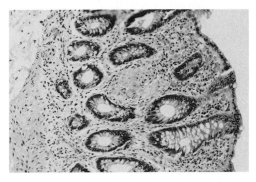

Fig. 9. There is a granuloma in the lamina propria between intact crypts; in the appropriate clinical setting, this finding is diagnostic for Crohn's disease.

epithelium, are of no value. These so-called "crypt granulomas" are reacting to mucin extruded from the crypt, and are not useful in establishing the diagnosis of Crohn's disease [5]. Metaplasia to a gastric antral type epithelium is frequent in Crohn's disease, more commonly in the ileum than in the colon. Biopsy of aphthous ulcers may show an early fissure ulcer characteristic of Crohn's disease.

Distinction of inflammatory bowel disease from lymphocytic colitis and collagenous colitis

Because these processes constitute the spectrum of chronic colitis, and because lymphocytic colitis and collagenous colitis do not share the cancer risk of ulcerative colitis and Crohn's disease, the distinction is of major importance. Like ulcerative colitis, these processes are limited to the mucosa of the colon. The key is paying close attention to the intercryptal surface epithelium, which is flatter than normal. The epithelial nuclei tend to lose their

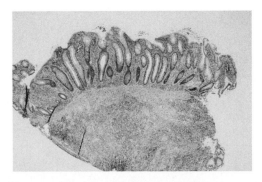

Fig. 10. This mucosal biopsy shows disproportionate inflammation of the submucosa in Crohn's disease.

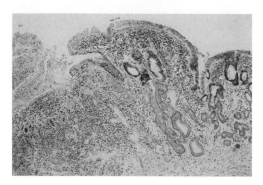

Fig. 11. The pale glands toward the center of the figure represent antral metaplasia characteristic of Crohn's disease.

basal orientation, and importantly, there is a clear increase in the surface of
intraepithelial T lymphocytes [4]. In addition, collagenous colitis has a thick
irregular collagen plate that entraps superficial lamina propria capillaries.
There may also be an increase in intraepithelial eosinophils in the surface.
The rectosigmoid may tend to be relatively spared in some cases of collagenous colitis. The presence of cryptitis and even crypt abscesses does not
preclude a diagnosis of lymphocytic colitis or collagenous colitis.

Dysplastic change in inflammatory bowel disease

Both ulcerative colitis and Crohn's disease predispose to colorectal carcinoma, and in both, dysplasia in involved mucosa is associated with and often precedes the development of invasion. The magnitude of the relative risk
between ulcerative colitis and Crohn's disease has been debated. Ulcerative
colitis has been considered to have a much higher risk than Crohn's disease,
but that has been questioned of late. Surveillance has been clearly

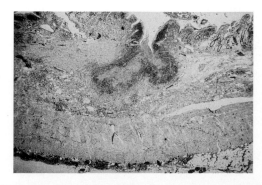

Fig. 12. This full-thickness segment of bowel from Crohn's disease shows a fissure ulcer extending into the submucosa.

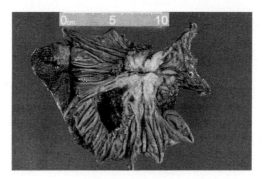

Fig. 13. A fistulous connection between colon and ileum is clearly seen in this gross specimen from a patient with Crohn's disease.

established to be effective in chronic ulcerative colitis, and is the standard of practice. Surveillance is being done more and more frequently in patients who have Crohn's disease.

The goal of surveillance is to identify dysplasia prior to invasion. The dysplastic epithelium in inflammatory bowel disease bears many histologic similarities to the epithelium seen in colonic adenomas (Figs. 14–21). This is no surprise, because adenomas of the colon are the form of dysplasia that gives rise to colorectal carcinoma in the population at large. The description and categorization of dysplasia in inflammatory bowel disease was codified in 1983 by a large group of distinguished pathologists led by Riddell [6]. A surveillance colonoscopy may reveal no dysplasia, reactive change, changes indefinite for dysplasia, dysplasia, or invasive carcinoma. The reproducibility of these categories is best at the ends of the spectrum. Dysplasia is further divided into low grade or high grade. The endoscopic appearance is also important. Dysplasia may occur in flat mucosa and not be endoscopically apparent, whether it be low or high grade. Great

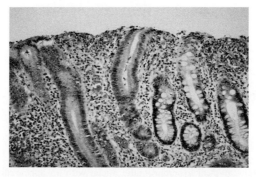

Fig. 14. This patient has quiescent ulcerative colitis involving the crypts to the right side of the photograph. The crypts to the left show evidence of dysplasia.

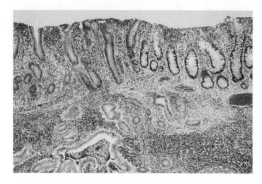

Fig. 15. A lower power view of this same biopsy shows invasive carcinoma beneath the muscularis mucosae arising from the dysplastic focus.

importance is attached to the presence of endoscopically visible lesions, referred to as dysplasia-associated lesions or masses (DALMs). The DALMs may be flat irregular plaques, or they may be more exophytic, resembling adenomas [7]. It may not be possible to separate an adenomalike DALM from a sporadic adenoma. The latter have an appearance endoscopically similar to adenoma occurring in patients who do not have inflammatory bowel disease. They are not associated with dysplasia on the stalk or in the adjacent flat mucosa. They occur in patients of typical adenoma-bearing age. The distinction may be of less significance than once thought, because both sporadic adenoma and adenomalike DALMs have been successfully treated with polypectomy. In contrast, dysplasia in the plaquelike DALMs is frequently associated with invasion, and is usually considered an indication for colectomy. Because the distinction between indefinite for dysplasia and dysplasia is so difficult, as is the distinction of low-grade from high-grade dysplasia (though to a lesser degree), it is recommended that the

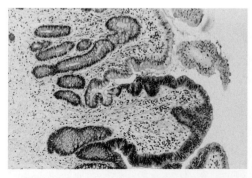

Fig. 16. Sections show atypical hyperchromatic nuclei with an appearance resembling those seen in an adenoma. This is low-grade dysplasia in ulcerative colitis. Note the sharp junction with the intact colonic mucosa.

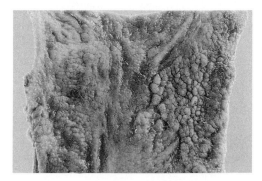

Fig. 17. The irregular plaque occupying the right half of this gross resection from a patient with ulcerative colitis is a dysplasia-associated lesion or mass (DALM).

diagnosis be confirmed by a pathologist with experience in gastrointestinal pathology before definitive therapy is undertaken.

The perioperative period: frozen sections

With carefully planning and proper clinical and pathologic information prior to surgery, frozen sections are rarely necessary. If there is an unexpected area suspicious for carcinoma, a frozen section can prove to be invaluable. At times the distinction of ulcerative colitis from Crohn's disease may not be clear, despite a complete preoperative workup. There may be unexpected operative findings casting doubt on the diagnosis of ulcerative colitis and raising suspicions for Crohn's disease. The frozen section may help in this distinction. In addition to the previously described differentiating histologic features, there is one more finding of practical importance that is particularly helpful in the frozen section situation. The transmural aggregated pattern of inflammation so characteristic of Crohn's disease

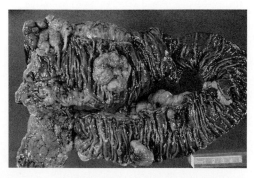

Fig. 18. Colon carcinoma may be multiple in patients with ulcerative colitis; four such neoplasms are seen here.

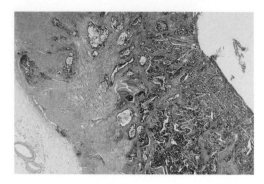

Fig. 19. The invasive carcinoma is transmural, although there is little in the way of an exophytic surface lesion.

has a striking predilection for the subserosal connective tissue, or for the junction of the longitudinal muscular layer with the mesenteric fat (Fig. 22). The lymphoid aggregates (or granulomas) often line up in this plane. The appearance has been likened to the beads of a rosary [8]. Given the difficulties in looking at full-thickness sections or of sampling sufficient mucosa with the frozen section technique, it is useful to orient the frozen section toward showing this area to maximum advantage.

When the involved segment of the gastrointestinal tract is removed, it should be sent to the pathology laboratory expeditiously. It is important for the pathologist to know the clinical problem. Was the colon removed because of the failure of medical control? Was the colon removed because of biopsy proven dysplasia? Was the colon removed electively because of the duration of colitis? Is the distinction between ulcerative colitis and Crohn's disease clearly established or not? The pathologist should open the colon shortly after it is received and pin it out flat in a container with abundant formalin. This will allow for good fixation for good histologic detail. It

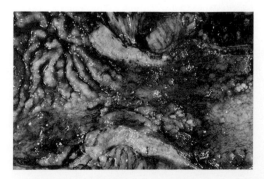

Fig. 20. An area of stricture appearing in ulcerative colitis is strongly suspicious for the presence of an invasive carcinoma; such was the case here.

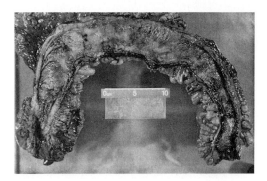

Fig. 21. Many times the carcinoma in ulcerative colitis is not readily grossly evident, as is true in this specimen.

will also allow for well-oriented sections, which idealize the important determination of the presence or absence of the transmural aggregated pattern of inflammation.

Gross pathology of inflammatory bowel disease

Overview

Gross examination of intestinal resection specimens can prove to be quite helpful in the evaluation of a patient who has idiopathic inflammatory bowel disease (Figs. 23–29). Likewise, endoscopic gross examination can provide this important information, which is critical to convey to the pathologist. Additional clinical history, especially in relation to prior sites of disease or resections, can be extraordinarily useful as well. The distribution

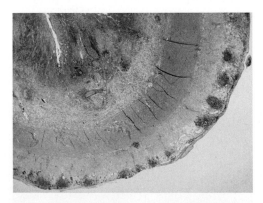

Fig. 22. The presence of multiple lymphoid aggregates in the subserosal connective tissue resembles beads on a string. This finding is particularly useful during the frozen section evaluation, in which the question of distinguishing Crohn's disease from ulcerative colitis arises.

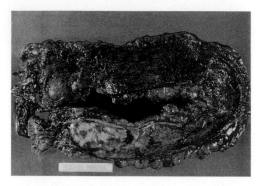

Fig. 23. This gross specimen shows a severe pancolitis in a patient with active ulcerative colitis. The usual haustral folds are no longer visible.

of disease, characteristic gross findings, and gross differential diagnoses of inflammatory bowel disease have been well-documented [9–12], and the salient points are summarized as follows.

Upon receipt of an intestinal resection specimen, often the primary pathologic diagnosis is known (or at least strongly suspected), and it is the goal of the pathologic examination to confirm this diagnosis. At other times, the resection is performed in an urgent manner, such as for fulminant colitis, intestinal perforation, obstruction, and so forth, and there is no established diagnosis. It is in these situations with no clinical history of chronic intestinal symptoms that one should be very wary of diagnosing inflammatory bowel disease, and keep a sharp eye for those entities that can mimic inflammatory bowel disease. Regardless of the situation leading to resection, it is the goal of the examination of expected cases of inflammatory bowel disease to categorize the pathologic process into one of the two specific diagnostic categories: ulcerative colitis or Crohn's disease. This is, of course, an important distinction, with many implications for the patient with regards to recurrence, surgical options, surveillance, and risk for associated diseases.

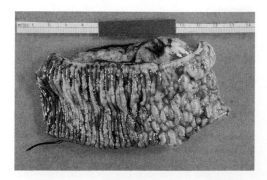

Fig. 24. Multiple shallow ulcers in an otherwise featureless mucosa are characteristic of ulcerative colitis.

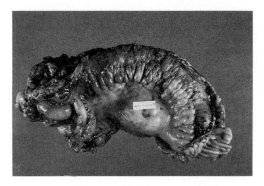

Fig. 25. Fat wrapping is a sign of Crohn's disease. In reality, it is evidence of transmural inflammation, regardless of the cause.

Before describing the classic findings in ulcerative colitis and Crohn's disease, it is helpful to review the basic terminology often used to describe the gross appearance of the intestine in inflammatory bowel disease. An ulcer is the loss of the mucosal layer (epithelium, lamina propria, and muscularis mucosae) of the gut wall, and can have specialized forms such as aphthous ulcers (small, round, well-demarcated ulcers surrounded by normal-appearing mucosa) or linear ulcers (longitudinally oriented ulcers). Parallel rows of linear ulcers can be seen and have been described as "bear-claw" ulcers, as if claws had been dragged along the mucosal surface, causing the characteristic injury. Deeper ulceration may lead to sinus tracts or fistulas; these are granulation-tissue–lined tracts that may connect the bowel lumen to adjacent bowel, other organs, the skin surface, or a peri-intestinal/mesenteric abscess. The mucosa may have long, wormlike polypoid projections, which are inflammatory polyps (also known as pseudopolyps). This is in distinction to "cobblestoning" of the mucosa that is characterized by multiple islands of intact mucosa separated by linear ulcerations. Bowel wall thickening is often

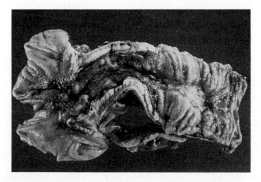

Fig. 26. The longitudinal ulcer, the thickened wall, and an area of stricturing of the terminal ileum with a distorted ileocecal valve are classic findings in Crohn's disease.

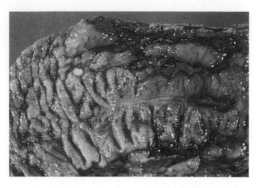

Fig. 27. The ileum shows a striking longitudinal ulcer in this patient who has Crohn's disease.

seen, and may take the form of a stricture (a localized, discrete, circumferential narrowing of the lumen). The mesenteric adipose tissue may migrate and surround the bowel wall in response to serosal inflammation, in a process referred to as "fat wrapping" or "creeping fat"; this finding correlates with the presence of transmural inflammation. The inflammatory process may be limited to the mucosa, or may be transmural, affecting the mucosa, submucosa, and serosa. In reference to the distribution of these gross features of inflammatory bowel disease, the involved anatomical segment of bowel is designated, and it may be affected in a diffuse, continuous pattern, or it may show distinct segments of disease separated by uninvolved areas (skip lesions).

Crohn's disease

The classical gross description of Crohn's disease is a segmental inflammatory disease affecting the bowel transmurally, with a preference for the

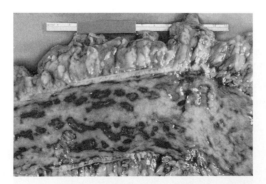

Fig. 28. This segment of ileum shows cobblestoning, particularly evident on the right side of the photograph. The cobblestoning results from the variable involvement with some sparing of adjacent mucosa typical of Crohn's disease.

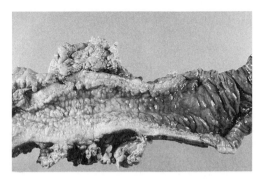

Fig. 29. The area of stricturing and cobblestoning in this colonic resection specimen was characteristic for Crohn's disease.

terminal ileum or right colon. Segmental disease refers to the presence of normal intervening mucosa between segments of affected bowel, which are often referred to as "skip lesions." There are instances where the gross impression of skip lesions may be misleading; this is elaborated on in the following section on ulcerative colitis. Distribution of disease is one of the major keys to differentiating Crohn's disease from ulcerative colitis; the preferential involvement of the terminal ileum in Crohn's disease is helpful in making this distinction. Any other portion of the gastrointestinal tract may be affected as well, and upper gastrointestinal tract involvement by Crohn's disease is usually accompanied by ileal disease. A minor percentage of Crohn's disease (10%–20%) presents as disease limited to the colon, and in these cases there is often relative rectal sparing.

The mucosa in Crohn's disease generally exhibits discrete ulceration with aphthous ulcers, linear ulcers, or bear-claw ulcers. This imparts a cobblestone appearance to the mucosa. Inflammatory polyps may also been seen. Although the hallmark of Crohn's disease is transmural inflammation, superficial Crohn's disease with disease limited to the mucosa has been identified. The characteristic deep inflammation leads to bowel wall thickening with possible stricture formation. Fissures and fistula tracts are common, and may connect the bowel lumen to other hollow viscera (small intestine, colon, urinary bladder, vagina), the skin surface, or to a pericolonic/mesenteric abscess. The serosal surface may show evidence of transmural inflammation with fat wrapping.

Ulcerative colitis

The classical gross description of ulcerative colitis is a continuous inflammatory disease affecting the mucosa of the rectum and extending proximally into the colon without skip lesions. The distribution may range from rectal disease only (ulcerative proctitis) to pancolitis. The terminal ileum is not involved, aside from what is often referred to as backwash ileitis, which should be a minor degree of inflammation limited to the distal 1 or 2 cm of the ileum. There are a number of caveats with regards to the distribution of ulcerative colitis and possible skip lesions. Rectal sparing and skip lesions that are recognized grossly at resection or endoscopically may not be confirmed as such when viewed through the microscope. Also, true rectal sparing and patchy disease have been reported in classic ulcerative colitis patients under therapy with both oral and topical medications. Pediatric patients who later develop classic ulcerative colitis have also been shown to have a higher predominance of rectal sparing on presentation. There has also been documentation of duodenitis as a related lesion in otherwise classic ulcerative colitis.

The mucosa in ulcerative colitis is usually hemorrhagic and granular appearing, and is less likely to exhibit the discrete ulceration seen in Crohn's disease. Inflammatory polyps may be seen. The bowel wall should not be significantly thickened, and any areas of stricture should be concerning for ulcerative colitis complicated by the development of carcinoma. No signs of serositis or fat wrapping should be seen; however, occasionally ulcerative colitis presents as fulminant colitis requiring emergency surgery, in which case transmural inflammation and ulcers with serositis may be seen.

Indeterminate colitis

Indeterminate colitis is not in itself a diagnostic entity, but rather it is terminology reserved for those cases that cannot be definitively categorized as ulcerative colitis or Crohn's disease. Often times cases presenting as fulminant colitis may fall into this category because of the transmural nature of the inflammatory process, discrete ulceration, and fissures, which obscure the typical features of ulcerative colitis. The term should be reserved for those cases in which the distinction cannot be made even with a resection specimen. It is inappropriate when used in the situation when mucosal biopsies have not allowed for the separation of ulcerative colitis from Crohn's disease [13].

Other diagnostic considerations

There are a limited number of entities that may grossly mimic inflammatory bowel disease. Ischemic lesions may resemble Crohn's disease; there is discrete ulceration with pseudomembrane formation and submucosal edema. The inflammation may be deep leading to perforation or stricture formation upon healing. The distribution of ischemic lesions preferentially affecting the watershed area of the splenic flexure is a helpful distinctive feature.

Infection may also lead to resection, and will occasionally be confused with inflammatory bowel disease. There are a number of organisms that may cause ulceration of the right-sided colon or terminal ileum, causing diagnostic confusion with Crohn's disease. These include bacterial infections such as yersiniosis, tuberculosis, and salmonellosis, and parasitic infections such as amebiasis. Histology as well as clinical history is helpful in arriving at the proper diagnosis.

The last common mimic of inflammatory bowel disease is diverticular-disease–associated colitis. The histology of these lesions may very closely mimic ulcerative colitis or Crohn's disease. Likewise, colovaginal/colovesicular fistulas, pericolonic abscess, and large masslike fibrous lesions may be seen. The key to recognition is the distribution of disease and finding the colitis limited to the area of diverticula.

Postsurgical period

Pouchitis

Pouchitis is an inflammatory condition of the ileal reservoir that is created in the ileal pouch anal anastomosis surgery, or its precursor, the continent ileal reservoir (Kock ileostomy). The ileal pouch anal anastomosis is now the surgical procedure of choice for patients who have familial adenomatous polyposis and ulcerative colitis, and is contraindicated in Crohn's disease. In the past, pouchitis has been difficult to precisely define, but it is now a well-studied condition and the subject of a number of thorough recent reviews [9,14–19] as well as surgical pathology reference texts [9].

Pouchitis is the most common long-term complication of ileal pouch anal anastomosis. Other possible complications include fistula, obstruction, incontinence/functional disorders, anastomotic leaks, other inflammatory/infectious disorders, or metabolic disorders. Interestingly, the incidence of pouchitis is much higher in patients who have ulcerative colitis (approximately half will experience at least one episode) as compared with familial adenomatous polyposis (probably less than 10%). A wide variation in the incidence of pouchitis is reported in the literature because of the historical lack of a standardized definition.

Proposed etiologies for pouchitis are variable, and illustrate the probable heterogeneous nature of the disease. One of the most popular models for disease is an offending bacterial agent or disruption of the resident bacterial flora of the gut. This is supported by the response of many cases to treatment with antibiotics, and also the use of probiotics in long-term maintenance for prevention and treatment of chronic pouchitis. Other possible etiologies or contributors include fecal stasis, genetic susceptibility, disregulation of the immune system, nutrition, ischemia, recurrent ulcerative colitis, missed Crohn's disease, or a novel type of inflammatory bowel disease.

Endoscopic/gross features

Upon endoscopy, the mucosa of the pouch in pouchitis may show ulceration or erosion with exudates, nodularity, erythema, granularity, friability, mucosal flattening, edema, loss of vascular pattern, mucosal hemorrhage, and contact bleeding. The neoterminal ileum proximal to the pouch should appear normal, with inflammation here being concerning for Crohn's disease. Also, assessment of the residual rectal mucosa at the distal anastomosis is critical in assessing the possibility of ongoing ulcerative colitis in this area (cuffitis). It is not unusual to see ulceration along the stapled anastomosis, and biopsy of this area should be avoided to prevent confusion and histologic overdiagnosis of pouchitis.

Histologic features

To avoid overdiagnosing pouchitis on histologic grounds, it is important to recognize the physiologic changes that the ileal reservoir naturally undergoes. The gut function changes from a primarily absorptive organ to an organ of fecal storage. This is accompanied by histologic changes that are identifiable in even the non-dysfunctional pouch. Villous blunting and crypt hyperplasia with increased crypt mitoses and increased lamina propria chronic inflammation are seen; rare neutrophils can also be seen. Varying levels of incomplete colonic-type metaplasia can be seen, but these changes are more associated with long-standing active inflammation.

The most consistent findings in pouchitis are neutrophilic inflammation with cryptitis and crypt abscess formation, and ulceration with granulation tissue. Pouchitis should not be diagnosed in the absence of acute inflammation. Often, reactive epithelium with mucin depletion is identified. At times histologic features may be seen that point to a more specific diagnosis. The granulomas of Crohn's disease may be identified, and the diagnosis of Crohn's disease is elaborated upon in the following section. Specific infectious etiologies may be identified, such as the characteristic cytologic inclusions of cytomegalovirus. Also, the nonspecific mucosal changes indicative of ischemia or prolapse are identifiable here, as they are anywhere in the gastrointestinal tract.

Crohn's disease

Crohn's disease is an important cause of postoperative pouch complication, and may cause strictures, decreased pouch compliance, and fistulas. It is important to recognize, however, that these may also be caused by mechanical/surgical or ischemic complications, and are not specific to Crohn's disease. Fistulas arising from the anastomosis are most often associated with surgical complication, whereas fistulas from the pouch and neoterminal ileum are more often associated with Crohn's disease. With suspected Crohn's disease in the pouch, the prior colectomy specimen should be reviewed to look closely for signs of possible unrecognized Crohn's disease at the time of the original surgery. The neoterminal ileum should be analyzed by endoscopy and biopsied if there are any signs of inflammation. Inflammation in this location is supportive of a diagnosis of Crohn's disease.

As can be imagined, it can be difficult to distinguish Crohn's disease from chronic long-standing pouchitis solely on histologic findings. The identification of the characteristic granulomas of Crohn's disease in biopsy specimens is helpful, but these are not often present; however, one must take care to exclude foreign body granulomas associated with the anastomosis site. The distribution of disease, review of the prior colectomy, and other clinical findings, such as fistulas, tend to be the most helpful in arriving at the proper diagnosis of Crohn's disease of the pouch.

Cuffitis

In patients who have ileal pouches, there is often 1 to 2 cm of residual rectal mucosa at the distal anastomosis site, which is often referred to as the rectal cuff (sometimes called the anal transition zone). This rectal mucosa may be involved by ulcerative colitis, and this process is designated cuffitis. Patients can present with the classical symptoms of pouchitis, and on endoscopy show only signs of inflammation in the rectal cuff with a normal pouch mucosa. Cuffitis may also be asymptomatic, but when it is symptomatic, rectal bleeding seems to be the most specific symptom. Pouchitis and cuffitis may also coexist, so it is important to sample both areas at endoscopy and designate the biopsy sites accordingly. The endoscopic and histologic features of pouchitis and cuffitis are very similar.

Irritable pouch syndrome

Irritable pouch syndrome is diagnosed when a patient presents with a dysfunctional pouch and the symptoms of pouchitis, but no endoscopic or histologic evidence of pouchitis is identified. This is a diagnosis of exclusion, because other causes of noninflammatory pouch dysfunction must be excluded (stricture, decreased pouch compliance, decreased pouch emptying, pelvic floor dysfunction, anal sphincter dysfunction, bacterial overgrowth, and long efferent limb). These patients may benefit from therapy with motility medications and antidepressants, analogous to patients who have irritable bowel syndrome.

Dysplasia and surveillance

Pouchitis may lead to dysplasia and adenocarcinoma, but it is a rare occurrence. It is the patients who have chronic pouchitis with constant severe acute inflammation who are at the greatest risk of developing dysplasia. There is also a risk of dysplasia in the residual rectal mucosa that may be involved by ulcerative colitis (cuffitis), and care should be taken to sample this area upon surveillance endoscopy. There are no universally agreed-on surveillance guidelines for detecting pouch dysplasia, but following similar guidelines as those used in ulcerative colitis patients seems reasonable.

This is especially true in the setting of chronic active pouchitis, or in patients who have dysplasia on their original resection specimen.

Diversion colitis

There is a peculiar form of mucosal inflammation that may appear in a segment of colon that is not exposed to the flow of feces. It is thought that this results because certain fatty acids in feces are necessary for maintaining mucosal integrity. The mucosal inflammation may mimic that seen in inflammatory bowel disease. This includes a prominent expansion of the lamina propria cellularity throughout the entire depth of the lamina propria, cryptitis, and even crypt abscesses. Diversion colitis can cause a great deal of difficulty in patients who have Crohn's disease when it must be distinguished from recurrence of Crohn's disease in the diverted segment. One should ensure that features essentially specific for Crohn's disease, such as granulomas, are not present. The key positive finding characteristic for diversion colitis is the presence of increased numbers of physiologic lymphoid aggregates related to the deep aspects of the colonic crypts, the so-called "lymphoglandular complexes" [20]. Restoring continuity provide effective therapy for diversion colitis.

Summary

Interpretation of biopsy and surgical specimens from patients who have inflammatory bowel disease is highly dependent on communication among the various specialties involved in caring for the patient. Clearly establishing the diagnosis of inflammatory bowel disease is of paramount importance. Historical information, particularly with regards to chronicity, is most important in this regard. Distinguishing ulcerative colitis from Crohn's disease is a major problem. Judicious sampling of the involved and uninvolved areas is key, as is conveying information as to the distribution of disease as seen endoscopically and radiographically. Access to this information is essential to minimize the possibility of confusing ulcerative colitis and Crohn's disease. Once again, careful systematic sampling with appropriate endoscopic information maximize detection and characterization of dysplasia. Close communication of surgeon and pathologist before, during, and after surgery maximize the contribution of pathology to patient management.

References

[1] Yantiss RK, Odze RD. Diagnostic difficulties in inflammatory bowel disease pathology. Histopathology 2006;48:116–32.
[2] Surawicz CM, Haggitt RC, Husseman M, et al. Mucosal biopsy diagnosis of colitis: acute self-limited colitis and idiopathic inflammatory bowel disease. Gastroenterology 1994; 107(3):755–63.

[3] Nostrant TT, Kumar NB, Appelman HD. Histopathology differentiates acute self-limited colitis from ulcerative colitis. Gastroenterology 1987;92(2):318–28.

[4] Lazenby AJ. Collagenous and lymphocytic colitis. Semin Diagn Pathol 2005;22(4):295–300.

[5] Mahadeva U, Martin JP, Patel NK, et al. Granulomatous ulcerative colitis: a re-appraisal of the mucosal granuloma in the distinction of Crohn's disease from ulcerative colitis. Histopathology 2002;41(1):50–5.

[6] Riddell RH, Goldman H, Ransohoff DF, et al. Dysplasia in inflammatory bowel disease: standardized classification with provisional clinical applications. Hum Pathol 1983;14(11): 931–68.

[7] Odze R. Diagnostic problems and advances in inflammatory bowel disease. Mod Pathol 2003;16(4):347–58.

[8] Day DW, Jass JR, Price AB, et al. Inflammatory disorders of the large intestine. In: Morson and Dawson's gastrointestinal pathology. 4th edition. Malden MA: Blackwell Publishing; 2003. p. 472–539.

[9] Petras R. Nonneoplastic intestinal diseases. In: Mills SE, Carter D, Greenson JK, et al, editors. Sternberg's diagnostic surgical pathology. 4th edition. Philadelphia, PA: Lippincott Williams & Wilkins; 2004. p. 1501–41.

[10] Greenson J, Odze R, Goldblum JR, et al. Inflammatory diseases of the large intestine. In: Surgical pathology of the GI tract, liver, biliary tract, and pancreas. Philadelphia PA: Saunders; 2004. p. 213–46.

[11] Kleer C, Appleman H. Surgical pathology of Crohn's disease. Surg Clin North Am 2001; 81(1):13–30.

[12] Burroughs S, Williams G. Examination of large intestine resection specimens. J Clin Pathol 2000;53:344–9.

[13] Martland GT, Shepherd NA. Indeterminate colitis: definition, diagnosis, implications and a plea for nosological sanity. Histopathology 2007;50:83–96.

[14] Mahadevan U, Sandborn W. Diagnosis and management of pouchitis. Gastroenterology 2003;124:1636–50.

[15] Macafee D, Abercrombie J, Maxwell-Armstrong C. Pouchitis. Colorectal Dis 2004;6: 142–52.

[16] Shen B, Fazio V, Remzi F, et al. Clinical approach to diseases of ileal pouch-anal anastomosis. Am J Gastroenterol 2005;100:2796–807.

[17] Pardi D, Sandborn W. Systematic review: the management of pouchitis. Aliment Pharmacol Ther 2006;23:1087–96.

[18] Sandborn W, Tremaine W, Batts K, et al. Pouchitis after ileal pouch-anal anastomosis: a pouchitis disease activity index. Mayo Clin Proc 1994;69:409–15.

[19] Heuschen U, Autschbach F, Allemeyer E, et al. Long-term follow-up after ileoanal pouch procedure: algorithm for diagnosis, classification, and management of pouchitis. Dis Colon Rectum 2001;44:487–99.

[20] Edwards CM, George B, Warren B. Diversion colitis—new light through old windows. Histopathology 1999;34(1):1–5.

ELSEVIER
SAUNDERS

Surg Clin N Am 87 (2007) 787–796

SURGICAL
CLINICS OF
NORTH AMERICA

Index

Note: Page numbers of article titles are in **boldface** type.

A

Abscesses
    in anorectal Crohn's disease, 622
    intra-abdominal, in Crohn's disease,
        590–591
        in children, 653
    perirectal, in Crohn's disease, in
        children, 653

Acquired immune responses, in intestinal
    immune system, 683

Adacolumn, in leukocyte filtration, for
    inflammatory bowel disease, 737–738

Adalimumab
    for Crohn's disease, 707
    for inflammatory bowel disease, 729
        adverse effects of, 719

Adenocarcinoma
    anorectal Crohn's disease and,
        624–625
    small bowel, Crohn's disease and, 667

Alternative and complementary therapies,
    for inflammatory bowel disease,
    735–737

5-Aminosalicylates
    for Crohn's disease, 699–701, 708
        in children, 651
    for inflammatory bowel disease,
        adverse effects of, 716–717
    for ulcerative colitis, 710–712, 714–715
        in children, 645
    to prevent colorectal cancer, in
        inflammatory bowel disease, 668
    to prevent dysplasia, in inflammatory
        bowel disease, 755–756

Anal fissures, in anorectal Crohn's disease,
    623–624

Ankylosing spondylitis, in Crohn's disease,
    675

Anorectal Crohn's disease. *See* Crohn's
    disease.

Anovaginal fistulas, in anorectal Crohn's
    disease, 623

Antibiotics
    for Crohn's disease, 701
        in children, 651
    for inflammatory bowel disease,
        adverse effects of, 717–718
    for pouchitis, in ulcerative colitis, 716
    for ulcerative colitis, 713

Antidepressants, for Crohn's disease, 678

Antigen-presenting cells, in intestinal
    immune system, 683

Antigen-specific adaptive immune
    responses, in intestinal immune
    system, 683

Anxiety, in Crohn's disease, 677

Aphthous ulcers, in Crohn's disease, 581

Appendectomies, and inflammatory bowel
    disease, 577

Arthropathy, in Crohn's disease, 675

Azathioprine
    for Crohn's disease, 705, 708
    for inflammatory bowel disease,
        adverse effects of, 718
    for ulcerative colitis, 713–714, 715
    to prevent recurrent Crohn's disease,
        604–605

B

Bacterial flagellin, in inflammatory bowel
    disease, 691

Balloon dilatation, of strictures, in Crohn's
    disease, 589–590
    of colon and rectum, 615

Barrett's esophagus
    and esophageal cancer, 660
    cytokines in, 660

Behçet's disease, in Crohn's disease, 676

doi:10.1016/S0039-6109(07)00063-1

Moving?

Make sure your subscription moves with you!

To notify us of your new address, find your **Clinics Account Number** (located on your mailing label above your name), and contact customer service at:

E-mail: elspcs@elsevier.com

800-654-2452 (subscribers in the U.S. & Canada)
407-345-4000 (subscribers outside of the U.S. & Canada)

Fax number: 407-363-9661

Elsevier Periodicals Customer Service
6277 Sea Harbor Drive
Orlando, FL 32887-4800

*To ensure uninterrupted delivery of your subscription, please notify us at least 4 weeks in advance of move.

ELSEVIER